MW01104144

TEXTBOOK OF

OCCUPATIONAL MEDICINE PRACTICE

3rd Edition

TEXTBOOK OF

OCCUPATIONAL
MEDICINE
PRACTICE

3rd Edition

edited by

David Koh
National University of Singapore, Singapore

Ken Takahashi
University of Occupational and Environmental Health, Japan

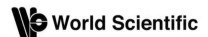 **World Scientific**

NEW JERSEY · LONDON · SINGAPORE · BEIJING · SHANGHAI · HONG KONG · TAIPEI · CHENNAI

Published by

World Scientific Publishing Co. Pte. Ltd.

5 Toh Tuck Link, Singapore 596224

USA office: 27 Warren Street, Suite 401-402, Hackensack, NJ 07601

UK office: 57 Shelton Street, Covent Garden, London WC2H 9HE

Library of Congress Cataloging-in-Publication Data
Textbook of occupational medicine practice / editor, David Koh ; co-editor,
    Ken Takahashi. -- 3rd ed.
    p. ; cm.
    Includes bibliographical references and index.
    ISBN-13: 978-981-4329-57-6 (hardcover : alk. paper)
    ISBN-10: 981-4329-57-6 (hardcover : alk. paper)
    1. Medicine, Industrial. I. Koh, David, 1956– II. Takahashi, Ken, 1956–
    [DNLM: 1. Occupational Diseases. 2. Occupational Health. 3. Occupational Medicine--
methods. WA 400]
    RC963.T53 2011
    616.9'803--dc22

                                                                   2011006436

British Library Cataloguing-in-Publication Data
A catalogue record for this book is available from the British Library.

Copyright © 2011 by World Scientific Publishing Co. Pte. Ltd.

All rights reserved. This book, or parts thereof, may not be reproduced in any form or by any means, electronic or mechanical, including photocopying, recording or any information storage and retrieval system now known or to be invented, without written permission from the Publisher.

For photocopying of material in this volume, please pay a copying fee through the Copyright Clearance Center, Inc., 222 Rosewood Drive, Danvers, MA 01923, USA. In this case permission to photocopy is not required from the publisher.

Typeset by Stallion Press
Email: enquiries@stallionpress.com

Printed by FuIsland Offset Printing (S) Pte Ltd. Singapore

For
Wan Tsyr, Nicola, Katherine, Elliot and Gregory
Yukari and Joe

Foreword

According to the best traditions of the medical profession, everything we do in occupational medicine should be based on a sound scientific foundation and on well-proven and feasible practice. It is also an ethical imperative of the medical profession throughout the world.

A very special feature of occupational medicine is that it synthesizes knowledge, methods and research results from several disciplines, such as basic biomedicine, physiology, toxicology, psychology, several clinical specialities, such as internal medicine, neurology, allergology, physiotherapy, just to mention a few. But even more, the competencies of occupational hygiene, ergonomics and safety are also needed for exposure assessment. Only by combining so many knowledge pools can a reliable diagnosis of occupational diseases be made and appropriate treatment, preventive and control actions be undertaken.

Today, the discipline of occupational medicine is being challenged from several different directions. First, the progress of basic research in several relevant fields provides new opportunities for practical solutions and the gap between the new research findings and practical applications needs to be bridged. On the other hand, the new demands and needs set by the rapid changes in working life, introduction of new technologies, new chemical substances and materials, new exposures and new working practices together with the traditional problems of occupational medicine call for new knowledge and new approaches. The demographic changes of working populations, such as ageing of workers and growing participation of women in working life, growing national and international mobility and changes in occupational structures and lifestyles of working people, also need new applications of scientific knowledge.

Since the first and second editions of this book, the world of work has changed substantially. Today the globalizing work life sets challenges to occupational health everywhere in the world. The human somatic and psychological responses to workplace exposures, workloads and stressors are, with only a few exceptions, largely the same among the workers of the world. So are our needs for knowledge for identification and assessment of risks and actions for risk prevention and management. This international textbook serves well such global needs.

The contributors to this book are well-known senior international experts in the research and practice of occupational medicine, who share their competence and experience with readers by bridging scientific knowledge and everyday practice and thus promote the development of modern occupational medicine.

The book will be a useful guide for all those who are interested in occupational medical practice, be they medical students at various levels, occupational health nurses, general practitioners or more senior professionals in occupational medicine. In other words, for all who have committed themselves to do the best for the health of the working people.

Professor Jorma Rantanen
Past President
International Commission on
Occupational Health

Preface to the Third Edition

The global economy has surged ahead in the last several decades due to advances in work technology and supported by a highly diligent and productive workforce. However, such successes have their dark sides. In the context of occupational medicine, these are the occurrence of occupational diseases, accidents and work-related diseases. Occupational medicine practice aims to protect and promote the health, safety and welfare of workers. Today, such practice must address a variety of issues that are old and new, universal and regional as well as clinical and multidisciplinary. This textbook aspires to bridge such gaps and elaborates on the practice of occupational medicine.

The first and second editions were well received, and this textbook has been utilized as a teaching text in many countries in East Asia and the Middle East. It has also been translated into a Korean edition. However, it has been 10 years since the second edition of this textbook. Advances in the science and practice of occupational medicine have necessitated the preparation of a third edition.

Similar to the past editions, the clinically oriented chapters form Section One, while Section Two comprises other issues of special interest to occupational health practitioners. This edition incorporates new chapters on metabolic disorders, male and female reproductive disorders, ethical and legal aspects of practice, and hyperbaric and aviation medicine.

As before, we are grateful to many people who have so generously helped us to produce this book. In particular, we appreciate the feedback from the many readers who have given us their very useful comments on the earlier editions of the book. Finally, we also wish to thank Dr. Lim John-Wah for his meticulous help in reading and indexing the draft, and the publishers, especially Ms. SC Lim.

We hope you find the textbook useful, and that its use will translate into the improvement of the health and safety of all who work.

David Koh, Singapore (e-mail: ephkohd@nus.edu.sg)
Ken Takahashi, Japan (e-mail: ktaka@med.uoeh-u.ac.jp)
January 2011

Preface to the Second Edition

It came as a pleasant surprise when the publishers informed us that it would be timely to prepare a new edition. We were told that the first edition was well received, and is now used as a standard text in occupational health training courses in several countries, such as Singapore, Malaysia, Indonesia, Vietnam and Jordan.

The second edition has allowed us to revise and update the contents and add new material. Several changes have directly resulted from feedback that some readers have very kindly given. Among these are the inclusion of new chapters on occupational infections, the health of corporate travelers, shiftwork and occupational health standards and legislation.

The contents of the book have been streamlined to appear in two sections. The approach of examining occupational health issues and concerns from the standpoint of clinical presentations of the different organ systems is retained. These clinically oriented chapters form Section One. Section Two comprises other issues of special interest to occupational health practitioners.

Case studies to demonstrate real-life situations and to make clear the relevant issues were appreciated by many readers, and we have responded by adding several more to the text. The formula of having chapters jointly written by occupational health specialists and clinicians also seemed to work well, and is continued in this edition.

As before, we are grateful to many people who have so generously helped us to produce this book. This time round, we also wish to thank the publishers, in particular Ms. SC Lim and Ms. Joy Quek, and the many readers who have given us their very useful comments and feedback on the first edition.

David Koh
Chia Kee Seng
J Jeyaratnam
Singapore, February 2001

Preface to the First Edition

In the recent past, there have been a large number of books published on occupational health. In the main, these books have focused on special issues and subjects in occupational health or addressed the needs of specialists in occupational health and medicine. However, there is a relative paucity of books which provide information on the interface between the health practitioners' needs and occupational medicine. This book hopes to improve this situation by providing information necessary for practitioners to better understand occupational medicine, and to better incorporate it into their daily clinical practice.

As this book aims to provide a link between occupational health and clinical practice, it is suitable for medical undergraduates, general practitioners and postgraduate students in occupational health. Further, this book will be a valuable starting point for clinicians with an interest in occupational medicine as well as those intending to specialize in occupational medicine. Other occupational health professionals, in particular occupational health nurses, will also find this book useful. The main approach of most chapters is to examine occupational health issues and concerns from the standpoint of clinical presentations of the different organ systems, e.g. respiratory disorders, musculoskeletal disorders, dermatological disorders. This book also contains chapters on screening and routine medical examinations, health promotion in the workplace, assessment of disability for compensation, medical planning and management of industrial disasters and prevention of occupational diseases. Where appropriate, case studies have been incorporated in the chapters to demonstrate real-life situations and make clear the relevant issues. The international and regional contributors to the book are experienced and respected occupational health specialists and clinicians.

We owe thanks to many people who have helped us to produce this book. This book would not have been possible if not for the contributors who so readily came forward to share their knowledge with us and our readers. We would further like to acknowledge and thank the publishers, in particular Ms. SC Lim for her interest and support; Ms. Saadiah Awek for her patience, meticulous typing and cheerful help in proofreading the earlier drafts of the chapters; and the MMed (Occupational Medicine) class of 1995/1996, National University of Singapore, for their comments and proofreading of the later drafts. Finally, to the many others who have helped in various ways, but are too numerous to mention, we offer our thanks and gratitude.

J Jeyaratnam, David Koh
Singapore, January 1996

About the Book

This book provides a link between occupational health and clinical practice. It aims to provide a valuable starting point for health professionals with an interest in, as well as those intending to specialize in, occupational medicine. It also serves as a useful guide for those who are involved in occupational health practice. These include medical students at various levels, occupational health nurses, general practitioners, or colleagues and professionals in occupational health and safety — in other words, all who have committed themselves to do their best for the health of working people.

The contents of the book have been streamlined into two sections. The approach of examining occupational health issues and concerns from the standpoint of clinical presentations of the different organ systems is retained. These clinically oriented chapters form Section One. Section Two deals with cross-cutting issues of special interest to occupational health practitioners such as screening and routine medical examinations, assessment of disability for compensation, medical planning and management of industrial disasters, occupational medicine practice and the law, and the prevention of occupational diseases.

Several changes have directly resulted from feedback from readers of the previous editions. Among these are the inclusion of chapters on metabolic disorders, and occupational medicine practice and the law. As before, case studies have been incorporated in the chapters to make clear the relevant issues that may be encountered on a day-to-day basis.

About the Editors

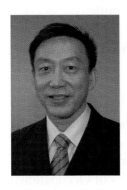 **David Koh,** MBBS, MSc, PhD, FFOM, FFOMI, FFPH, FAOEM, FAMS
Director, Centre for Environmental and Occupational Health Research
Professor, Department of Epidemiology and Public Health
Yong Loo Lin School of Medicine, National University of Singapore

David Koh is Professor of Occupational Medicine in the Department of Epidemiology and Public Health of the School of Medicine; and Director of the Centre for Environmental and Occupational Health Research, National University of Singapore (NUS). Prior to joining NUS, he was the Assistant Director of the Division of Occupational Safety and Health of the then National Productivity Board, and Medical Director in a multinational insurance company.

Dr. Koh has been engaged by the World Health Organization as a consultant in occupational health to several countries. He serves on the advisory boards of several international occupational and environmental health journals, and has undertaken international consulting work with several large organizations and multinational companies.

Within Singapore, he is Chairman of the Ministry of Health Specialist Training Committee (Occupational Medicine), and Program

Director of the National Residency Program in Preventive Medicine. He is also a past President of the Society of Occupational Medicine and the Occupational and Environmental Health Society. He currently holds Visiting Consultant appointments at the National Skin Centre, the Singapore General Hospital, Changi Hospital and the Singapore Armed Forces.

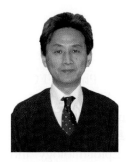

Ken Takahashi, MD, MPH, PhD
Professor of Environmental Epidemiology
Acting Director of the WHO Collaborating
Centre for Occupational Health
University of Occupational and Environmental
Health (UOEH), Kitakyushu, Japan

Ken Takahashi is Professor of Environmental Epidemiology in the Department of Environmental Epidemiology and Acting Director of the WHO Collaborating Center for Occupational Health at the Institute of Industrial Ecological Sciences, University of Occupational and Environmental Health, Japan. He is Committee Chair and Course Leader of the international courses sponsored by the Japan International Cooperation Agency (JICA).

Dr. Takahashi has been serving as a consultant/advisor to the World Health Organization and the International Labour Organization as well as an expert for JICA. He has been engaged by a number of academic/research institutes in the Asia-Pacific as an examiner and advisor. He has served twice as elected Board Member of the ICOH, is current Fellow of the Collegium Ramazzini and editorial board member of several international/domestic scientific journals.

Within Japan, he has been involved in national committees at the ministerial level, appointed as a Consulting Occupational Health Physician to the Prefectural Labor Bureau designated by the Ministry of Health Labor and Welfare, Japan, and chairs a municipal committee on asbestos diseases.

Contributors

Aw Tar Ching PhD, FRCP, FRCPC, FFOM, FFOMI, FFPH
Professor and Chair
Department of Community Medicine
Faculty of Medicine and Health Sciences, UAE University
Al-Ain, United Arab Emirates

Aw Lee Fhoon Lily MBBS, GDFM, GDFP(Derm), MCFP
Senior Family Physician and Designated Factory Doctor
Lily Aw Pasir Ris Family Clinic and Surgery, Singapore

Iain Blair MA, MB, BChir
Associate Professor
Department of Community Medicine
Faculty of Medicine and Health Sciences, UAE University
Al-Ain, United Arab Emirates

Jens Peter Bonde MD, PhD, DrMedSs
Professor of Occupational Medicine
University of Copenhagen
Bispebjerg Hospital, Copenhagen, Denmark

Gregory Chan PP, MBBS, MMed(Occup Med)
Dip Geriatric Med, Dip FP Derm, Cert DHM, GCIA,
FSIArb Head, Division of Occupational Health
Senior Occupational Health Physician and Dive Control Officer
Office of Safety, Health and Environment
National University of Singapore

Chia Kee Seng MBBS, MSc(Occup Med), MD, FAMS
Professor and Head, Department of Epidemiology and Public Health
Yong Loo Lin School of Medicine
National University of Singapore
National University Health System, Singapore

Chia Sin Eng MBBS, MSc(Occup Med) MD, FFOM, FAMS
Associate Professor, Department of Epidemiology
and Public Health
Yong Loo Lin School of Medicine
National University of Singapore
National University Health System, Singapore

Alphonsus KS Chong MBBS, MRCS, MMed, FAMS
Consultant Hand Surgeon
University Orthopaedics, Hand and Reconstructive
Microsurgery Cluster
National University Health System, Singapore

Kenneth KY Choy MBBS, MMed(Occup Med)
MSc(HFE), FAMS
Senior Specialist (Occupational Medicine)
Occupational Safety and Health Specialist Department
Ministry of Manpower, Singapore

Goh Chee Leok MBBS, MD, FRCP
Senior Consultant, National Skin Centre, Singapore
Clinical Professor, Yong Loo Lin School of Medicine
National University of Singapore

Malcolm Harrington CBE, MD, FRCP, FFOM FFPH, FMedSci
Emeritus Professor of Occupational Medicine
University of Birmingham
Edgbaston, Birmingham, United Kingdom

Noor Hassim Ismail MD, MSc(Occup Med) FFOMI, FAOEM, AM
Professor and Head, Department of Community Health
Faculty of Medicine, Universiti Kebangsaan Malaysia
Kuala Lumpur, Malaysia

David Koh MBBS, MSc(Occup Med), PhD, FFOM
FFOMI, FFPH, FAOEM, FAMS
Professor, Department of Epidemiology and Public Health
Yong Loo Lin School of Medicine
National University of Singapore
National University Health System, Singapore
Visiting Consultant, National Skin Centre, Singapore
Visiting Consultant, Singapore General Hospital and
Changi General Hospital, Singapore

Kua Ee Heok MBBS, MD, FRCPsych, PBM
Professor and Senior Consultant Psychiatrist
Yong Loo Lin School of Medicine
National University of Singapore
National University Health System, Singapore

Naresh S Kumar MBBS, MS(Orth), DNB(Orth), FRCS(Ed)
FRCS(Orth & Trauma), DM(Orth-Nottingham)
Associate Professor, Senior Consultant and Spine Surgeon
University Orthopaedics, Hand and Reconstructive
Microsurgery Cluster
Yong Loo Lin School of Medicine
National University of Singapore
National University Health System, Singapore

Lee Eng Hin MD, FRCS(C), FRCS(Ed), FRCS(Glas), FAMS
Professor and Senior Consultant
University Orthopaedics, Hand and Reconstructive
Microsurgery Cluster
Yong Loo Lin School of Medicine
National University of Singapore
National University Health System, Singapore

Lee Hock Siang MBBS, MSc(Occup Med), FAMS
Director, Occupational Safety and Health Specialist Department
Ministry of Manpower, Singapore
Adjunct Associate Professor
Department of Epidemiology and Public Health

Yong Loo Lin School of Medicine
National University of Singapore

Lee See Muah MBBS, MSc(Occup Med), FAMS
LLB(Hons), PG Dip Diab
Adjunct Associate Professor
Department of Epidemiology and Public Health
Yong Loo Lin School of Medicine
National University of Singapore
Occupational Health Physician, Diabetes Clinic
Khoo Teck Puat Hospital, Singapore

Lim John-Wah MB BCh (UK), MPH(Occup Med)
Registrar, Department of Epidemiology and Public Health
Yong Loo Lin School of Medicine
National University of Singapore
National University Health System, Singapore

Laurence Lim MBBS, MRCS
Registrar, Singapore National Eye Centre

Lim Meng Kin MBBS, MSc(Occup Med)
FRCP, FFOM, FFPH, FAMS
Associate Professor, Department of Epidemiology
and Public Health
Yong Loo Lin School of Medicine
National University of Singapore
National University Health System, Singapore

Marja-Liisa Lindbohm PhD
Senior Research Scientist, Adjunct Professor
Finnish Institute of Occupational Health, Helsinki, Finland

Roberto Lucchini MD
Professor, Department of Experimental and Applied Medicine
Section of Occupational Health and Industrial Hygiene
University of Brescia, Brescia, Italy

Ng Tsun Gun MBBS, FRCP, FAMS
Consultant, Department of Renal Medicine
Tan Tock Seng Hospital, Singapore

Ng Wee Tong MBChB, MMed(Occup Med), Dip Av Med
Dip Geriatric Med
Medical Director (Clinical Services)
Singapore Aeromedical Centre

Ong Hean Yee MBBS, FRCP, FAMS, FESC
Consultant Cardiologist
Khoo Teck Puat Hospital, Singapore

Krishna Gopal Rampal MBBS, MPH, PhD, FFOMI, FFOM
FAOEM, AM
Professor of Community Medicine
Perdana University Graduate School of Medicine
Kuala Lumpur, Malaysia

Ailin Razali MBBS, MSc(Audiological Medicine)
Assistant Professor, Department of ORL-HNS
International Islamic University Malaysia
Kuantan, Malaysia

Judy Sng MBBS, GDFM, GDOM, MMed (OM)
Assistant Professor, Department of Epidemiology and
Public Health
Yong Loo Lin School of Medicine
National University of Singapore
National University Health System, Singapore

Sum Chee Fang MBBS, FRCPE, FAMS, FACE
Senior Consultant Endocrinologist
Khoo Teck Puat Hospital, Singapore
Clinical Associate Professor
Yong Loo Lin School of Medicine
National University of Singapore

Ken Takahashi MD, MPH, PhD
Professor of Environmental Epidemiology
University of Occupational and Environmental Health
Kitakyushu City, Japan

Tan Keng Leong MBBS, FAMS, FCCP, FRCP
Senior Consultant
Department of Respiratory and Critical Medicine,
Singapore General Hospital
Adjunct Assistant Professor
Yong Loo Lin School of Medicine
National University of Singapore

Helena Taskinen MD, PhD, Specialist in Occupational Medicine
Professor, Chief Medical Officer, Team Leader
Finnish Institute of Occupational Health
Faculty of Medicine, Hjelt Institute, University of Helsinki
Helsinki, Finland

Ken Ung MBBS, MRCPsych
Senior Consultant Psychiatrist
Adam Road Hospital, Singapore

Wong Hee Kit MBBS, MMed(Surg), FRCS(Glas)
MChOrth(Liv), FAMS
Professor and Head, Department of Orthopaedic Surgery
Yong Loo Lin School of Medicine
National University of Singapore
Chair, University Orthopaedics
Hand and Reconstructive Microsurgery Cluster
Head, University Spine Centre
National University Health System, Singapore

Michael Wong MBBS, MMed(Family Med), GDGM, FCFP
Director, Health for Life
Khoo Teck Puat Hospital, Singapore

Wong Tien-Yin MBBS, FRCSE, FRANZCO, FAFPHM, PhD
Professor, National University Health System
Director, Singapore Eye Research Institute
Senior Consultant, Singapore National Eye Centre

Contents

Section 1

Clinical Occupational Medicine

Chapter 1

Work and Health

David Koh* and Judy Sng*,†

Occupational Health, Occupational and Environmental Medicine

The International Labour Office (ILO) and World Health Organization (WHO) define occupational health as the promotion and maintenance of the highest degree of physical, mental and social well-being of workers in all occupations. Occupational health service provision is a means to achieving this objective.

Occupational and environmental medicine, as defined by the American College of Occupational and Environmental Medicine, is the medical specialty devoted to the prevention and management of occupational and environmental injury, illness and disability, and the promotion of health and productivity of workers, their families, and communities.

A crucial concept in occupational health is the recognition of a two-way relationship between work and health.

WORK ⇔ HEALTH

Work may have an adverse impact on health; on the other hand it can be beneficial to health and well-being. The health status of a worker

*Department of Epidemiology and Public Health, Yong Loo Lin School of Medicine, National University of Singapore.
†Corresponding author: E-mail: ephjsgk@nus.edu.sg

will have an impact on his work. A worker who is healthy is more likely to be more productive than an unhealthy worker. Workers with impaired health are not only less productive but could also pose a risk to themselves as well as to other workers, the community and the environment.

Case Study 1

An oil company had known for years that the captain of one of its oil tankers had a serious drinking problem, but nonetheless left him in command of oil tankers. On one of the tanker journeys, the captain was drunk on duty and left an inexperienced officer in charge of navigating the tanker through hazardous icy conditions. The tanker ran aground on a reef and spilled millions of liters of crude oil, which coated thousands of kilometers of coastline and killed thousands of birds and marine mammals.

History of Occupational Medicine

The discipline of occupational medicine is a relatively recent development in the history of modern medicine. If modern medicine evolved from Hippocratic times which date back 2500 years, occupational medicine became a recognized discipline from the time of Bernardino Ramazzini, who lived in the 18th century. Certain historical features in the development of occupational medicine have had a serious impact on it. First, its developmental direction was influenced by the fact that it was intimately linked to the legislative process, with legislation such as the Factories Act and Compensation Act. Even today, legislation is an important component of occupational medicine. Second, during the Industrial Revolution, much attention was focused on workers in mines and factories, as these workers were at obvious health risk as a consequence of their work. This led to the discipline being known in the early days as industrial medicine or even factory medicine. With the recognition of other hazards in the workplace, however, the focus was enlarged to include all persons at work, and the term "occupational medicine" was given.

The specialty has since evolved and become known as occupational health, for the reason that it is concerned not only with preventing disease but also with promoting health among people who work. The term "occupational health" also implies a multidisciplinary responsibility as well as a mechanism for the provision of health services for the working population.

Work and Health

A worker may suffer the full spectrum of diseases: (i) diseases that are prevalent in the community; (ii) work-related diseases; and (iii) occupational diseases. This means that an occupational health physician must recognize the relationship between work and disease, whichever the category of disease. For instance, many people who have diabetes are still in the workforce. Their health condition would have an impact on work performance (as illustrated in Case Study 2). Equally, work may adversely affect their health condition (Fig. 1).

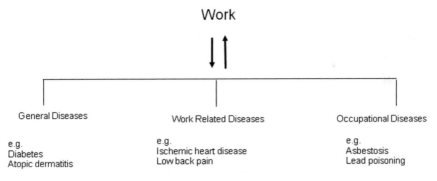

Fig. 1.   Categories of disease at the workplace.

Occupational diseases are more commonly seen in developing nations where the more hazardous occupations such as mining and traditional forms of agriculture are predominant. Work-related diseases generally become increasingly important as a country becomes more industrialized and phases out industries which are associated with the "traditional" occupational diseases. There is also a group of countries that underwent rapid economic growth in a short span of time, termed the newly industrializing countries (NICs). Such countries face a unique blend of traditional occupational diseases, emerging occupational diseases as well as work-related diseases.

Case Study 2

Mr. B is a factory supervisor who has to be placed on shift work after the restructuring of the company's production and work processes. In addition, the recent acquisitions of new factories in overseas locations requires that he travel frequently.

Mr. B is an insulin-dependent diabetic and is concerned about his diabetic control in relation to the changes in the work situation. He wants to learn about diabetic control with regard to traveling through several time zones, access to medical care in the developing countries where the new factories are located, and vaccination requirements for the travel.

Occupational Diseases

Occupational diseases occur as a result of exposure to physical, chemical, biological or psychosocial factors in the workplace (Table 1).

Table 1.   Occupational Health Hazards and Adverse Effects

Hazard	Adverse Effect
Physical hazards	
e.g. noise	Noise-induced hearing loss
vibration	Vasospastic disease
extremes of temperature	Heat stress, cold-induced disorders
fire, explosion, accidents	Burns, injuries
Chemical hazards	Intoxications, cancers, allergies
Biological hazards	Infections, allergies
Ergonomic hazards	
e.g. repetitive movements	Repetitive strain injuries
poor work organization	Lowered productivity and work quality
Psychosocial hazards	Stress, work dissatisfaction, conflicts, burnout, depression

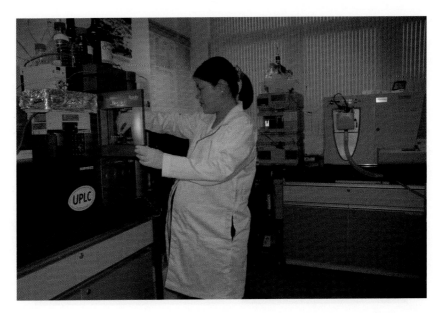

Fig. 2. A pregnant laboratory technologist may be exposed to various chemicals in her workplace.

These factors in the work environment are necessary in the causation of occupational diseases. For example, exposure to lead in the workplace is essential for lead poisoning, and exposure to silica is necessary for silicosis to occur. It must, however, be recognized that other factors such as individual susceptibility may play a varying role in the development of disease among exposed workers (i.e. workplace exposures are necessary but not sufficient to cause occupational diseases).

Occupational diseases occur exclusively among workers exposed to specific hazards (Figs. 2 and 3) and are cause-specific; for example, asbestos causes asbestosis. However, in some situations these diseases may also occur among the general community as a consequence of contamination of the environment from the workplace, e.g. lead, pesticides.

Work-related Diseases

The World Health Organization categorizes work-related diseases as "multifactorial" in origin. These are diseases in which workplace

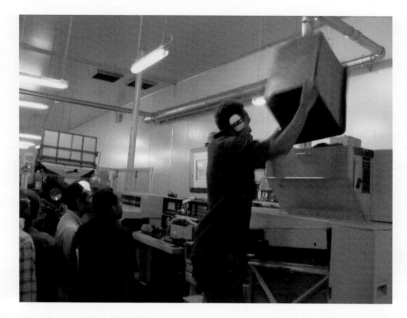

Fig. 3.   This worker who has to repeatedly lift cartons above shoulder height may develop neck and shoulder complaints.

Table 2.   Differences between Occupational and Work-related Diseases

Work-related Diseases	Occupational Diseases
Occurs largely in the community	Occurs mainly among working population
"Multifactorial" in origin	Cause-specific
Exposure at workplace may be a factor	Exposure at workplace is essential
May be notifiable and compensable	Notifiable and compensable

factors may be associated in their occurrence but need not be a risk factor in each case. These are diseases that are frequently seen in the general community. Such work-related diseases include (i) hypertension; (ii) ischemic heart disease; (iii) psychosomatic illness; (iv) musculoskeletal disorders; and (v) chronic non-specific respiratory disease/chronic bronchitis.

In these diseases, work may be associated in their causation or may aggravate a pre-existing condition. The main differences between occupational diseases and work-related diseases are shown in Table 2.

Clinical History Taking

It was only in the 1700s that Bernardino Ramazzini (Fig. 4), a physician and professor of medicine in Modena and Padua, Italy, recommended that physicians enquire about a patient's occupation. Previous to this, the standard three questions recommended by Hippocrates were about the patient's name, age and residence.

The routinely asked question "What is your job?" often provides inadequate information. It is important to obtain an adequate occupational history in order to assess the extent to which the illness has been caused or is related to the patient's job. For example, a patient's

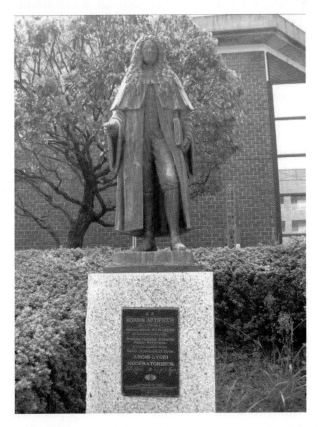

Fig. 4. Statue of Ramazzini at the University of Occupational and Environmental Health in Kitakyushu, Japan.

anemia may be a consequence of exposure to lead; while a "malingering" patient may be in some way related to a highly stressful or hostile work environment.

Another reason for taking a good occupational history is to assess the patient's fitness to return to work. In this connection, four factors need to be considered: (a) the long-term effects of the disease; (b) the nature of the job the patient is returning to; (c) whether the return to work is likely to cause a recurrence of disease or to aggravate the disease; and (d) whether the return to work is likely to cause damage or ill-health to other work colleagues or the general community.

For instance, if the patient was seen for a condition which was clearly the result of occupational exposure, e.g. occupational asthma, occupational dermatitis or musculoskeletal disorders due to poor ergonomic factors, then obviously his return to the same work situation will only result in a recurrence of the condition. Here, corrective measures need to be taken at the workplace to prevent such recurrences.

There are other situations where return to work may aggravate the worker's illness. For instance, a diabetic patient's regular mealtime and medication may be adversely affected if he returns to shift work, particularly as a diurnal variation exists with medication and insulin. Similarly, a patient after myocardial infarction may not be able to return to work requiring heavy physical exertion or work in a high-stress environment. Finally, return to work may have an impact on work colleagues or the general community. One instance is the problem of a patient with a chronic infectious disease returning to work, such as a healthcare worker with hepatitis B or HIV. Another situation would be one where a worker's residual clinical condition may pose a danger to himself as well as fellow workers; for example, an epileptic working at a conveyor belt or alone at the worksite. As for the general community, again there exist some concerns, e.g. a worker with an infected wound on his finger returning to work as a food vendor, or a pilot with psychological problems, or as illustrated in the scenarios painted in Case Studies 1 and 3.

Case Study 3

Mr. C has just been discharged from the hospital after a cerebrovascular accident. He has responded well to treatment and has only a mild residual left-sided paresis. He decides to return to work as a taxi driver after a further two weeks of rest. This is not in contravention of any law, as there are no legislative requirements for a return-to-work medical assessment, and no approved guidelines for medical assessments for fitness to work as a taxi driver in his country.

Finally, asking a patient about his job will provide a good indication of the patient's educational and socio-economic status. This information is of considerable value in providing holistic care as well as appropriate advice to the patient which he is able to appreciate.

Challenges in History Taking

End occupations

Most patients would give their current occupations when a healthcare worker asks about their job. However, the patient could have retired or changed job and his current health problems may be associated with a previous job. Therefore it is important to ask patients about their entire occupational history, as far as possible. In some situations this may be tedious, but it is crucial so that proper diagnosis and management can be instituted, particularly if there is even the slightest likelihood of the illness being linked to an occupational exposure, as in Case Study 4.

Case Study 4

A 63-year-old retiree consults his general practitioner about his chronic respiratory complaints which started two years ago, and has worsened since then. He also complains of tinnitus, which keeps him awake at night. His case notes record that he worked as a general worker for 20 years before retiring three years ago.

He is a non-smoker, and has no other past medical or surgical history of note. His previous consultations were infrequent and unremarkable.

At this consultation, further enquiry reveals that he had worked as a general worker in a shipyard, doing a variety of jobs. One of his main duties was sandblasting paint off the ships. The patient also recalls having removed the insulation on the ships' boiler pipes several times a year in the course of his work.

Job titles

Most patients usually provide a job title that may not be of much value, unless the physician is familiar with the workplace and the potential hazards of the job. This is particularly so when a worker gives his job title as "factory worker". It is obviously necessary to follow up with questions about the nature of the job hazards. Further, a job description that may seem relatively safe may still have relevance to the causation of the illness.

For instance, a young lady was seen with a rash over the malar region of the face. She worked as a clerk. The rash had been persistent and was better during weekends and holidays, indicating a relationship to work. On detailed enquiry, it was revealed that her work desk was directly below the air-conditioner vent. Her rash was diagnosed as low humidity dermatitis — a condition that disappeared as soon as her desk position was changed. Similarly, backache is a common problem. If an office worker or a nurse complains of it, the likelihood of ergonomic factors contributing to the illness must be considered.

Multiple jobs

Another potential pitfall in taking an occupational history is that some patients may be holding more than one job. In such situations, the patients may choose only to reveal what they consider to be their main occupation, and not inform the physician of the other jobs. Thus, it is often appropriate to ask if they hold other jobs as well.

In summary, the components of an occupational history include:

- job description/nature of job;
- hours of work/shift work;

- types of hazards;
- past occupations;
- other concurrent jobs;
- domestic exposures; and
- hobbies.

In taking an occupational history, as many details as possible must be obtained regarding the job. Quite naturally, the details would depend on the circumstances. It is important to know the possible hazards the worker may be exposed to, the type of job and the hours of work. Equally important would be to take a history of past occupations, as the present health problem may be a consequence of an earlier job, particularly if the disease has a long latent period between exposure and onset of disease, e.g. asbestosis, silicosis, toxic neuropathies and occupational cancers.

To complete the picture with regard to the illness being associated with a specific hazard, enquiry must be made about whether the patient holds other jobs and whether there is the possibility of exposure to hazards in domestic tasks or hobbies.

Additional information in an occupational history should include:

- smoking history/alcohol intake/drugs;
- similar complaints among other workers;
- time relationship between work and symptoms;
- relationship of illness to periods away from work;
- degree of exposure;
- use of protective devices; and
- methods of materials handling.

These are additional items that may be useful in an occupational history. For instance, a history of smoking is of particular relevance. Workers who smoke are at a higher risk of developing certain occupational diseases such as asbestosis and lead poisoning, as well as many cancers including that of the lung and bladder. Similarly, alcohol consumption may increase the risk of hepatitis in a solvent-exposed worker.

Another important question is the temporal sequence of the onset of symptoms and exposure. This is of particular importance in occupational diseases of acute onset, such as pesticide poisonings, and occupational asthma. Occupational diseases also tend to improve when the patient is away from work, such as during long weekends or on vacation.

Asking about whether other workers suffer similar problems can often provide a valuable hint as to whether the current illness is due to occupational factors or otherwise.

The degree of exposure (e.g. whether the workplace is very dusty, hot or noisy) may give a clue as to the possibility of the illness being related to work. Finding out about the use of protective devices such as masks or gloves is also useful. One pitfall is that often the workers may use such devices inappropriately or incorrectly. Thus, even if the worker reports that protective devices are used, it does not automatically exclude occupational disease.

Walk-through Assessment of the Workplace

An occupational physician should be able to undertake, in a systematic way, a complete evaluation of a workplace for occupational hazards. In occupational health practice, such an evaluation may be needed because of concerns expressed by the workforce or management about possible health effects related to the work environment, as in Case Study 5. Alternatively, it may arise in the course of a regular inspection to ensure compliance with health and safety legislation. It can also occur because of a request to audit a work area in order to identify potential problem areas, and to recommend appropriate preventive action to reduce occupational ill-health.

Most experienced occupational physicians have their own methods for evaluating workplaces. This would have been developed over years of practical experience of visiting places of work. The methods include using a mental checklist, a written aide-mémoire or a blank sheet of paper to record observations. In order to ensure that any evaluation is complete, some form of a written checklist is needed. This allows for a reduced likelihood of error and/or omission. A standardized basic form can be used to record findings when evaluating a workplace for occupational hazards.

Case Study 5

Eighteen workers in a warehouse complained of rashes on their limbs, neck and trunk within a period of two weeks after their workplace was chemically treated for termites. One day after the chemical treatment, the central air-conditioning unit, which cooled about two thirds of the warehouse, ceased functioning. The workers felt that the chemical exposure and the poor ventilation were responsible for the outbreak of skin rashes.

A list of chemicals used for the treatment was obtained, and the major chemicals used were identified as borax, arsenic trioxide and iron oxide. The contractor who performed the treatment had not encountered similar problems in his previous operations. A workplace investigation showed that the majority of workers with rashes worked in areas where the air-conditioning was not functioning, and that the rashes had the appearance of miliaria rubra (Figs. 5 and 6). A walk-through survey of the warehouse showed that the ventilation was poor in the non-air-conditioned areas.

The diagnosis was that it was an outbreak of heat rashes, and a recommendation (after the walk-through survey) was made for the air-conditioning to be restored urgently. Heat stress measurements were taken at various sites the following day (Fig. 7), and all the readings were within the threshold limit values recommended by the ACGIH. In order to allay the workers' concern about arsenic exposure, environmental samples were collected and analyzed for arsenic, but none was detected.

The problem was resolved within two weeks after the repair of the air-conditioner.

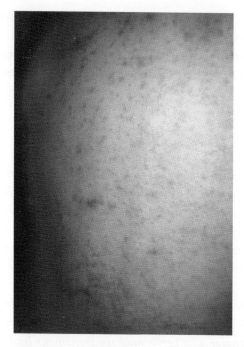

Fig. 5.   Miliaria rubra of the back in a worker in the warehouse.

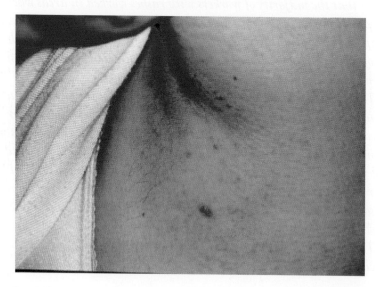

Fig. 6.   Miliaria rubra of the axillary region in another worker in the warehouse.

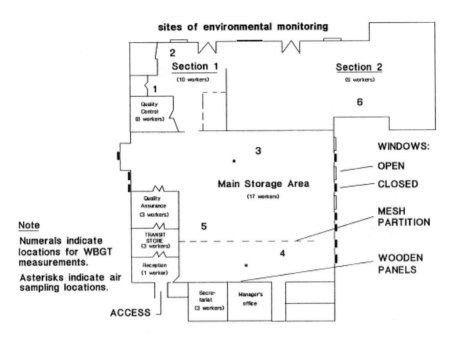

Fig. 7.   Plan of warehouse, showing distribution of sites of environmental monitoring.

The form

The contents of the form are shown in Box 1. This requires the recording of identification data on the workplace visited. It is analogous to a hospital patient record where identification data is needed for future reference. Information about names and telephone numbers of contacts is best recorded as they are provided. This avoids having to contact the factory again to re-establish the identity of the key people met with during the visit, but whose names and telephone numbers have been forgotten or not written down by the end of the visit. Furthermore, if further contact with the factory is required, knowledge of the key names invokes a sense of concern and interest on the part of the caller.

Information on the history of the workplace — whether it has been recently built, if it is part of a larger conglomerate, what it does, how it has developed over time in relation to its activities and

Box 1. Workplace Visit Checklist Contents

1. Identification data:
   a. Name of workplace
   b. Address and phone number

2. Contacts (name and telephone no.):
   a. Personnel manager/managing director
   b. Union representative
   c. Doctor
   d. Other, e.g. supervisor

3. Workplace:
   a. History
   b. Geography and site plan
   c. No. of workers
      Age
      Sex
      Race
      Shifts
      Turnover
   d. Services
      Medical
         — staff
         — procedures
      Canteen/shower
      Protective equipment
      Hygiene and safety

Raw materials → Finished product

1. Physical
2. Chemical
3. Biological
4. Mechanical/Ergonomic
5. Psychosocial
6. Safety issues

the surrounding community and environment, and its record on health and safety — is useful as a background to understanding that particular workplace. The analogy in the clinical situation is a patient's social, family, personal and past history. The geographical location of the factory can be recorded, for example, by obtaining a map that shows the way to the workplace. A site plan helps to ensure that any work area visited is put in the context of the rest of the worksite, and that all relevant areas are eventually visited and evaluated.

Two other sections of importance are:

- Data on the workforce: The characteristics of the workforce give an indication of the population "exposed" to the work environment. This will also be of use if epidemiological investigations are contemplated.
- Services provided and available to the workforce: This enables an assessment of the health, safety and welfare provisions in relation to any workplace hazards that may be identified.

All the above information may be obtained before or during the visit to the workplace.

Findings on whether an occupational hazard exists are recorded in the next section. This requires that the occupational physician using the format visits each section of the factory, starting from raw materials to storage and distribution of the finished product(s).

Although it would be ideal to systematically go through the various stages of production, in practice, because of the location of the different parts of the processes, these may not necessarily be shown to the visiting physician in any systematic order. Hence, the usefulness of a site plan to indicate what has been seen and what has not.

At each part of the process, the occupational physician needs to determine and record the presence of any hazards according to whether these are physical, chemical, mechanical and ergonomic, biological or psychosocial. This is based on an etiological classification of occupational hazards. The procedure allows a complete and thorough evaluation to be made; and it ensures that important hazards at each stage of the work activities are not missed out. The analogy to clinical medical practice is that in the examination of a patient, the doctor systematically goes through inspection, palpation, percussion and auscultation.

Physical hazards would include exposure to extremes of temperature, poor lighting, noise, pressure, vibration, electricity and radiation.

Chemical hazards may be present in solid, liquid, semi-solid or gaseous form. Identification of the presence of a chemical may require that the information on the label of the container or packaging be recorded, so that the chemical composition of a trade substance and its known health effects can be subsequently ascertained. If necessary, arrangements can then be made for industrial hygiene measurements to be taken to determine compliance with current airborne standards.

Mechanical hazards are often obvious to the trained safety professional, who will readily spot the unguarded sections of factory machinery. Ergonomic problems may be anticipated by observing the way in which posture and repeated movements of limbs and joints occur in the course of work.

Biological hazards are relevant to workplaces such as laboratories and hospitals. These may be classified according to etiological agent into viruses, bacteria, fungi and so on.

Psychosocial problems in the workplace may be difficult to identify, and one approach is to gather information by talking to workers on the production line in the course of the factory visit, or to consider other indirect indicators such as labor turnover rate, industrial relations difficulties, poor quality control or sickness absence.

An extended version of this form can be prepared to give further items to be recorded for an audit on occupational health services. The additional checklist is shown in Box 2.

Box 2. Additional Items in Workplace Visit Checklist

Additional Checklist for Occupational Health Services

1. Staff
Medical
Nursing
First aiders
Industrial hygiene staff
Safety officer/adviser
Welfare officer

2. Facilities
Rooms for OHS services
Equipment
  Medical
  Hygiene
  Safety
OH records
  (computerized or files?)
Library or information
  source
Other amenities
  Canteen
  Showers/Changing room
  Laundry

3. Activities
Health examinations/assessments
Periodic
Post-sickness
Special groups
  — statutory
  — non-statutory
Immunization
Health education/counselling
Treatment activities
Rehabilitation
Compensation
Disaster planning
Food hygiene
Ergonomics
Environmental health
  Waste management
  Waste disposal

From Occupational Health to Environmental Health

Previously, public interest in environmental health was not matched by a well-developed specialty in the health field which could respond to its needs and concerns. Occupational health practice today has gradually evolved to encompass environmental health issues.

This is for several reasons. First, many sources of pollution originate from the workplace. Second, in many other instances, the

Table 3.   Comparison of Occupational Health and Environmental Health

Occupational Health	Environmental Health
Hazards in workplace environment	Hazards in community environment
Hazards largely in air	Hazards in air, soil, water and food
Hazards are physical, chemical, biological and psychosocial	Hazards are physical, chemical, biological and psychosocial
Route of exposure: inhalation and dermal	Route of exposure: ingestion, inhalation and dermal
Exposure period: 8 hr/day for working life	Exposure period: lifelong
Exposed population: adults, usually healthy	Exposed population: children, adults, elderly, sick persons

distinction between the work environment and the home environment may not be clearly defined. This is particularly seen in agriculture and small-scale industries, where a clear demarcation does not exist between the workplace and home.

Furthermore, there are several areas of common ground between occupational and environmental health. Table 3 compares factors in the work environment that influence the health of the working population (occupational health) and that of the general environment affecting the health of the community (environmental health). Several areas of similarity between the work environment and the general environment affecting health exist.

Occupational health practitioners and physicians have the necessary skills in clinical medicine, toxicology, hygiene, epidemiology and preventive health to position themselves for the management of environmental health concerns, as illustrated in Case Study 6.

Case Study 6

Villagers living along a river began to complain of skin disorders a few months after a pulp mill was sited upstream from their villages. The residents, who were mainly fishermen and farmers, bathed in the river and used river water for many of their domestic activities. They claimed that pollutants discharged from the pulp mill caused the skin disorders. An occupational health team was consulted to resolve the matter.

Workplace assessment revealed some occupational health and safety issues that needed to be addressed. The plant utilized modern "state of the art" technology, with a closed-mill system. Monitoring of the effluent from the mill revealed that the quality of the discharge was within internationally accepted limits.

Examination of a group of the most severely affected villagers revealed that the main skin disorders were fungal infections of the skin, endogenous eczema and irritant contact dermatitis at specific sites (e.g. from application of topical medicaments, hand dermatitis from use of detergents).

A comparison of the existing health records of the village showed no increase in the proportion of cases of skin disorders before and after the pulp mill commenced operations. The main health problems were malaria and gastroenteritis.

The conclusion was that the villagers' health concerns (with regard to dermatological disorders) were unrelated to the pulp mill. The mill management, however, provided supplementary community health care through its health care department, in conjunction with the local health authorities. This gesture was appreciated by the villagers.

Conclusion

This chapter introduces the concept of occupational health, emphasizing that occupational health is concerned with the total health of all persons at work. The three categories of illnesses affecting the working population are: general diseases, work-related diseases and occupational diseases. General diseases and work-related diseases of a working population are usually covered in the undergraduate and postgraduate training programs of medical education.

This book specifically focuses on occupational diseases that affect the working population. Nevertheless, the reader should remember that occupational diseases are only one of the three components of the total health concern of the working population.

The book addresses occupational diseases in a manner that they are likely to be dealt with by practitioners. For instance, if a worker is diagnosed to be anemic, the question that arises is the relationship of this condition to his work. To this end the book covers medical conditions on the basis of organ systems affected and thereafter examines their relationship to work. This book also explores other issues of interest to the occupational health practitioner.

In the practice of occupational health, prevention of work-related and occupational disease is a major objective. Primary prevention should be the main priority in occupational health practice. When this fails, secondary prevention activities are undertaken to contain the damage.

However, health protection is not the only occupational health concern. Health promotion in the working population is another important activity. The workplace is an ideal setting for health promotion activities, and appropriate lifestyle interventions can prevent many of the common causes of morbidity in society.

Finally, the practice of occupational health today has extended beyond the domain of the workplace, into the general environment. Hence, the term "occupational and environmental medicine" might more accurately describe this important aspect of health care.

References

Baxter PJ, Aw TC, Cockcroft A, *et al.* (eds). (2010) *Hunter's Diseases of Occupations*, 10th edn. London: Hodder Arnold.

LaDou J. (ed). (2007). *Current Occupational and Environmental Medicine*, 4th edn. McGraw Hill.

Levy BS, Wegman DH, Baron SL, Sokas RK. (2011) *Occupational and Environmental Health*, 6th edn. Oxford University Press, New York, US.

Rom WN, Markowitz S. (eds.) (2007) *Environmental and Occupational Medicine*, 4th edn. Philadelphia: Lippincott Williams & Wilkins.

Rosenstock L, Cullen M, Brodkin C, Redlich C. (eds.) (2004) *Textbook of Clinical Occupational and Environmental Medicine*, 2nd edn. Philadelphia: Elsevier Health Sciences.

Stellman JM, *et al.* (eds). (1998) *ILO Encyclopaedia of Occupational Safety and Health*, 4th edn. Vol 1–4. Geneva: International Labour Office.

Chapter 2

Renal Disorders

Judy Sng*,‡, Tsun-Gun Ng† and Kee-Seng Chia*

Introduction

The renal system plays a key role in homeostasis by removing the waste products of metabolism and regulating electrolyte, fluid as well as acid-base balance. Renal blood flow is nearly a quarter of the cardiac output, and the average glomerular filtration rate (GFR) of 180 l/day is equal to 15 times the extracellular fluid volume and 60 times the plasma volume. This physiological process is highly effective in excreting waste products and maintaining water and electrolyte balance, but may also allow toxic xenobiotics (substances that are foreign to the body or exogenous toxins) to be concentrated in the kidneys. For this reason, the kidneys in man are highly vulnerable to xenobiotics. In fact, the concentration of some xenobiotics in the kidneys may reach toxic levels even when serum levels are within acceptable limits.

The kidneys and urinary tract are subject to a wide range of pathologies either as a direct or indirect result of external insults.

*Department of Epidemiology and Public Health, Yong Loo Lin School of Medicine, National University of Singapore.
†Department of Renal Medicine, Tan Tock Seng Hospital, Singapore.
‡Corresponding author. E-mail: ephjsgk@nus.edu.sg.

Apart from catastrophic events such as acute poisoning resulting in acute renal failure, it is not usually possible to isolate occupational exposures as the major causative factor. This makes it difficult to define the epidemiology of occupational renal disorders. It is more often the case that work-related factors hasten the onset or worsening of renal disease, such as diabetic nephropathy in a shift worker whose irregular mealtimes contribute to poor glycemic control, or the progression of primary glomerulonephritis to frank renal failure through lead or solvent exposure. This will be discussed in more detail in a later section.

The prevalence of chronic kidney disease (CKD) and end-stage renal disease (ESRD) is increasing in many countries. Although mortality among renal failure patients requiring dialysis is still high, improved medical care, dialysis access and renal transplantation is gradually allowing more ESRD patients to have longer and better lives. Physicians will thus need to consider the employability of patients with CKD or ESRD, especially those in the younger age groups.

Singapore has the fifth highest incidence of renal failure in the world. More than 1000 people were diagnosed with ESRD in 2006, with the age-standardized rate rising from 231 to 253 per million persons among Singapore residents (data from *Singapore Renal Registry Report* 2005/6). The commonest cause of ESRD in Singapore is diabetic nephropathy, followed by primary glomerulonephritis and hypertension. The proportion of ESRD cases that can be attributed to occupational toxins is unknown, as etiologic information is lacking and exposures to nephrotoxins are not frequently documented. Furthermore, few nephrotoxins produce clinically unique, recognizable syndromes or specific histological changes in renal biopsies. Histological changes in the end-stage kidney look very much alike with nonspecific glomerulosclerosis, tubular atrophy and interstitial fibrosis.

Many nephrotoxins are still used in industries, potentially exposing a large number of workers to them. The identification of these agents may not help in the clinical management of a patient with ESRD, but will help in controlling and regulating the agents' use in industries to protect workers as well as the general public.

Occupational Factors Contributing to Renal Disease

Acute Kidney Injury

Acute kidney injury in the occupational health setting is often associated with acute high-dose exposure to nephrotoxins. Cadmium is probably the best known occupational cause of acute kidney injury. There have been a number of reports on welders who were exposed to cadmium oxide fumes while cutting cadmium-containing metals or cadmium alloys and who later developed acute kidney injury following respiratory manifestations. Mercury and chromium have also been associated with acute tubular necrosis at high exposure levels. Apart from heavy metals, some organic solvents such as chloroform, carbon tetrachloride, trichloroethylene and toluene, as well as phosphorus and arsine, have also been known to induce acute kidney injury. Other occupational exposures which may precipitate acute kidney injury include hyperthermia. Rhabdomyolysis (muscle injury, from various causes such as mechanical trauma or electrocution) can lead to myoglobinemia and haemoglobinemia, which are predisposing factors for acute tubular necrosis.

Chronic Kidney Disease

Commonly cited occupational causes of chronic kidney disease include heavy metals such as cadmium, lead and mercury, organic solvents as well as silica. However, chronic kidney disease that is directly or mainly caused by an occupational exposure (occupational renal disease) is encountered much less frequently than primary non-occupational chronic kidney disease. It is also important to recognize that work-related renal disease, in which work exposure is not the sole or main cause but plays an important contributory role, is also fairly common. For example, in the case of an insulin-dependent diabetic who has difficulty maintaining good glycemic control due to irregular shift-work hours and subsequently develops diabetic nephropathy, it could be said that the nephropathy is work-related. In the same way, hypertensive nephropathy could be deemed work-related in a worker who faces very high work stress which results in uncontrolled blood pressure. However, it is often difficult to determine the degree of work-relatedness of CKD cases in the population. Analgesics and medical conditions like diabetes mellitus, glomerulonephritis or hypertension most likely contribute more to chronic kidney disease than occupational or environmental lead exposure. Furthermore, the toxicity of lead may be influenced by other dietary and lifestyle factors. Therefore, it is difficult to demonstrate the extent of the contribution of low-level occupational lead exposure to cases of chronic kidney disease.

Urinary Tract Malignancy

Workers in the rubber and dye-manufacturing industries who were exposed to aromatic amines (2-naphthylamine, 4-aminobiphenyl, benzidine) have an increased risk of bladder cancer. A number of other substances including polychlorinated biphenyls, solvents and polycyclic aromatic hydrocarbons have also been linked to bladder cancer risk. Chlorinated aliphatic hydrocarbons, a class of organic solvents, have also been associated with increased renal cancer risk.

Other Work-related Disorders

Working in hot environments or where the work schedule does not permit sufficient toilet breaks may contribute to persistent dehydration and predisposes the worker to developing urinary tract infections or to urinary calculi formation.

Nephrotoxins

Heavy Metals

Cadmium

Cadmium-containing compounds are widely used in electroplating, manufacturing of pigments, plastics, glass, metal alloys and electrical equipment. The growth in cadmium use was temporarily halted in the early 1970s due to environmental concerns. However, due to the demand for rechargeable batteries, cadmium production was further increased in the late 1970s.

It has been estimated that prior to 2001, only 50% of cadmium-containing batteries sold in Sweden and other European countries were recycled. The remainder was to a large extent burned among household waste, resulting in general environmental pollution. The European Union has since passed a law to increase the recycling of batteries containing cadmium as well as mercury and lead.

In the 1950s, industrial effluents containing cadmium polluted the river water used for rice cultivation in Japan. The painful bone disease "itai-itai" ("ouch-ouch") that resulted was also associated with a reduction in the glomerular filtration rate.

Acute poisoning

As mentioned earlier, acute occupational cadmium poisoning is commonly due to inhalation of cadmium oxide fumes from welding and cutting cadmium-plated metal or cadmium-containing alloys. In such circumstances, the first clinical manifestation is usually respiratory distress from severe chemical pneumonitis, often quickly followed by acute tubular necrosis and renal failure. Chelation therapy may be considered in cases with severe exposure.

Chronic poisoning

For chronic cadmium poisoning, renal effects are by far the best documented, manifesting as increased urinary excretion of low molecular weight (LMW) proteins. The level of β_2-microglobulin, widely used as a marker, rises after long-term exposure when the urinary cadmium level is above 10 $\mu g/g$ creatinine. Levels of other LMW proteins and enzymes are raised after shorter durations of exposure and with lower urinary cadmium levels. The critical urinary cadmium level is proposed to be at 5 $\mu g/g$ creatinine, below which no kidney dysfunction is likely to develop.

Tubular proteinuria, once established, is irreversible even when the workers are removed from further exposure. Decrease in GFR, renal functional reserve capacity and increased incidence of nephrolithiasis have been reported upon long-term follow-up, especially among workers who experienced heavy exposure.

Despite the association of chronic cadmium exposure with a number of renal disorders, there is little literature reporting excess in deaths due to renal diseases among cadmium-exposed subjects. This could have been influenced by how the deaths were reported. Patients with chronic kidney disease, for example, are at high risk of cardiovascular morbidity and mortality which may not be reflected as directly related to cadmium nephrotoxicity.

Lead

Case Study 1

During a periodic medical examination, a lead-exposed worker was found to have a blood lead (PbB) level of 750 µg/l. He had been working in the same factory for the last 14 years and had repeated episodes where his PbB level exceeded 500 µg/l. He was noted to be mildly hypertensive four years ago. Further investigations showed mild anemia (hemoglobin of 13.4 g/dL) with slightly elevated serum creatinine (1.6 mg/l) and low creatinine clearance of 74 ml/min/1.74m² (the normal is 80–140 ml/min/1.74m²). There was also microalbuminuria and β₂-microglobulinuria.

The worker was removed from further exposure. Six months later, his PbB was slightly lower at 610 µg/l, but a repeat measurement of serum creatinine and creatinine clearance showed no further improvement.

Though lead is a well-known nephrotoxic agent, there are no early markers of lead nephropathy. The diagnosis of lead nephropathy is at best circumstantial. Irreversible renal damage would have already occurred by the time serum creatinine and creatinine clearance become abnormal. In this case, a past history of high exposure to lead coupled with historical records of high PbB levels suggests lead as the causative agent. However, in the presence of hypertension, diabetes mellitus or a past history of glomerulonephritis, it is often impossible to identify the contributory role of each factor.

Lead was previously widely used in the manufacture of lead-acid storage batteries, ammunition, polyvinyl chloride stabilizers, paints and glazes. Its use has declined greatly in many countries due to increasing awareness of lead toxicity not only on exposed workers but also on others, especially children, from environmental exposures. However, it can be said that much of the problem has not been eliminated but merely transferred to developing countries, resulting in the continued exposure of both the workforce as well as the general population through environmental contamination with lead-containing waste. The renal effects of lead exposure are seen with its inorganic compounds, whereas organic lead compounds such as tetraethyl and tetramethyl lead found in some anti-knock agents affect mainly the central nervous system.

The renal effects of lead are primarily tubular or tubulointerstitial, and may extend from reversible tubular dysfunction and ultrastructural changes (Stage I reversible nephropathy) to chronic nephropathy (Stage II irreversible nephropathy) and possibly to a third stage of renal failure. Collated data has shown that chronic low-level lead exposure (corresponding to blood lead levels below 5 μg/dl) can contribute to nephropathy, especially in susceptible persons with pre-existing diabetes or chronic kidney disease.

Acute reversible lead nephropathy

Acute exposure to high levels of inorganic lead has been reported to cause proximal tubular impairment which is apparently reversible, associated with intranuclear inclusion bodies composed of a lead-protein complex. The resultant clinical picture is similar to Fanconi syndrome, with aminoaciduria, glycosuria and hyperphosphaturia. Acute lead poisoning is usually associated with gastrointestinal and neurologic symptoms, although in cases with large exposures acute renal failure may develop.

Chronic lead nephropathy

The pathological mechanism in chronic lead nephropathy is chronic tubulointerstitial nephritis. Progression to the chronic irreversible stage occurs over months or years, usually with continual exposure, as renal tubular atrophy and interstitial fibrosis become more prominent. Until 50% to 75% of nephrons have been destroyed, blood urea nitrogen and serum creatinine remain normal. By then, there would already be irreversible nephropathy. Recent increases in blood lead level, and not merely current blood lead levels or the cumulative lead burden, may contribute to the toxicity of lead on the kidneys.

Bone is the main storage organ for inorganic lead. The half-life of inorganic lead in compact bone has been reported to be several decades long. Measurement of bone lead content by X-ray fluorescence therefore better reflects the total body burden of lead, but is not necessarily a good surrogate measure of lead in the kidneys.

Mercury

Though elemental mercury is preferentially accumulated in the kidneys, the neurologic rather than the renal effects are more prominent. Nephrotoxicity of mercury depends on its chemical form. Mercuric chloride ($HgCl_2$) is highly nephrotoxic, while mercurous chloride (Hg_2Cl_2) is relatively non-toxic and is used as a medicinal agent. Organic mercury produces mainly acute irritative effects or central nervous system toxicity, but may also induce renal injury. Occupations at risk of mercury exposure include chemical industry workers, dentists, dental assistants and some pharmaceutical industry workers.

Acute tubular necrosis

With the ingestion of as little as 0.5 gm of $HgCl_2$, acute renal failure from proximal tubular necrosis occurs rapidly, provided the victim does not first succumb to gastrointestinal sequelae. If performed before the onset of oliguria, chelation therapy using intravenous British anti-Lewisite (BAL) has been shown to limit the extent of renal damage. Following full recovery, even when renal function becomes normal, the kidneys will show residual interstitial nephritis.

Nephrotic syndrome

Many studies have reported an association between mercury exposure and proteinuria/nephrotic syndrome, most often with histologic features consistent with membranous nephropathy. The dose-response relationship is however inconsistent. In most instances, the proteinuria appears to be self-limiting and disappears spontaneously when mercury exposure is stopped, although it may take several months.

Statutory medical examinations

Under Singapore's labor laws, cadmium, mercury and lead are classified under health hazards requiring statutory medical examinations by suitably qualified and registered factory doctors. This is indicated when workers are likely to be exposed to airborne concentrations greater than 10% of permissible exposure levels (for cadmium: 0.05 mg/m^3, lead: 0.15 mg/m^3, inorganic mercury: 0.025 mg/m^3) or have a significant risk of ingesting the substance during the work processes.

Pre-employment and annual examinations for cadmium-exposed workers include blood cadmium and urine β_2-microglobulin estimations. Serum urea and creatinine are not included in routine statutory medical examinations but may be added if indicated. It is important to remember that β_2-microglobulin is highly pH-sensitive and rapidly degrades when the urine pH is less than 5.5, even within the bladder. As much as 80% of the original concentration can be lost within two hours at a pH of 5 and a temperature of 37°C.

For persons handling lead at the workplace, pre-employment and six-monthly periodic examinations are performed which include measurement of blood lead and hemoglobin levels. It is also important to evaluate the renal function of workers with long exposure history or repeated episodes of high blood lead levels. If evidence of nephropathy such as proteinuria is documented, these workers should be protected from further exposure and provided with long-term follow-up. Functional tests such as creatinine clearance should also be carried out.

For mercury-exposed workers, pre-employment and annual medical examinations are conducted which include urine mercury level estimation. Workers are routinely advised to avoid consuming seafood for three days before the urine collection.

Organic Solvents and Petroleum Hydrocarbons

Petroleum hydrocarbons and organic solvents contain several sub-groups of chemically related compounds. Those that are of significance as nephrotoxic agents include halogenated hydrocarbons (e.g. trichloroethylene, carbon tetrachloride and chloroform), certain glycols (e.g. ethylene glycol), alcohols (e.g. methyl, ethyl and isopropyl alcohol), aromatic hydrocarbons (benzene, toluene and xylene) and other complex aromatic naphthas. Organic solvents such as toluene, xylene and a number of petroleum products have recently also been implicated by some researchers in the progression of pre-existing primary glomerulonephritis to end-stage renal disease.

Acute kidney injury

Acute renal failure caused by halogenated hydrocarbons and glycols has been reported. It is probably a result of direct toxic effect (acute tubular necrosis) rather than via immunological mechanisms. Some researchers believe that the hydrocarbon may act as a "solvent" for the membrane structure of the proximal tubules or that metabolic activation of the hydrocarbon may release metabolites of greater nephrotoxic action.

Chronic kidney disease and chronic glomerulonephritis

The renal lesion induced by complex petrochemical hydrocarbons is characterized by excessive hyaline droplets accumulation in the cytoplasm of epithelial cells of the proximal convoluted tubules. Though these lesions are not unique to petroleum products, they appear to be consistently produced by them. Further studies have indicated that it is the alkane fraction that is primarily responsible for the nephrotoxic activity.

There have been several case reports on Goodpasture's syndrome or anti-GBM disease with exposures to various hydrocarbons including gasoline and jet fuel.

Statutory medical examinations

Currently, under Singapore's labor laws, only workers exposed to trichloroethylene and perchloroethylene are required to undergo statutory medical examinations which focus mainly on the liver and central nervous system. This is due to the severe hepatotoxicity and neurotoxicity that these solvents are associated with. Nonetheless, it is important to bear in mind the potential nephrotoxicity of organic solvents and petroleum products, especially for workers with known primary glomerulonephritis, diabetes and hypertension. Screening for proteinuria is simple, non-invasive and inexpensive and should be considered in the routine follow-up of solvent-exposed workers.

Silica

There is both animal and human evidence that silica is nephrotoxic. Raised levels of urinary albumin and α_1-microglobulin suggest the presence of glomerular and tubular dysfunction. The abnormalities appear to be confined to those who had prolonged and heavy exposure. The abnormalities were probably irreversible as they were present among silicotics who had ceased exposure for many years. The clinical significance of these findings is unclear. Based on mortality studies of silica-exposed workers, few studies reported data on deaths due to renal diseases.

Investigations for Renal Dysfunction

Proteinuria

The glomerular basement membrane (GBM) is a size- and charge-selective barrier to circulating plasma proteins. Due to this selectivity, high molecular weight (HMW) plasma proteins such as albumin can only be found in very small amounts in the urine under normal circumstances. When there is an increase in glomerular permeability, such as in chronic glomerulonephritis, HMW proteins appear in the urine.

On the other hand, LMW plasma proteins (molecular weight of less than 40,000 daltons) pass freely into the glomerular ultrafiltrate and are very efficiently reabsorbed by the proximal tubules. The high efficiency of this reabsorption process ensures that the excreted urine is virtually protein-free. Thus, LMW proteinuria indicates tubular dysfunction or possibly overflow proteinuria, such as in the case of paraproteinemias. As a LMW protein, urinary β_2-microalbumin (β_2m) is widely used for evaluating the nephrotoxicity of various drugs and chemicals, although it is highly sensitive to pH changes. In addition, β_2m is a membrane antigen that is synthesized by nearly all nucleated cells, especially lymphoid cells like monocytes and macrophages. Serum levels can increase in malignancy, systemic inflammatory processes and acquired immunodeficiency syndrome.

Urinary retinol binding protein (RBP: a LMW plasma protein that transports retinol from the liver to the epithelial tissues) and α_1m are more stable than β_2m in acidic pH, and an increase in urinary RBP and α_1m in the absence of a decrease in GFR can be interpreted as a direct measure of tubular function. The urine α_1m concentration appears to be unaffected by the presence of urinary infection, hematuria or tissue breakdown products in bladder cancer and was shown by some occupational studies to be a sensitive biomarker of tubular damage in cadmium-, lead- or silica-exposed workers. Some researchers have therefore suggested that urinary retinol binding protein and α_1-microglobulin (α_1m: a glycosylated plasma protein) may be more sensitive and practical than urinary β_2m for the monitoring of nephrotoxicity. These tests are, however, not widely available in clinical practice currently.

Albumin is quantitatively the major HMW serum protein found in the urine. It is widely used as an index of glomerular damage as it is easier to assay in normal unconcentrated urine.

Screening for proteinuria can be done with a 24-hour urine collection for total protein quantification or with a random urine sample for urine protein to creatinine ratio estimation. Differentiation of the various types of proteinuria (e.g. glomerular, tubular, etc.) can be done in consultation with the renal physician. The significance of microalbuminuria in occupational renal diseases has not yet been established.

Assessment of Renal Function

The commonest methods used to assess renal function in clinical practice are serum creatinine concentration, the creatinine clearance test and GFR estimating equations.

Although serum creatinine is convenient and the commonest method of assessing renal function in routine clinical practice, it is not a very sensitive marker and an initial small rise in serum creatinine usually reflects a marked fall in absolute GFR. This phenomenon is due to an increase in proximal tubular creatinine secretion when GFR has effectively decreased, leading to only a slight increase in the absolute serum creatinine concentration. Variations in dietary intake (e.g. vegetarian diet versus increased protein diet or the use of creatine supplements), muscle mass, medications and other factors also need to be taken into account for an accurate interpretation of serum creatinine values.

A 24-hour urine collection for creatinine clearance can also be used to assess renal function. Creatinine clearance represents an overestimation of the true GFR as a result of tubular secretion of creatinine. This is more significant in patients with CKD as the proportion of tubular secretion of creatinine versus filtered creatinine increases in CKD. An accurate representation of the creatinine clearance requires a complete 24-hour urine collection which can be difficult to obtain. As a result of the difficulties with 24-hour urine collections, GFR estimating equations based on the serum creatinine concentration are becoming a popular method of assessing renal function. GFR equations are better than the use of serum creatinine alone as they incorporate demographic and clinical variables which are known to affect the serum creatinine concentration. The commonest equations are the Cockcroft–Gault and Modification of Diet in Renal Disease (MDRD) study equations. It should be noted however that these equations are not validated for use in all populations and that equations based on serum creatinine are not reliable for an estimation of GFR in individuals with significant variations in dietary intake or muscle mass. In such cases, creatinine clearance testing would offer a more accurate assessment of the renal function.

Chronic and End-stage Renal Disease: Fitness to Work Issues

Case Study 2

Mr. K is a middle-aged man. He suffers from longstanding diabetes complicated by nephropathy-induced renal failure and is on continuous ambulatory peritoneal dialysis. He is the sole breadwinner of his family of four and was previously working as a taxi driver but found it impossible to cope after starting dialysis. Moreover, he had encountered a series of near-miss driving mishaps, brought on by deteriorating vision from diabetic retinopathy.

Fortunately, Mr. K was able to find a job as a gardener in a club and has been working there for more than a year. He now works 9.5-hour days, inclusive of two half-hour breaks for dialysis, and performs garden maintenance tasks such as grass cutting. He is well provided with personal protective equipment (safety boots, gloves, goggles) as well as loose-fitting overalls that can both protect and conceal his peritoneal dialysis catheter. Despite a smaller salary, he is satisfied and very appreciative of his employer who has set aside a room for him to perform his dialysis in during break times and also allowed him time-off to go for his medical reviews every month.

Mr. K's case scenario shows us that while it may not always be easy, it is still possible for patients who are on dialysis to remain employed. Being employed is important to dialysis patients as it provides a sense of purpose, generates income, allows social interaction in the workplace and maintains self-esteem. Frequently, employers also provide health insurance and medical benefits. Many dialysis patients feel well enough to work and want to be employed. Unfortunately many of them are unable to find a job or lose their jobs very quickly once their medical condition is disclosed. In fact, many patients feel they can work, but not all of them are employed.

A careful assessment of fitness to work (pre-employment) or fitness to return to work would require a good understanding of the modality and schedule of dialysis, concomitant medical problems as well as adequate knowledge of the job requirements. Patients can occasionally request the assistance of nephrologists or the occupational healthcare team to speak to employers who are hesitant to keep dialysis patients on their payroll. With a proper assessment of the patient's suitability to remain in employment, physicians are in a good position to reassure the employer of the patient's ability to contribute to the company's operations. Prior communication with the employer is very important. Employers are often understanding and would allow employees temporary leave of absence from work for access surgery, time to adjust to dialysis in the initial stages, clinic visits for follow-up as well as understanding the need for unexpected hospitalizations for complications of the disease.

It is important to choose a work-friendly treatment schedule for patients on dialysis. Hemodialysis sessions can be arranged in the evenings after work to minimize disruptions to their jobs. Alternatively, patients could arrange with their employers to work longer hours on their non-dialysis days to make up for the loss of working hours on dialysis days. Frequently patients can also work on their laptops during dialysis sessions. It would also help if patients choose a dialysis center near to their residence or working place to reduce traveling time and costs. For patients who are on continuous ambulatory peritoneal dialysis, they can perform their mid-day exchanges during their break or lunchtime. Thirty minutes would suffice for the exchange which needs to be done in a clean environment. Patients who are on automated peritoneal dialysis usually find the least disruption to their work as dialysis is performed at night during their sleep hours with a cycler.

Patients with an arteriovenous fistula or graft should avoid lifting heavy objects with the access arm and avoid constrictive clothing and accessories on that arm. Peritoneal dialysis patients must avoid occupations that would not allow them to keep the Tenckhoff catheter exit site clean and dry.

Hemodialysis patients may experience fatigue after dialysis sessions, with a "washed out" feeling. It is important to advise patients not to engage in strenuous, laborious activities immediately post-dialysis. A large interdialytic weight gain can also result in intradialytic hypotension, resulting in a longer recovery period post-dialysis.

Patients should therefore be advised on the need for salt and fluid restrictions accordingly.

Physicians should counsel patients on the need to maintain their health in an optimal state to ensure that they remain employable. Measures include reinforcing the need to remain compliant with their treatment schedules, medications, dietary and fluid restrictions as well as clinic visits where appropriate. Physicians should also ensure that the patient's hemoglobin levels are within the target range so as to avoid the symptoms of anemia which could affect their functional status.

If full-time employment is not possible, dialysis patients could consider part-time employment. Alternatively jobs that allow them to work from home would be ideal in some cases. A multi-disciplinary approach would certainly help to keep more dialysis patients in employment. Patients could also be referred to the various renal failure support groups and non-governmental organizations in Singapore and other countries that collaborate with employment agencies to help patients with renal failure find suitable employment.

References

Ekong EB, Jaar BG, Weaver VM. (2006) Lead-related nephrotoxicity: A review of the epidemiologic evidence. *Kidney Int* **70**: 2074–2084.

Jacob S, Hery M, Protois JC, Stengel B. (2007) New insight into solvent-related end-stage renal disease: Occupations, products and types of solvents at risk. *Occup Environ Med* **64**: 843–848.

National Registry of Diseases Office, Health Promotion Board. (2009) *Sixth Report of the Singapore Renal Registry* 2005/2006.

Palmer KT, Cox RAF, Brown I. (2007) *Fitness for Work: The Medical Aspects*, 4th edn. Chapter 4, Renal and urological disease. New York: Oxford University Press.

Scélo G, Brennan P. (2006) The epidemiology of bladder and kidney cancer. *Nat Clin Prac Urol* **4**(4): 205–217.

Chapter 3

Cardiovascular Disorders

Hean-Yee Ong* and See-Muah Lee[†,‡]

Cardiovascular diseases (CVDs) are a group of disorders of the heart and blood vessels. CVDs are common causes of morbidity and mortality worldwide (Box 1). Such disorders include those affecting the heart and the central nervous system.

> **Box 1. The World Health Organization Report 2008 (WHO, 2008)**
>
> **Facts about Cardiovascular Diseases (CVDs)**
>
> CVDs are the number one cause of death globally: more people die annually from CVDs than from any other cause.
>
> An estimated 17.5 million people died from CVDs in 2005, representing 30% of all global deaths. Of these deaths, an estimated 7.6 million were due to coronary heart disease and 5.7 million were due to stroke.
>
> Over 80% of CVD deaths take place in low- and middle-income countries and occur almost equally in men and women.
>
> By 2015, almost 20 million people will die from CVDs, mainly from heart disease and stroke. These are projected to remain the single leading causes of death.

*Department of Cardiology, Khoo Teck Puat Hospital, Singapore.
†Department of Epidemiology and Public Health, Yong Loo Lin School of Medicine, National University of Singapore, Diabetes Clinic, Khoo Teck Puat Hospital, Singapore.
‡Corresponding author. E-mail: ephlsm@nus.edu.sg

Singapore, with a total population of 4.6 million, experienced 17,140 deaths in 2007. Of these, 3394 (19.8%) were attributed to ischemic heart disease, the second most common cause of mortality after cancer (MOH, 2009).

Many affected individuals are in the prime of their lives. Suffering from ischemic heart disease has a profound impact on work, income and family.

This chapter will consider the implications of coronary heart disease — the disease of blood vessels supplying the heart muscle — and work, as well as some of the specific cardiogenic occupational exposures.

Risk Factors for Coronary Heart Disease

Coronary heart disease presents clinically as either stable or unstable ischemic heart disease. Ischemic heart disease is stable when the cholesterol plaques build up slowly and gradually. Stable ischemic heart disease is deemed to be present when the patient has demonstrable ischemia during exertion. This is usually due to blockage of a major coronary artery and may be discovered during a stress electrocardiogram (ECG).

Workers with stable ischemic heart disease who work in sedentary occupations may not be at risk. However, if the occupation is physically demanding, then the increased physiological demands on the heart during such work may put the worker at high risk of plaque rupture and an acute coronary syndrome. Workers who complain of exertional chest symptoms should be advised to seek treatment. However, many cases of pain due to ischemic heart disease may be atypical in nature, and some, especially among those with diabetes mellitus, may be completely asymptomatic, giving rise to what is known as silent myocardial ischemia (Xanthos, Ekmektzoglou and Papadimitriou, 2008).

Unstable ischemic heart disease develops when there is an acute unpredictable obstruction (either transient or persistent) of a coronary artery by a platelet-rich plug over a vulnerable cholesterol plaque. This occurs during a plaque rupture.

The risk of developing a plaque rupture resulting in an acute coronary syndrome (which may present as sudden cardiac death, acute myocardial infarction or unstable angina) does not correlate with the degree of luminal stenosis of the coronary arteries but instead is related to the number of "cardiovascular risk factors" present (Falk, Shah and Fuster, 1995).

These risk factors were originally developed in the Framingham Study. They include age, gender, blood pressure, cholesterol level and smoking history. The cardiovascular disease risk score can be derived and classified as very low, low, moderate, high or very high. Such scoring systems are freely available on the internet (NHLBI, 2009).

Diabetes mellitus is considered to be a coronary risk equivalent by many (Haffner *et al.*, 1998; Bulugahapitiya *et al.*, 2009). It is also increasingly recognized that those with metabolic syndrome (high blood pressure, obesity, insulin resistance and lipidemia), because of the clustering of these cardiovascular risk factors, have an amplified cardiovascular risk. Its presence is in essence also a call for action to reduce the likelihood of developing both diabetes (if not already present) and cardiovascular disease (see chapter on metabolic disorders and work).

Employers should be encouraged to assist their employees in lowering their modifiable risk factors, such as providing healthy food options at the canteen (two servings of fruits, salt not exceeding a teaspoon a day and reduced intake of trans fat) and helping to manage stress and work — life balance. Physical activity should be encouraged (30 minutes a day for most days of the week) and, where resources permit, provision of facilities be made for exercise. Non-smoking policies at work and opportunities to attend smoking cessation services should be encouraged. Health screening and follow-up management could also be offered (Box 2).

Box 2.   Modifiable Cardiovascular Risk Factors

Total cholesterol:
    LDL (<3.40 mmol/l)
    HDL (>1.55 mmol/l)
    TG (<1.77 mmol/l)
Body mass index (18–25 kg/m^2)
Blood pressure (<140/90 mmHg)
Physical activity (30 minutes, 3 times per week)
Diet (low fat, low salt)
Smoking (cessation)

Fitness to Work

Employing a Person with Ischemic Heart Disease

The majority of occupations can be undertaken by persons with or without cardiovascular diseases. In most of these cases, for example, working at a desk-bound job, in sales, teaching or other sedentary occupations, there is no unacceptable increased risk to the cardiovascular health of the person concerned. These occupations generally do not require a sustained high aerobic effort, during which a person with compromised cardiovascular health may be adversely affected. In fact, the discovery of a heart condition may not have a significant impact on the way work is performed, and only leads to the individual and his doctor taking steps to improve his health.

For others, perhaps some job modifications and accommodations may be required. This may be in the form of avoiding strenuous activities like lifting heavy loads and being assigned to different tasks.

Stress and cardiovascular risk

Stress can occur in any job situation. There are many workplace factors that can cause stress. They range from hostile organizational climate, hazards at work, poor interpersonal relationships, inappropriate skill match for the job, overwork or underwork, among many others. These stress factors can cause a variety of adverse health problems, including heart attacks. The signs of stress are not always obvious, and both workers and employers have a responsibility to jointly address and manage such issues.

Jobs where a minimum level of cardiovascular fitness is required, and evaluation of fitness

For some workers in certain occupations, the presence of cardiovascular problems may, however, pose an increased risk to health. The assessment of cardiovascular fitness in relation to work can thus be considered in the following ways:

1. Physically demanding work for which a person with compromised cardiovascular health may be at increased adverse health risk (e.g. firefighting).
2. Work which may not necessarily be physically demanding, but for which a cardiovascular event may have extensive impact on personal risk or public interest and have further implications. The acceptability of a worker's personal health risk of a cardiovascular event in such circumstances is a question that has to be examined (e.g. airline pilots).
3. Special occupation-specific cardiovascular risk factors and their assessment.

Cardiovascular Assessment

Case Study 1: Fitness for Work in Remote Locations

You have assessed a 51-year-old man, Mr. X, as fit for a job as an operations manager. He is also being posted to a remote location by the company, which deals in mining. Three months into the job, he suffers an acute coronary event. The medical facilities in the location are very basic and he dies while being transported to the capital for further management.

The company has now written to you requesting an explanation, wanting to know, in particular, if his heart condition could have been uncovered earlier during the pre-employment medical evaluation, which could have averted the tragic turn of events.

On recall, aided by the clinical notes, you remember that Mr. X was a pleasant man of nondescript appearance. A quick calculation, based on height and weight, which thankfully was recorded by the nurse, but which obviously was not much heeded during such examinations, revealed a BMI of 29 kg/m². Resting ECG was normal. There was no clinical history of ischemic heart disease. There was no history of chest pains, but this could have been easily withheld by the applicant, or might have been dismissed as trivial and unworthy of mention by him. He did not have diabetes. His total cholesterol was 5.7 mmol/l, HDL was 1.0 mmol/l, and he was under treatment for hypertension, with repeated systolic readings of 150 mmHg. He was also a smoker.

Risk Assessment

An assessment of his cardiovascular risk, using the Framingham risk score, establishes his risk at about 25% over the next 10 years. This means that for 100 people with similar risk factors, comparable in sex and age, 25 will have a cardiac event, whilst 75 will not. A risk of such magnitude is considered high. Given the circumstances of his job in a remote environment where access to medical care can be a problem, it would have been prudent for the physician to discuss this risk and its management in greater detail with the employer and the applicant. Employers are of course ultimately free to employ or reject any prospective applicant, but the physician entrusted to do a pre-employment medical examination will need to discuss any special risk considerations with all parties concerned to enable them to make informed decisions (Lee and Koh, 2008).

There are limitations of a resting ECG in the prediction of future cardiac events (Mulcahy *et al.*, 1997; Stone *et al.*, 1997). This patient, with his multiple risk factors, would have benefited from a more detailed cardiac evaluation and intensification of therapy.

Framingham risk score

The National Cholesterol Education Panel defines high risk as a 10-year predicted risk of >20%, intermediate risk as a predicted risk of 10–20%, and low risk as a predicted risk of <10%. All patients with diabetes, and anyone who has already had a myocardial infarction (or heart attack), are considered to be at high risk.

Case Study 2: Fitness for Firefighters

Captain Tan is a 46-year-old firefighter veteran, having joined the service since the age of 22 years. He has gained some weight through the years. His last BMI was 28 kg/m². His cholesterol was top normal. His blood pressure was 140/90, on treatment with medication. He is asymptomatic.

He does not smoke and is a teetotaler. At the last medical examination done six months ago, he was cleared as fit. One month ago, during a firefighting mission, he experienced a heart attack. Fortunately, he was able to alert his colleagues in time and was sent to the hospital where he was treated successfully.

He appears to be rehabilitated and is eager to go back to work after resting at home for four weeks.

What are the medical tests that should have been done?

Firefighters at recruitment are probably self-selected: they are generally younger and fitter. But there is no reason to believe that these attributes will not, like for the rest of the general population, deteriorate with time. The idea of periodic health screening with the potential of loss of livelihood for affected workers may not be an attractive one. Such problems will have to be sensitively addressed and handled. There is, however, a need for mandatory periodic medical evaluations for firefighters. Unfortunately, in most organizations, consensus medical guidelines have yet to be established. Medical history, physical examinations, lipid biochemistry and resting ECG all have a role, but may not be sensitive enough to pick up ischemic heart disease in a 46-year-old.

Firefighting is a hazardous job. Episodic demands on the body caused by high-surge activities can be deleterious to health. In a study of the data between 1990 and 2000 in the United States, coronary heart disease was responsible for 44% of on-duty deaths, followed by trauma at 27%. Firemen above 35 years old were more likely to die from a heart attack as opposed to death from the fire or disaster they were fighting. Most of the deaths (60%) occur in those over 40 years old (FEMA, 2002).

A separate study by Kales *et al.*, also of US firefighters from 1994 to 2004, determined that 449 deaths were due to coronary heart disease. The highest risk was during fire suppression activities, which, though only accounting for 2% of working time, were associated with 144 (32.1%) of the coronary deaths (Kales *et al.*, 2007).

For firefighters above 35 years old, an exercise stress ECG for a formal evaluation of the exercise capacity will be necessary. Besides being a risk indicator for sudden cardiac death, a low exercise capacity, in the absence of ischemia, will also have implications on a firefighter's ability to complete his job safely. One useful test is by evaluating the VO_2 max. The VO_2 max is the maximum energy that a person consumes and is expressed in ml/kg/min or metabolic equivalents (METs). 1 MET, equal to approximately 3.5 ml of O_2 per kg of body weight per minute, is the amount of energy expended at rest by an average person. According to National Fire Protection Association (NFPA) guidelines, firefighters must be able to achieve at least 12 METs before they can be considered fit. Measuring VO_2 max directly is expensive and can only be done in specialized laboratories. However, a normal treadmill test will allow us to estimate a person's exercise capacity based on the stage achieved or duration on the treadmill. If Captain. Tan can complete stage 4 of the Bruce protocol without any problems he would have reached an exercise capacity of 12.9 METs.

Return to Work

There have been instances of firefighters returning to unrestricted duty, only to have a relapse and die during fire suppression activities. There has to be a fitness to return to work assessment, and planned rehabilitation with definite end points to be achieved before a return to full duty can be allowed. Considering the nature of such work, it is not surprising that more stringent standards would apply, compared to, for example, working as a bank manager. However, employers in organizations like the fire service are unique. Their activities can have profound impacts on the lives of their employees and the communities they serve. Perhaps more so than other employers, their role in raising and improving the fitness of their employees is a non-delegable and critical duty and must complement any health screening measures that are adopted.

While all efforts must be directed at enabling physicians to accurately identify firefighters who are at risk, it must also be remembered that the most specific and sensitive of laboratory tests in the doctor's office may not be able to reproduce the conditions during which the cardiovascular risk is most pronounced. Fire suppression activities and rescue work take place under highly charged environments. Heat, arduous physical activities that involve lifting, hoisting, wearing protective gear including respiratory protection, and potential contamination by carbon monoxide and other products of combustion are additional stressors.

Post-myocardial infarction and following appropriate risk stratification, patients in sedentary jobs can return to work after four weeks. For patients such as Captain Tan in physically demanding occupations, a normal exercise stress test at the end of the four-week rest period is advised as a prerequisite to returning to frontline work.

Case Study 3: Fitness to Drive

Captain Tan, the firefighter veteran in the previous case study, was found to be unfit for fire suppression activities. He has decided to opt for retirement on grounds of ill health, and will retrain as a bus driver.

Different countries would differ in the regulations and laws pertaining to fitness to drive heavy vehicles or passenger vehicles like buses. The main concern is the safety implications in the event of a heart attack occurring while driving. Passenger vehicles often ply busy thoroughfares while heavy goods vehicles may be loaded up with hazardous materials, e.g. hydrofluoric acid and petroleum products.

Coronary bypass arterial grafting and angioplasty need not be contraindications to driving fitness if other functional test require-ments are met.

Unstable symptomatic angina, a left ventricular ejection fraction of less than 40% and failure to reach stage 3 of the standard Bruce protocol (equivalent to 10.1 METs) safely are contraindications to driving heavy vehicles and buses. The use of cardiac devices for man-agement of the heart condition may also affect fitness to drive, but is more often related to the underlying nature of the cardiac disease than the use of the devises per se. Both local and international guide-lines may serve as a useful guide to helping physicians advise patients (SMA, 1997; DVLA UK, 2008).

Case Study 4: Fitness to Dive

A 36-year-old diving specialist was assessed for fitness to dive after an episode of decompression sickness, from which he recovered after treat-ment. No details are available on this. It happened on an overseas diving mission. He is a vocational diver and has to dive repeatedly to depths of 50 meters for work assignments repairing pipes laid on the seabed.

A physical examination revealed a systolic murmur with a split second heart sound. A resting ECG also demonstrated a right bundle branch block (Fig. 1). An echocardiogram confirmed a small atrial septal defect (Fig. 2).

How should you advise the patient? He is otherwise physically very fit.

The normal pressures in the chambers of the heart favor blood flow-ing from left to right in those with an atrial septal defect (ASD) or patent foramen ovale (PFO). However, there are periods in which this flow is reversed. Doppler studies have shown that most divers will have venous bubbles after a dive of significant depth and bottom time. These usually pose no significant threat, and the diver remains symptom-free. Dives of less than 15 meters are thought to be safe regardless of the presence of a shunt.

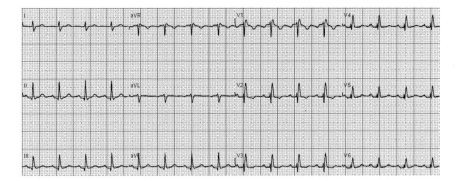

Fig. 1. Resting ECG. Note right bundle branch block.

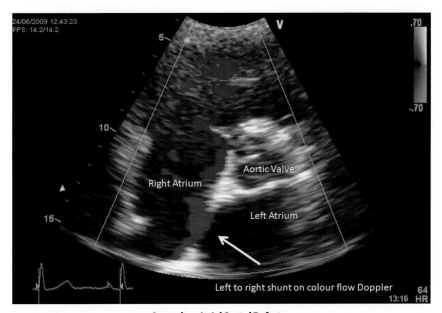

Fig. 2. Atrial septal defect on echocardiogram.

However, if bubbles were to flow from right to left, harm could result from air embolism occurring in the brain, spinal cord and other tissues. Several studies have demonstrated that the rate of divers with ASDs and PFOs treated for decompression illness is higher than the rate in the general population.

Should there be widespread screening of all divers for ASD or PFO? The incidence of ASD is 1 in 1500; that of PFO is higher at about 25%. It may be difficult to justify such a step as the risk of paradoxical embolus in these patients is still very low (see chapter on health screening). However, in cases like that of the professional diver, where the diving profile of the particular incident was unable to account for the decompression illness or in someone with recurrent decompression sickness, the search for a defect may be justified. The risk can then be explained to him. Can the risk be mitigated by measures to reduce bubble load or by surgical closure of the defect? At present, there are no clinical trials to support this approach and expert opinion should be sought (UKSDMC, 2009).

Case Study 5: A Security Guard with Ischemic Heart Disease

Mr. Chan is a 58-year-old with a history of ischemic heart disease. He is currently under treatment and has applied for a job as a security guard. He also has diabetes mellitus. He is on various medications. His employer requires him to undergo a medical evaluation for fitness for the job.

Additional information that will be required

If his job requires him to carry firearms and encounter potentially safety-sensitive circumstances, then the additional risk may be found to be unacceptable. Diabetic patients, particularly those in whom diabetes has been going on for years, can also have silent ischemia because of concomitant cardiovascular autonomic neuropathy.

However, many security jobs are not so onerous. The standard operating procedure often requires no more that the guards be vigilant, make rounds and be able to summon help when the situation arises. The fitness requirements in such circumstances would be less stringent than those of the earlier job where firearms are carried and there is a risk of violent encounters. In fact, it might be foolhardy for unarmed security guards, even if fit and young, to give chase and put themselves in danger in burglary situations.

Automated External Defibrillators (AEDs) in the Workplace

Rapid defibrillation in a non-hospital setting for ventricular fibrillation can be life-saving. The American Heart Association considers early defibrillation to be an important link in the chain of survival. Certainly, its use in occupational situations like the firefighting service is a given, in this case, not only for the rescue and resuscitation of victims, but also for the firefighters themselves working in such high-risk environments. The remote location of workplaces is another indicator that such instruments may come in very useful, and in these places, workers should be trained in basic life support as well as in the use of these AEDs.

Cardiogenic Chemicals in the Workplace

Carbon Disulphide

Occupational epidemiological investigations have also revealed a number of chemical exposures leading to excessive heart diseases. Carbon disulphide is one of these, and was identified as early as the 1960s, when exposures were less well controlled. However, its actual role and clinical importance remains uncertain (Sulsky *et al.*, 2002).

Nitrate Compounds

Sudden deaths due to mixtures of nitroglycerine and nitroglycol were first reported in 1952. Such deaths tend to occur after an absence from work of one or two days, giving rise to the name "Monday morning deaths".

Chronic exposure results in the development of tolerance to the cardiovascular effects of nitroglycerin. A break in chronic exposure of one to three days can result in malaise, severe chest pains, palpitations and even sudden death (Clayton and Clayton, 1993; OSHA, 2009).

Halogenated Hydrocarbons and Dysrhythmias

Many halogenated hydrocarbons have been known to cause cardiac dysrhythmias. Exposure to trichloroethylene, an industrial degreaser, has been reported to cause ventricular fibrillation in workers (Kaufman, Silverstein and Moure-Eraso, 1994).

Cobalt and Cardiomyopathy

Quebec beer-drinkers' cardiomyopathy was first described in 1967. The cardiomyopathy was noted to affect heavy beer drinkers who drank mainly beer treated with cobalt. A review of the recent literature does lend support to the belief that cobalt-exposed workers may have a higher risk for cobalt accumulation in the myocardium, affecting myocardial function (Seghizzi *et al.*, 1994; Linna *et al.*, 2004).

Other Environmental Agents Affecting the Heart

Besides the usual culprits like carbon monoxide and tobacco smoke, other environmental agents believed to play a role include poly-aromatic hydrocarbons, aldehydes and metals such as arsenic and lead which have been reported to elevate CVD risk by affecting atherogenesis, thrombosis or blood pressure regulation (Mastin, 2005).

> **Box 3. Summary of Points for Assessing Cardiovascular Fitness for Work**
>
> 1. Assess the worker's complete cardiovascular risk profile and look for warning symptoms.
> 2. Assess the job requirements. Does the job require special cardiac fitness? Does it impose additional cardiovascular burden when the duties are performed?
> 3. Can the risk be lowered, either by improving cardiac fitness of the worker, or by reducing workplace risk factors?
> 4. Are there any chemical substances at the workplace that might put the worker at risk?

References

Bulugahapitiya U, Siyambalapitiya S, Sithol J, Idris I. (2009) Is diabetes a coronary risk equivalent? Systematic review and meta-analysis. *Diabet Med* **26**: 142–148.

Clayton G, Clayton F. (1993) *Patty's Industrial Hygiene and Toxicology*, 4th edn, Vol I, Part A and Part B, General principles. New York, NY: John Wiley & Sons.

Driver and Vehicle Licensing Authority United Kingdom. (2008) *At a Glance: Guide to the Current Medical Standards of Fitness to Drive.* http://www.dvla.gov.uk/media/pdf/medical/aagv1.pdf (accessed 18 May 2009).

Falk E, Shah PK, Fuster V. (1995) Coronary plaque disruption. *Circulation* **92**: 657–661.

Federal Emergency Management Agency (FEMA), United States Fire Administration, National Fire Data Center. (2002) *Firefighter Fatality Retrospective Study.* http://www.usfa.dhs.gov/downloads/pdf/publications/fa-220.pdf (accessed 18 May 2009).

Haffner SM, Lehto S, Ronnemaa T, *et al.* (1998) Mortality from coronary heart disease in subjects with Type 2 diabetics and in non-diabetic subjects with and without prior myocardial infarction. *N Engl J Med* **339**: 229–234.

Kales SN, Soteriades ES, Christophi CA, Christiani DC. (2007) Emergency duties and deaths from heart disease among firefighters in the United States. *N Engl J Med* **356**: 1207–1215.

Kaufman JD, Silverstein MA, Moure-Eraso R. (1994) Atrial fibrillation and sudden death related to occupational solvent exposure. *Am J Ind Med* **25**(5): 731–735.

Lee SM, Koh D. (2008) Fitness to work: Legal pitfalls. *Ann Acad Med Singapore* **37**: 236–240.

Linna A, Oksa P, Groundstroem K, *et al.* (2004) Exposure to cobalt in the production of cobalt and cobalt compounds and its effect on the heart. *J Occup Environ Med* **61**(11): 877–885.

Mastin JP. (2005) Environmental cardiovascular disease. *Cardiovasc Toxicol* **5**(2): 91–94.

MOH: Ministry of Health Singapore. (2009) *Health Facts Singapore, Principal Causes of Death.* http://www.moh.gov.sg/mohcorp/statistics.aspx?id=5526 (accessed 18 May 2009).

Mulcahy D, Husain S, Zalos G, *et al.* (1997) Ischemia during ambulatory monitoring as a prognostic indicator in patients with stable coronary artery disease. *JAMA* **277**: 318–324.

National Heart Lung and Blood Institute (NHLBI). (2009) *10-year CVD Risk Calculator.* http://hp2010.nhlbihin.net/atpiii/calculator.asp (accessed 18 May 2009).

Occupational Safety and Health Administration (OSHA), United States Department of Labor. (2009) *Guideline for Nitroglycerin.* http://www.osha.gov/SLTC/healthguidelines/nitroglycerin/recognition.html (accessed 20 June 2009).

Seghizzi P, D'Adda F, Borleri D, *et al.* (1994) Cobalt myocardiopathy: A critical review of literature. *Sci Total Environ* **150**(1–3): 105–109.

Singapore Medical Association. (1997) *Fitness to Drive.* http://www.sma.org.sg/references/SMA_Medical_Guidelines_Fitness_to_Drive_1997.pdf (accessed 18 May 2009).

Stone PH, Chaitman BR, Forman S, *et al.* (1997) Prognostic significance of myocardial ischemia detected by ambulatory electrocardiography, exercise treadmill testing, and electrocardiogram at rest to predict cardiac events by one year (the Asymptomatic Cardiac Ischemia Pilot [ACIP] study). *Am J Cardiol* **80**: 1395–1401.

Sulsky SI, Hooven FH, Burch MT, Mundt KA. (2002) Critical review of the epidemiological literature on the potential cardiovascular effects of occupational carbon disulfide exposure. *Int Arch Occup Environ Health* **75**(6): 365–380.

UKSDMC. (2009) *UK Sport Diving Medical Committee Standards.* http://www.uksdmc.co.uk/standards/Standards.htm (accessed 18 May 2009).

World Health Organization. (2009) *The World Health Report 2008.* http://www.who.int/whr/2008/whr08_en.pdf (accessed 18 May 2009).

Xanthos T, Ekmektzoglou KA, Papadimitriou L. (2008) Reviewing myocardial silent ischemia: Specific patient subgroups. *Int J Cardiol* **124**(2): 139–148.

Chapter 4

Respiratory Disorders

Hock-Siang Lee*, Ken Takahashi[†,§] and Keng-Leong Tan[‡]

Introduction

Recognizing the Occupational Relationship

The following case histories are representative of the spectrum of occupational respiratory diseases that may be encountered by the general practitioner, chest physician, occupational physician, the doctor in the accident and emergency unit or the medical ward. Besides the treatment of the symptoms, it is important to make an etiological diagnosis of the disease so that definitive treatment can be given and preventive measures taken to prevent recurrences and to protect other workers.

Occupational or environmental factors that play a role in the etiology, whether causal or contributory, should be identified for proper management of the case. This requires not only a knowledge of respiratory medicine, the common environmental or occupational etiologies of respiratory disorders, how these occupational respiratory

*Occupational Safety and Health Specialist Department, Ministry of Manpower, Singapore, Department of Epidemiology and Public Health, Yong Loo Lin School of Medicine, National University of Singapore.
†University of Occupational and Environmental Health, Kitakyushu City, Japan.
‡Department of Respiratory and Critical Medicine, Singapore General Hospital, Yong Loo Lin School of Medicine, National University of Singapore.
§Corresponding author. E-mail: ktaka@med.uoeh-u.ac.jp

diseases present and the occupations at risk, but also a good occupational history and a high index of suspicion.

Case Study 1

A 42-year-old female cleaner was carrying out her usual work of cleaning toilets. She used a chemical disinfectant which was acidic to mop the toilet floors. The mops were normally rinsed with water and soaked in chlorox solution overnight. On that particular occasion, she inadvertently mixed the chlorox (sodium hypochlorite) with the chemical disinfectant while in the relatively confined space of a toilet. Immediately, she smelt an irritating pungent smell and started tearing and coughing. She became acutely breathless and was admitted to hospital.

On admission she was found to be dyspnoeic. Rhonchi and crepitations were heard on auscultation. Her chest X-ray showed slightly increased lung markings but was otherwise normal. Blood gas analysis showed a slightly reduced paO_2 of 75 mmHg. When she was reviewed three weeks later, she had a forced expiratory volume in the first second (FEV_1) of 2.1 liters and a forced vital capacity (FVC) of 2.3 liters which was about 80% of her predicted values. She had no further attacks of bronchospasm and no past history of asthma. She still had a persistent cough and a mild degree of bronchial hyperreactivity on histamine inhalational testing.

Sometimes the occupational relationship is quite obvious as in Case 1 where her symptoms were immediately consequent to the specific incident of mixing the chlorox and the disinfectant. A knowledge of basic chemistry would tell us that the chemical reaction between an acid and a hypochlorite generates chlorine gas which is pungent and acutely irritating to the eyes and respiratory system, causing bronchospasm or even pulmonary edema, depending on which part of the respiratory tract is affected and the concentration of the gas. She had an acute lung injury from inhaling chlorine gas. Should her airway hyperreactivity have persisted and developed into symptoms of asthma subsequently, she might have had what is called a reactive airways dysfunction syndrome. She was handling common household chemicals and similar accidents can be prevented through public education.

Case Study 2

A 39-year-old woman was admitted to hospital for an acute attack of asthma. This was her first admission for asthma. She started having symptoms of cough, breathlessness and wheezing about six months earlier. She had a history of allergic rhinitis for many years but no asthma. Her attacks were nocturnal. She noted improvement on days she was not working. She was pregnant at the time of admission. When she was on her maternity leave for two months, she did not have any attacks of asthma. One week after returning to work, the asthma recurred. When examined at the outpatient clinic, her lungs were clear on auscultation. She monitored her peak expiratory flow rate (PEFR) every three hours for a total of three weeks, inclusive of one week when she was resting at home. Her PEFR record was normal during the week at home but showed an asthmatic pattern during the weeks at work (Fig. 1). Her job was to supervise the finishing process in the manufacture of wooden doors. Often she would herself fill up cracks in the doors with a glue which

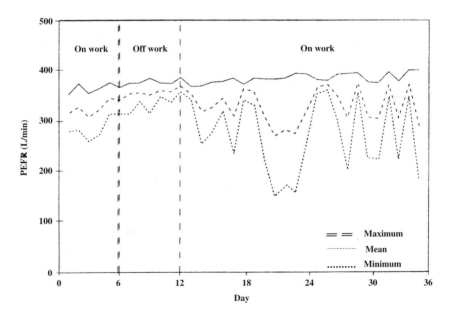

Fig. 1. Serial PEFR record of patient in Case Study 2.

contained cyanoacrylate, after which she would smoothen the surface with a portable sanding machine. A specific bronchial provocation test (specific inhalation challenge (SIC) test) to the glue was carried out in hospital. She developed immediate rhinitis and a delayed asthmatic reaction 12 hours after exposure to the glue. She improved after transferring to another section not using the glue.

An occupational relationship is also fairly obvious in Case 2, based on the recent onset of asthma and the temporal relationship between her symptoms and exposure at work. Her symptoms of asthma improved when she was away from work (e.g. weekends and maternity leave) and recurred when she returned to work. However, various investigations had to be carried out (e.g. the serial PEFR recording, the workplace visit and the specific bronchial provocation test) before the diagnosis of occupational asthma due to cyanoacrylate glue could be confirmed.

Case Study 3

A 55-year-old man consulted his general practitioner about the vague chest pain and shortness of breath on climbing up stairs for the past two to three years. A chest X-ray was done and it showed bilateral scattered opacities throughout the lung fields. There were also "eggshell calcifications" in the hilar areas (Fig. 2). The X-ray was classified as 2/2 pqr according to the International Labour Organization (ILO) classification of pneumoconiosis.

Clinically, no abnormalities were detected. His FEV_1 was 84% and FVC was 79% of the predicted values. He had been working as a tombstone engraver for the past 36 years. He was exposed to dust from the cutting, grinding, polishing and engraving of tombstones. He had smoked 10 cigarettes a day for the past 30 days with no history of tuberculosis. A repeat chest X-ray done six months later showed a similar picture.

Case Study 4

A 54-year-old man was admitted for breathlessness. He had been experiencing shortness of breath on exertion for the past two years only. His

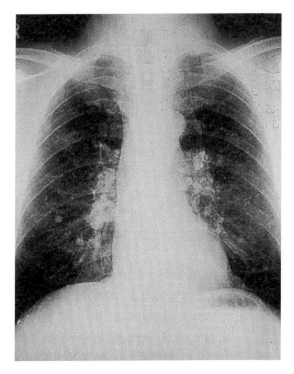

Fig. 2. Chest X-ray of the patient, a tombstone engraver. It shows diffuse nodular opacities in both mid and upper zones and "eggshell-calcifications" of the hilar nodes, consistent with silicosis.

effort tolerance was about 20 meters. He had a slight cough on and off with white sputum but no chest pain or haemoptysis. He had smoked 12 cigarettes a day for the past 40 years. He was dyspnoeic at rest and air entry was poor in both lungs. Fine crepitations were heard in both lungs. He had gross clubbing of his fingernails. Blood gas analysis showed a paO_2 of 53 mmHg, a pCO_2 of 47 mmHg, a pH of 7.45 and an oxygen saturation of 88%. The chest X-ray showed severe reticular nodular shadowing in both the mid and lower zones, giving a "honey-combed" appearance (Fig. 3). There was also evidence of calcification of the left diaphragmatic pleura and evidence of bilateral pleural thickening. He gave a history of having worked in an asbestos-cement factory about 35 years ago for a period of 10 years. His condition

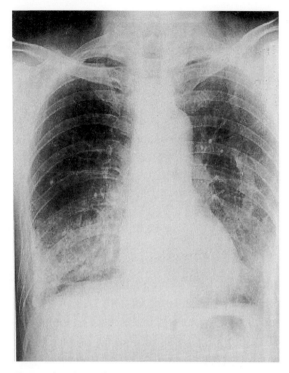

Fig. 3.   Chest X-ray of patient who previously worked in an asbestos-cement factory. It shows diffuse reticular nodular shadowing in both the mid and lower zones and bilateral pleural thickening consistent with asbestosis and asbestos-related pleural disease.

deteriorated and he was on home oxygen therapy before he passed away one year later.

In Cases 3 and 4, there was no temporal relationship between the symptoms and any particular incident or exposure due to the insidious onset and long latent period of the diseases. Case 4 had already ceased exposure to asbestos for more than 20 years before he started to have symptoms. The diagnosis of asbestosis in Case 4 and silicosis in Case 3 was based on the chest X-rays and clinical pictures, the definite and prolonged exposures to asbestos or silica and the exclusion of other causes of reticular-nodular shadowing in the chest X-rays.

Epidemiology

According to the 2005 study of the global burden of occupational diseases, a study virtually endorsed by the WHO, the annual number of deaths due to occupational lung diseases is estimated at 318,000 for chronic obstructive pulmonary diseases (COPD), 38,000 for asthma, 30,000 for pneumoconiosis, 102,000 for lung cancer and 43,000 for malignant mesothelioma. The corresponding DALY (or "disability-adjusted life years",) defined as the sum of Years of Life Lost (YLL) and the Years of Life Disabled (YLD), the latter for which is weighted by the serverity of the disability, is 3.73 million (M) for COPD, 1.62 M for asthma, 1.29 M for pneumoconiosis, 0.97 M for lung cancer and 0.56 M for malignant mesothelioma (Driscoll *et al.*, 2005).

There is an increasing recognition that a large proportion of adult-onset asthma is attributable to occupational exposures: a review of papers published during 1999–2007 reported the proportion at 16.3% (Toren and Blanc, 2009). Earlier papers reported the corresponding figure at 9–15% in industrialized countries (Mapp *et al.*, 2005) and 29% for men and 17% for women in Finland (Karjalainen *et al.*, 2001). Caution is warranted, however, as occupational asthma remains underrecognized (hence the population burden underestimated) due to difficulties in accounting for the "healthy workers effect" in population studies (Le Moual *et al.*, 2008). Nevertheless, occupational asthma is regarded as the most common occupational lung disease in industrialized countries, and the second most common occupational lung disease reported after pneumoconiosis in developing countries (Schuitemaker *et al.*, 2007).

COPD, with smoking as the established prime risk factor, is now recognized as a global health issue. Other than smoking, occupational exposures are listed among the important risk factors for COPD together with indoor (e.g. smoke from biomass fuel) and outdoor air pollution and infections (Mannino and Buist, 2007; Salvi and Barnes, 2009).

The population attributable fraction (PAF) of occupational exposure factors for lung cancer, the leading cause of cancer death world-wide, has been evaluated. Based on 32 epidemiologic studies which evaluated occupational exposures to suspected/known lung carcinogens among men and controlled for smoking, the PAFs ranged between 0 to 40%. The wide range in time and place is primarily due to the variable prevalence of hazardous industries (De Matteis, Consonni and Bertazzi, 2008).

For example, it can be expected that countries and regions which record high levels of asbestos use will eventually shoulder a proportionate burden of asbestos-related diseases. Such relationships have been demonstrated as plausible correlations using national-level data, accounting for latency time. This supports the premises for the need to eliminate asbestos use as a national policy (Lin *et al.*, 2007). Indeed, the WHO recognizes that asbestos is one of the most important occupational carcinogens, causing about half of the deaths due to occupational cancer.

To address the question of whether screening by low-dose computed tomography (LDCT) is justified for detecting occupational lung cancer, a literature review concluded that it is unclear whether LDCT reduces mortality from lung cancer in view of the absence of randomized, controlled studies needed to address biases commonly encountered in observational and population-based studies (McCunney, 2006).

Clinical Tools Useful in the Investigation of Respiratory Disorders

History

A complete history should include a careful review of respiratory symptoms, the smoking history, the history of atopy and allergies, including family history, and occupational and environmental exposures. The review of symptoms should include questions on cough, sputum production, shortness of breath, chest tightness, wheezing and chest pain. Other related symptoms such as rhinitis, eye irritation, rashes, fever and muscular pains may also be relevant.

For positive symptoms, details on the onset, duration, severity, aggravating or relieving factors and time relationship to work or any particular exposures or activities should be sought. For occupational asthma, it is particularly useful to ask if the symptoms improve during periods away from work (e.g. during weekends, holidays or leave) and recur when back at work. Some workers may even be able to identify the particular substance or activity which provokes their asthmatic attacks. For chronic diseases such as silicosis and asbestosis, a detailed and accurate occupational history, starting from the patient's very first job, is important to document possible exposure to silica or asbestos. Both the intensity and duration of exposure should be documented as far as possible. It is also useful to ask whether other workers have been similarly affected.

Physical Examination

In most cases there is a relative absence of physical signs. This should not imply that this crucial step should be omitted or that a cursory examination would suffice. A general observation of the patient may reveal a patient who is dyspnoeic at rest or after performing a lung function test. There may be clubbing of the digits in the case of asbestosis, berylliosis or lung cancer. Auscultation of the lungs may reveal fine crepitations at the lung bases of a patient with asbestosis or silicosis. There may be wheezing and rhonchi in a patient with work-related asthma. Extrapulmonary manifestations of chronic beryllium disease, lung cancer or malignant mesothelioma should be sought where indicated. It is also important in the differential diagnosis or in the detection of complications, e.g. heart failure or mitral stenosis, which may not be work-related.

Imaging Techniques for Occupational Lung Disease

Correlation of imaging features with the history of exposure, clinical features and sometimes pathology is needed for the diagnosis of occupational lung disease.

Chest X-ray

The chest radiograph has been for many decades and remains the basic investigation for the detection and characterization of occupational lung disease. However, the sensitivity and specificity of chest radiographs for the diagnosis of occupational and environmental lung disease are low (Akira, 2008).

A full-sized chest X-ray of good quality is important, especially in the diagnosis of early asbestosis or silicosis. Comparison with the standard films for pneumoconiosis, e.g. the International Labour Organization (ILO) classification of radiographs of pneumoconiosis, is very helpful when looking for evidence of nodular or linear profusions suggesting silicosis or asbestosis. The ILO classification system has been extensively validated by comparison with the duration and intensity of dust exposure, and outcome. Hilar lymph node calcifications, i.e. "eggshell calcifications", may be seen in some cases of silicosis. Asbestos-exposed workers may show evidence of pleural thickening or calcifications or effusions, e.g. blunting of the costophrenic angle. There may also be a "shaggy heart" appearance.

Complications such as tuberculosis, progressive massive fibrosis and pneumothorax may be associated with some cases of silicosis. A chest X-ray is always useful in a worker with chronic respiratory symptoms, e.g. cough and breathlessness, to screen for tuberculosis, other infections or malignancy. Often serial chest X-rays may be required. The diagnosis of silicosis or asbestosis should not be based on a single film; it is usually based on at least two consistent films several months apart. It should be noted that the chest X-ray does not provide information on disability or impairment. There is little correlation between the chest X-ray findings and the lung function results. The chest X-ray is also useful in acute respiratory conditions, as illustrated in Case Study 1, to exclude the presence of pneumonitis and pulmonary edema.

Pleuropulmonary changes related to asbestos dust exposure include asbestosis, pleural plaques, benign pleural effusion, diffuse pleural thickening, round atelectasis, lung cancer and mesothelioma. Except for benign pleural effusion, asbestos-related pleuropulmonary complications usually occur after 20 or more years of exposure. Pleural plaques are localized thickenings of the parietal pleura which usually develop 20 years after asbestos exposure and serve only as a marker of asbestos dust exposure (Fig. 4). Malignant pleural mesothelioma may manifest as unilateral pleural effusion, diffuse pleural thickening or both on the plain chest radiograph (Fig. 5).

Computed tomography (CT)

CT is more sensitive than chest X-ray in the detection of pleuro-parenchymal abnormalities in pneumoconiosis and is able to demonstrate plaques along the mediastinum, paravertebral areas and diaphragm which are difficult to assess by conventional chest X-ray.

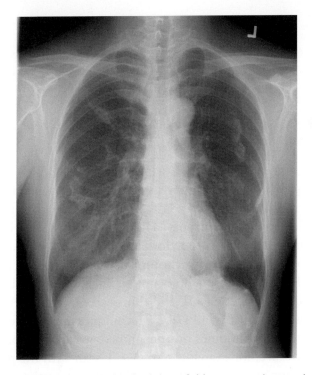

Fig. 4. Pleural plaques scattered in both lung fields, representing previous asbestos dust exposure.

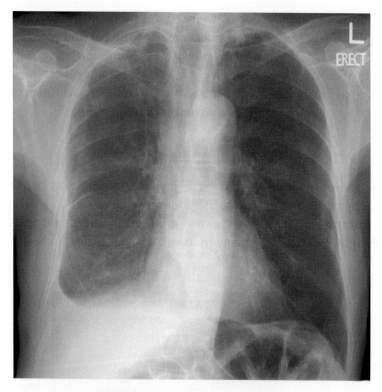

Fig. 5.   Previous shipyard worker presenting with right-sided chest pain. A chest X-ray revealed a right pleural effusion.

Chest X-ray has a low sensitivity (8.3% to 40.3%, depending on the detection criteria and population) for plaque detection, particularly for non-calcified pleural plaques. High-resolution CT (HRCT) is a more sensitive diagnostic tool for demonstrating the parenchymal lesions in occupational and environmental lung disease. The optimal technique for detecting pneumoconiosis includes a combination of conventional thick-section CT and thin-section HRCT. A combination of conventional CT and HRCT techniques are used for the early detection of micronodules in pneumoconiosis. In workers with asbestos exposure, for example, a spiral CT scan with the patient in a supine position may be performed for the detection of pleural plaques, pleural tumors and other pathologies, followed by HRCT imaging with the patient prone for the early diagnosis of lung and pleural disease.

CT plays a key role in the diagnosis of mesothelioma and is likely to be the initial study for the determination of resectability in most cases (Fig. 6). The CT findings of rind-like pleural involvement, mediastinal pleural involvement, pleural nodularity and pleural thickness greater than 1 cm are independent findings for the differentiation of malignant pleural disease from benign pleural disease.

Magnetic resonance imaging (MRI)

MRI is useful for the diagnosis and staging of mesothelioma. MRI is superior to CT in identifying local invasion by mesothelioma into the

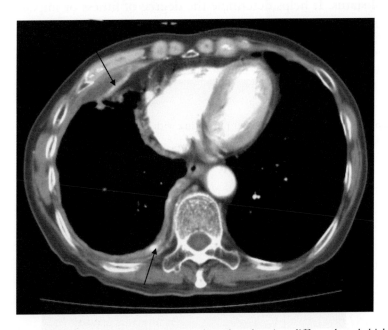

Fig. 6. CT thorax of the previous shipyard worker showing diffuse pleural thickening within the smaller right hemithorax, associated with pleural calcification (arrows), which were not visualized on his chest X-ray in Fig. 5. A video-assisted thoracoscopic biopsy of the pleura confirmed the diagnosis of a sarcomatoid (desmoplastic) mesothelioma.

diaphragm, endothoracic fascia or chest wall in selected patients who have potentially resectable mesothelioma. T2-weighted MRI may discriminate between pleural plaques and malignant mesothelioma.

Positron emission tomography (PET)

PET imaging with fluororodeoxyglucose may be useful in distinguishing benign from malignant asbestos-related pleural disease. PET, in conjunction with CT scanning, has improved the diagnosis and staging of pleural mesothelioma (Fig. 7).

Pulmonary Function Tests

The evaluation of lung function provides information on the functional status. It helps determine the degree of fitness or impairment. The most basic of these tests are the forced vital capacity (FVC), forced

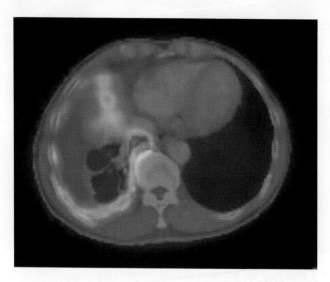

Fig. 7. F-18 fluorodeoxyglucose PET imaging with contrast-enhanced CT showing fluorodeoxyglucose-avid enhancing nodular thickening of the right pleura with pleural effusion. A pleural biopsy confirmed the diagnosis of sarcomatoid mesothelioma.

expiratory volume in the first second (FEV_1) and the ratio of these two measurements (FEV_1/FVC). The FVC is the total volume of air which can be forcefully expelled from the lungs after a maximum inspiration, and the FEV_1 is the volume of air expelled during the first second of the maneuver.

To be reliable, the maneuver requires the patient to start from total lung capacity (TLC) before blowing out. Thus the patient has to cooperate by inspiring maximally to TLC. For this reason, demonstration of the reliability of the test result is essential and it is usual to require three comparable measurements to be made. The test can be performed on a spirometer in a physician's consultation room or in the lung function laboratory of a large hospital. The values of these tests differ between males and females, and vary with age, height and race. The individual results must be interpreted by comparison with predicted normal values for someone of the same sex, age, height and race. Generally, the FEV_1 increases with growth of the lungs up to about 20–25 years of age, following which it declines by 25–30 ml/year. Cigarette smokers and occupational groups exposed to certain irritant dust or gases have been shown to have an accelerated decline in the FEV_1. Females have lower values of FEV_1 and FVC. Asians have lower values than Caucasians. Among the Asians, the Chinese have higher values than the Malays or Indians (Chia *et al.*, 1993; Poh and Chia, 1969).

While predicted normal values have been established for various populations, such values may need to be re-established from time to time. With improvements in the socio-economic and developmental status of a nation, succeeding generations would be expected to have higher normal values for the FEV_1 and FVC. Where baseline or serial measurements are available for the individual, a comparison with previous results is also informative. Based on the American Thoracic Society (ATS)/European Respiratory Society (ERS) Task Force 2005 recommendations (Pellegrino *et al.*, 2005) on the interpretation of lung function tests, for each lung function index, values below the 5th percentile of the frequency distribution of values measured in the reference population are considered to be below the expected "normal range" (i.e. below the lower limit of the reference range). The practice of using a predicted 80% as the fixed value for the lower limit of normal may lead to important errors when interpreting lung function in adults.

Chronic bronchitis, emphysema and asthma cause narrowing of the intrapulmonary airways. The FEV_1 is affected more than the FVC, and the ratio of FEV_1/FVC, which is normally more than 70–75%, is reduced. This is referred to as an obstructive defect. The ATS/ERS 2005 guidelines define an obstructive pulmonary defect as an FEV_1 to vital capacity (VC) ratio below the 5th percentile of the normal distribution (rather than a fixed value of 0.7). The obstructive defect in asthma can be distinguished from that of chronic bronchitis or emphysema by a significant immediate improvement in the FEV_1 following the inhalation of a standard dose of a bronchodilator. This is termed "reversible airway obstruction" to distinguish it from the irreversible airway obstruction seen in chronic obstructive pulmonary disease (COPD). By the ATS/ERS 2005 guidelines, an increase in the FEV_1 and/or FVC of $\geq 12\%$ of the control and ≥ 200 ml constitutes a positive bronchodilator response.

Diseases which cause inflammation and thickening of alveolar walls such as fibrosing alveolitis, asbestosis and hypersensitivity pneumonitis also cause stiffening of the lungs with impairment of gas transfer. Increased stiffness of the lungs reduces the volume of air which can be taken into the lungs but not the rate at which air can be expelled. Indeed, the FEV_1/FVC ratio is often greater than normal (>90%) because the FVC is reduced to a greater degree than the FEV_1 (Fig. 8). Maximal flows at low lung volumes are similarly increased. The supranormal flow rates may be due to the increased elastic recoil that characterizes interstitial lung disease. This is described as a restrictive defect. The associated impairment of gas transfer can be demonstrated by a diminution in the uptake of carbon monoxide (CO) from the inspired air.

A pre- and post-work shift FEV_1 and FVC can be measured in the same individual to study any cross-shift changes resulting from occupational exposures, e.g. byssinosis and occupational asthma. However, they may not be sensitive enough to detect those cases where the reaction is delayed beyond the normal shift. Serial PEFR

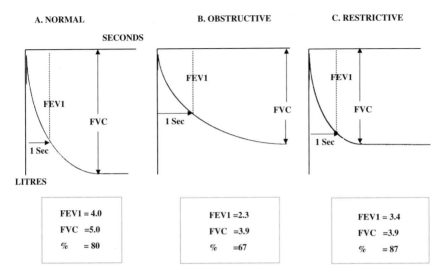

Fig. 8. Measurement of forced expiratory volume in one second, FEV_1, and forced vital capacity, FVC. In obstructive disease such as bronchial asthma, the FEV_1 is reduced much more than the FVC, giving a low FEV_1/FVC ratio. In restrictive diseases such as pulmonary fibrosis, both the FEV_1 and FVC are reduced but characteristically, the FEV_1/FVC ratio is normal or increased.

measurements done during periods at work and away from work have been found to be useful in the investigation for occupational asthma.

Methacholine/Histamine Inhalational Testing

The presence and degree of non-specific bronchial hyperreactivity can be documented by measuring the concentration or dose of histamine or methacholine that causes a 20% fall in the pre-test FEV_1 (PC20 or PD20, i.e. the provocative concentration or dose that causes a 20% fall in the FEV_1).

For the patient's safety, the test is normally done only when the FEV_1 is at least 60% of the predicted values. In the appropriate clinical setting, a positive test is strongly suggestive of asthma. Figure 9 and Table 1 illustrate the test and sample results.

A negative histamine or methacholine test result does not exclude sensitizer-induced occupational asthma if performed when the patient

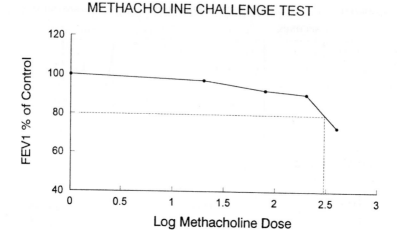

Fig. 9.   The FEV_1 % of control vs the log methacholine dose is plotted. In this example, the log methacholine dose when the FEV_1 is 80% of the control value is 2.49. The PD20 is thus anti-log (2.48), or 300 µg/ml.

Table 1.   Methacholine Challenge Test: Sample Results

Methacholine Dose (µg/ml)	Log Dose	FEV_1 (l)	FEV_1 % Control
—	—	1.91	100
20	1.3	1.87	97
80	1.9	1.76	92
200	2.3	1.72	90
400	2.6	1.40	73

is off work and free of symptoms. As it has been shown in studies of diisocyanate asthma, both methacholine reactivity and symptoms can resolve in workers who have been away from active work exposure for just a brief period. It may be necessary to re-expose workers to the causative agent at work before asthma and methacholine reactivity return. A negative histamine or methacholine test result has a good negative predictive value, i.e. a negative test excludes active asthma in an actively exposed worker.

Serial changes in non-specific bronchial hyperreactivity following removal or exposure may be used to support the diagnosis of sensitizer-induced occupational asthma. Guidelines for the diagnosis of sensitizer-induced occupational asthma have recommended a methacholine or histamine challenge be performed toward the end of a work week and be repeated at the end of a period (usually 10 to 14 days) away from the exposure. A worsening of the PC20 at work compared to that off work beyond the normal variability of the test (defined as a threefold or greater change in PC20) would provide additional evidence to support the diagnosis of sensitizer-induced asthma (Tarlo *et al.*, 2008).

Serial Peak Expiratory Flow Rate (PEFR) Monitoring

Serial PEFR monitoring is now an established tool in the investigation for occupational asthma. Patients are instructed on the proper use of a portable PEF meter and told to record their PEFR every two to three hours during waking hours for about three weeks. This should include periods at work and away from work. The period away from work should be about 7 to 10 consecutive days. Each time the best of three readings is taken. The daily maximum, minimum and mean readings are plotted on a graph (as in Fig. 1).

A diurnal variation of 20% or more is evidence of asthma. The diurnal variation is calculated as the difference between the maximum and minimum PEFR expressed as a percentage of the maximum for each day. Look for evidence of PEFR improvement during the period the patient is away from work, and deterioration during the period he is at work. Deterioration is shown by the falling mean and the widening diurnal variation, as demonstrated in the serial PEFR recording of Case 2.

Specific Inhalation Challenge

The specific inhalation challenge (SIC) involves exposing workers who are suspected of sensitizer-induced occupational asthma to suspected agents in a safe and controlled manner. SIC is intended to demonstrate a direct relationship between exposure to a suspected agent and an asthmatic response. SIC is considered to be a "reference standard" and is performed in only a few centers with specialized facilities and expertise.

SIC may be useful in confirming new workplace agents as a cause of sensitizer-induced asthma. SIC may confirm the diagnosis of sensitizer-induced occupational asthma when other testing has been non-conclusive, may make the diagnosis expeditiously or may identify the specific agent if the worker is exposed to more than one occupational asthma-causative agent.

Description of Common Occupational Respiratory Diseases

Tables 2 and 3 show the common acute and chronic respiratory tract responses to toxic agents, respectively.

Fitness to Work

The major cause of disability both in the common chronic bronchitis, emphysema and asthma and the less common pulmonary fibrosis is loss of ventilatory reserve, limiting the ability of the lungs to cope with the increased demands of exercise. The impact of these diseases on the capacity for work will, therefore, primarily occur in those whose work is physically demanding. It is therefore important for the physician to know both the patient's work capacity and the job demands.

Assessments for Specific Types of Work

There may be requirements (legal or administrative) for workers to undergo pre-employment and periodic medical examinations to determine fitness to work for certain specific occupations or work. An examination of the respiratory system may be required as part of determining cardiorespiratory fitness for physically demanding work, e.g. firemen, rescue workers and commercial divers. This may also be

Table 2. Common Acute Respiratory Tract Responses to Toxic Agents

Disease	Definition	Causative Agents/ Occupations at Risk	Clinical Presentation/ Diagnosis	Management	Additional Comments
1) Occupational asthma	Disease characterized by variable airflow limitation and/or airway hyper-responsiveness due to causes and conditions attributable to a particular occupational environment and not to stimuli encountered outside the workplace (Bernstein, 1993). Asthma caused by non-allergic mechanisms (e.g. inflammation) are included.	Common agents in industrialized countries are isocyanates, e.g. toluene diisocyanate (TDI) and diphenylmethane diisocyanate (MDI). Related industries are manufacture of polyurethane foam mattresses, cushions, insulation, paints, varnishes and adhesives. Other common agents include grain dust, wood dust, soldering and welding fumes, acid anhydrides and amines (used in epoxy resin systems) and antibiotics.	Look initially for work-related pattern of symptoms, including cough, breathlessness, chest tightness and wheezing with variable severity. Nocturnal pattern of symptoms is an important clue. The only symptom may be nocturnal cough in the early stages. Other evidence include clinical documentation of asthmatic attack or rhonchi on auscultation with improvement following treatment, obstructive pattern on spirometry with positive bronchodilator response, positive histamine or methacholine inhalational challenge test, or diurnal variation of 20% or more in PEFR measured over a period.	Symptoms are provoked whenever exposure occurs so medical treatment alone is insufficient. Consider implementing serial peak expiratory flow rate (PEFR) monitoring, workplace visit and specific bronchial provocation test (BPT). Once diagnosis is confirmed, transfer patient permanently away from the pertinent exposure. Symptoms may persist for variable lengths after transfer. Pharmacological treatment is similar to non-occupational asthma.	Presence of pre-existing asthma should not preclude this diagnosis. Important to identify aggravating work factors and take preventive action. Common causative agents vary by country reflecting industrial composition. Many patients are young and recommendation of job transfer may affect career prospects and pay. Early diagnosis and prompt removal from exposure are key to successful management.

(Continued)

Table 2.　(*Continued*)

Disease	Definition	Causative Agents/ Occupations at Risk	Clinical Presentation/ Diagnosis	Management	Additional Comments
2) Acute respiratory reactions to irritant gases	Acute upper respiratory tract irritation, chemical pneumonitis or pulmonary edema caused by exposure to high levels of irritant gases; sometimes lethal if exposure is massive or as a consequence of development of bronchiolitis 4–6 weeks later.	Gases, e.g. chlorine, ammonia, sulphur dioxide, ozone, nitrogen oxides, irritate mucous membrane and inflame respiratory tract. Exposures occur at work or in the community, by leakage during maintenance, in accidents or through chemical reactions from accidental mixing of chemicals.	Effects depend on concentration of gases and solubility of gas. 1) Highly soluble irritants act on upper respiratory tract within seconds. Epiglottic edema due to exposure to ammonia. Bronchospasm can occur with high doses. Lower respiratory tract is usually spared. Lung function tests shortly after exposure may show bronchoconstriction. CXRs are usually normal unless there is pulmonary edema.	Remove immediately from further exposure and give oxygen. Overnight observation is warranted for development of pulmonary edema, especially with low solubility irritants or delayed complications. Treatment essentially supportive, i.e. sufficient ventilation and treating complications.	For low solubility irritants, i.e. delayed onset of symptoms, large doses may be inhaled without many irritant symptoms. Following recovery from acute episodes, some patients may have persistent non-specific bronchial hyperreactivity which may manifest as chronic cough or asthma ("reactive airways dysfunction syndrome").

(*Continued*)

Table 2. (*Continued*)

Disease	Definition	Causative Agents/ Occupations at Risk	Clinical Presentation/ Diagnosis	Management	Additional Comments
		Exposure may also occur when entering a confined space contaminated with gas, e.g. storage silos (nitrogen dioxides) or where arc welding is performed (nitrogen oxides and ozone).	2) Moderately soluble irritants (e.g. chlorine, fluorine and sulphur dioxide) affect both upper and lower respiratory tract within minutes, producing upper respiratory tract irritation and bronchoconstriction. 3) Low solubility irritants (e.g. ozone, oxides of nitrogen and phosgene) penetrate to the lower respiratory tract and cause pulmonary edema 6–24 hours later.		

(*Continued*)

Table 2. (*Continued*)

Disease	Definition	Causative Agents/ Occupations at Risk	Clinical Presentation/ Diagnosis	Management	Additional Comments
3) Acute systemic reactions to metal fumes, polymer fumes and organic dusts	Acute, self-limiting febrile illness associated with myalgia and minor respiratory tract symptoms caused by inhalation of variable agents, i.e. metal fume fever, polymer fume fever and organic dust syndrome.	Agents/Occupations: 1) Metal fume fever: freshly generated fine particulate metallic oxides of various metals, e.g. copper, zinc, magnesium, aluminium, cadmium, chromium, iron, tin, selenium, silver, vanadium and antimony/welders, braziers, foundry workers, shipyard workers, metal cutters and burners, galvanizers, smelters.	Onset 1–8 hours following exposure characterized by fever, chills, headache, myalgia and general malaise. Possible respiratory tract irritation, e.g. cough, chest discomfort or dyspnea. Possible sweating, nausea, vomiting and abdominal colic. Temporal relationship of symptoms after specific exposure is key. Repeated exposure may lead to a tolerant state, with possibly no clinical signs	No specific treatment. Most patients recover after overnight rest.	Attend to possible complications, e.g. pneumonitis or pulmonary edema, which require more aggressive treatment. Important to prevent similar exposures in future.

(*Continued*)

Table 2. (*Continued*)

Disease	Definition	Causative Agents/ Occupations at Risk	Clinical Presentation/ Diagnosis	Management	Additional Comments
		2) Polymer fume fever: combustion products of fluorocarbon polymers, e.g. polytetrafluoroethylene, fluorinated ethylene propylene/workers engaged in fabricating fluorocarbon polymer products including extrusion, moulding, sintering and soldering, cutting or welding of metal parts coated with such polymers.	except for fever. There is no specific diagnostic test. Polymorph leucocytosis. CXR usually normal. Lung function test shows normal to mild obstructive signs.		
		3) Bacterial endotoxins and possibly mycotoxins/ cotton textile workers, cotton ginners, grain handlers, weavers and possibly farmers.			

(*Continued*)

Table 2. (*Continued*)

Disease	Definition	Causative Agents/ Occupations at Risk	Clinical Presentation/ Diagnosis	Management	Additional Comments
4) Hypersensitivity pneumonitis	A group of allergic lung diseases due to sensitization and recurrent exposure to inhaled organic dusts; also called allergic alveolitis. Diffuse, predominantly mononuclear inflammation of the lung parenchyma, particularly terminal bronchioles and alveoli. Inflammation often organizes into granulomas and may progress to fibrosis.	List of causative agents include those of bacterial, fungal, serum protein, chemical and dust origin. Unique disease names given. Handling of mouldy vegetable compost (e.g. farmers, sugar cane workers, mushroom compost handlers), often contaminated with thermophilic actinomycetes, poses risk. Non-occupational exposures possible, e.g. bird fancier's lung and pituitary snuff taker's disease.	Initial respiratory symptoms characterized by shortness of breath and non-productive cough but wheezing is uncommon. Possible to present in a dramatic form with sudden onset accompanied by fever and chills (4–10 hours after antigen exposure) or in an insidious form. Physical exam may show rapid breathing and fine basal crepitations. Lung function test may show marked restrictive pattern with reduced FEV_1	Corticosteroids can be used for acute episodes. Avoid further exposure to the specific agent.	Demonstration of specific serum precipitating antibodies to offending dust provides evidence of exposure. Suspected diagnosis can be confirmed by workplace challenge or inhalational challenge in hospital. Recovery usually complete but possible recurrence on re-exposure. Chronic repeated episodes may lead to chronic interstitial fibrosis.

(*Continued*)

Table 2. (*Continued*)

Disease	Definition	Causative Agents/ Occupations at Risk	Clinical Presentation/ Diagnosis	Management	Additional Comments
			and FVC and normal or increased $FEV_1/$FVC ratio. Reduced lung diffusing capacity (DLCO). CXR may show patchy infiltrates, similar to pulmonary edema or diffuse micronodular opacities. Leukocytosis present in acute phase.		
			Recognition of consistent clinical picture with temporal relationship after exposure to specific dust is key.		
5) Byssinosis	Acute or chronic airways disease caused by occupational exposure to dusts of	Offending agents are known but exact etiology is unknown.	Major symptoms are shortness of breath and chest tightness prominent	Mild or early byssinosis is probably reversible but the severe form is not.	Subjective and objective signs, i.e. respiratory symptoms and decreased FEV_1,

(*Continued*)

Table 2.   (Continued)

Disease	Definition	Causative Agents/ Occupations at Risk	Clinical Presentation/ Diagnosis	Management	Additional Comments
	cotton, flax and hemp, and possibly jute.	Exposure to raw cotton dust is highest near blowing and carding machines, thus strippers and grinders are at highest risk.	on first day of the work week ("Monday morning tightness"). Cough may accompany and become productive. Lung function test may reveal post-shift fall in FEV_1 (10%+), conducted after 6 hours of exposure on day 1 after a weekend, and considered objective evidence. As physical exam does not reveal typical or characteristic signs, diagnosis is based on clinical and exposure histories. Chronic effects are characterized by airway obstruction, clinically indistinguishable from chronic bronchitis and emphysema.	Transfer to non-exposed area required for patients with i) typical symptoms and a post-shift fall of 10%+; and ii) moderate or severe chronic airway obstruction, i.e. $FEV_1 < 60\%$ of predicted value.	respectively, usually diminish on day 2 of work week, but may aggravate and persist throughout work week with prolonged exposure. Degree of fixed airway obstruction assessed from pre-shift FEV_1 after 2 days of non-exposure. Older workers with many years of exposure may present with history of exertional dyspnea.

Table 3.   Common Chronic Respiratory Tract Responses to Toxic Agents

Disease	Definition	Causative Agents/ Occupations at Risk	Clinical Presentation/ Diagnosis	Management	Additional Comments
1) Silicosis	Fibrotic lung disease due to inhalation of dust containing free silica. Usually takes chronic form, requiring many years to develop, but can also present as an acute form under conditions of intense exposure.	Dust containing free silica or silicon dioxide. High-exposure industries include mining, quarrying and tunneling of granite or rock with high quartz content. At-risk industries include sandblasting, rubber milling, manufacture of abrasive detergent, pottery making, brickworks, foundry work, jade polishing.	Chronic simple silicosis is usually asymptomatic or has mild symptoms of cough and sputum. Lung function is normal to mildly restrictive. Progressive massive fibrosis (PMF) presents with progressive exertional dyspnea with deterioration of lung function and possible respiratory failure. Important complications include tuberculosis (especially so in low-income countries) and pneumothorax.	Treat symptomatically. Aggressively treat complicating tuberculous infection. Advise smokers to quit.	In acute silicosis, onset of symptoms and breathlessness may occur within months to a few years of intense exposure and may progress rapidly to massive fibrosis and respiratory failure. Even mild forms after ceasing exposure to silica may progress to fibrosis. Crystalline silica is a lung carcinogen (IARC). Lung cancer risk is elevated among silicotics.

(Continued)

Table 3. (*Continued*)

Disease	Definition	Causative Agents/ Occupations at Risk	Clinical Presentation/ Diagnosis	Management	Additional Comments
			CXR shows diffuse nodular shadows in both lung fields, predominantly in the mid and upper zones and should be read with reference to standard films, e.g. ILO.		
			Occupational history of exposure to dust containing silica is key. Occasional calcification of hilar lymph nodes is known as eggshell calcification.		
2) Coal workers' pneumoconiosis (CWP)	Chronic fibrotic lung disease due to inhalation of carbonaceous dust.	Coal miners and other surface workers; trimming or leveling of coal.	Asymptomatic at early stages. Early symptoms are progressive exertional dyspnea and associated bronchitis. Diagnosis is based on CXR showing diffuse	Directed at complications or associated conditions. Advise smokers to quit.	Simple CWP is usually not disabling but may progress to progressive massive fibrosis — which may lead to premature disability and death.

(*Continued*)

Table 3. (*Continued*)

Disease	Definition	Causative Agents/ Occupations at Risk	Clinical Presentation/ Diagnosis	Management	Additional Comments
			nodular opacities or PMF in absence of other differential diagnosis and presence of definite and prolonged exposure to coal dust. Differentiation from silicosis is based on job history.		
3) Asbestosis and other asbestos-related diseases (ARDs), excluding cancer	Chronic diffuse interstitial fibrosis of lung parenchyma due to inhaled asbestos fibers. Other ARDs except for cancer, include pleural plaques (calcified or non-calcified) and	Production of asbestos-cement (AC) products, asbestos-spraying, construction using AC, production of asbestos textiles, mining and processing of asbestos fibers, building, maintenance and scrapping of	1) Asbestosis: Shortness of breath on exertion and cough; dyspnea, crepitations on lung bases and finger clubbing. CXR shows diffuse interstitial fibrosis, evidenced by irregular streaky opacities in mid	Smoking cessation is imperative to maintain lung function and lower risk for cancer. Treatment is symptomatic.	Primary prevention, i.e. exposure elimination or reduction, through substitution, enclosure, local exhaust, ventilation and respiratory protection, is key.

(*Continued*)

Table 3.   (*Continued*)

Disease	Definition	Causative Agents/ Occupations at Risk	Clinical Presentation/ Diagnosis	Management	Additional Comments
	benign pleurisy. Other ARDs may or may not be associated with asbestosis.	ships, building demolition and renovation, and insulation work (e.g. boiler, furnace, plumbing). Industrial applications utilizing/ historically utilized asbestos reach several thousands, including brake lining, clutch pads, gaskets, and any type of machinery with anti-friction, heat-resistant, sound-proof capacities. Workers in power plants and oil refineries also at risk.	and lower zones. Lung function restrictive and DLCO restrictive. 2) Pleural plaques (PP): Found by simple CXR but more efficiently by CT. Calcification present or absent; circumscribed or diffuse. Diffuse pleural thickening may cause reduction in lung volume and restrictive impairment. It is considered a marker of asbestos exposure but does not predict development of MM.		

(*Continued*)

Table 3. (*Continued*)

Disease	Definition	Causative Agents/ Occupations at Risk	Clinical Presentation/ Diagnosis	Management	Additional Comments
			3) Benign pleurisy: Radiographic or thoracocentesis confirmation of effusion in first 10–20 years following asbestos exposure.		
4) Asbestos-related cancer, especially lung cancer and malignant mesothelioma (MM)	Lung cancer and malignant mesothelioma are the predominant types of asbestos-related cancers. IARC recently added laryngeal cancer and ovarian cancer as asbestos-related cancers.	Same as above. Note all types of asbestos fibers, including chrysotile, are carcinogenic (WHO, IARC). Amphibole fibers (e.g. crocidolite and amosite) may have higher potency for MM.	1) Lung cancer: Clinical presentation/ diagnosis is no different from general lung cancer so a careful job history is key (latency period 20–40 years). 2) Malignant mesothelioma (MM): Pleural MM is the predominant type,		There is a synergistic effect between asbestos exposure and smoking for risk of lung cancer. 80%+ of MM is attributable to asbestos exposure with no known relation to smoking. Primary prevention through substitution, enclosure, local

(*Continued*)

Table 3. (*Continued*)

Disease	Definition	Causative Agents/ Occupations at Risk	Clinical Presentation/ Diagnosis	Management	Additional Comments
			especially in men, but peritoneal MM is not rare, especially in women. Pleural MM presents commonly with chest pain and breathlessness, often progressive. Peritoneal MM presents diffuse abdominal pain, swelling and loss of weight. Biopsy is required for the confirmation of malignancy and cell type.		exhaust, ventilation and respiratory protection is key.
5) Hard metal lung disease	A group of respiratory diseases caused by job	Hard metal usually consists of 80–90% tungsten carbide	Patients with interstitial fibrosis develop cough, sputum and dyspnea on exertion.	Early diagnosis and removal from exposure arrest disease progression.	

(*Continued*)

Table 3. (*Continued*)

Disease	Definition	Causative Agents/ Occupations at Risk	Clinical Presentation/ Diagnosis	Management	Additional Comments
	exposure to "hard metal" (mixture of tungsten carbide, cobalt and other metals) dusts. Cobalt plays an etiological role but affects only susceptible individuals. Diseases include asthma (acute), fibrosing alveolitis (subacute) and diffuse interstitial fibrosis (chronic).	and 10% cobalt with traces of other metals. Used for making high-speed tools for machining metals, stone and wood. Workers may be exposed in the sintering process to produce alloy or in manufacture and servicing of cutting tools (grinding).	Crepitations may be audible in lung bases. CXR shows diffuse bilateral interstitial shadowing. Fibrosis develops in some workers within 2 years but usually occurs after 10 years of work. Clinical, physiologic and CXR features are similar to other types of diffuse interstitial fibrosis. Rare cases progress to respiratory failure. Diagnosis is based on the job history, radiologic, clinical features and pulmonary function	Engineering control measures, e.g. enclosure and local exhaust, are warranted to lower the exposure and to control exposures to within permissible exposure limits. Pre-employment and periodic CXR and urinary cobalt measurements are useful in early detection and monitoring exposure.	

Table 3.   (*Continued*)

Disease	Definition	Causative Agents/ Occupations at Risk	Clinical Presentation/ Diagnosis	Management	Additional Comments
			results consistent with diffuse interstitial fibrosis and exclusion of other causes.		
			Demonstration of tungsten and cobalt in lung tissue is helpful.		
6) Beryllium disease	Acute (rare) or chronic (exposure length months to years; latent period of 10–15 years or up to 25 years) forms of beryllium disease are due to inhalation of beryllium compounds. Acute form presents with nasopharyngitis, tracheitis, bronchitis or pneumonitis, with possible accompanying conjunctivitis and dermatitis.	Extraction, smelting, production and use of beryllium or its alloys. Most widely used alloy is beryllium-copper in non-spark tools, electrical switch parts, watch springs, cams and bushings. Applied in aircraft and aerospace industry.	Severity varies from asymptomatic to respiratory failure and cor pulmonale. Symptoms include exertional dyspnea, cough, fatigue, weight loss and chest pain. Signs: Basal crepitations, peripheral lymphadenopathy, hepatosplenomegaly,	Long-term oral corticosteroid treatment.	

(*Continued*)

Table 3. (*Continued*)

Disease	Definition	Causative Agents/ Occupations at Risk	Clinical Presentation/ Diagnosis	Management	Additional Comments
	Chronic form presents as pulmonary and systemic granulomatous disease, and is well-known for its striking clinical, radiological and histological resemblance to sarcoidosis.	Occult exposure may occur during refining of scrap metal, machining or welding of nonferrous alloys and in dental laboratories.	skin lesions and clubbing. Lung function tests may show obstructive or restrictive patterns or reduced DLCO. CXR typically shows diffuse infiltrates (granular, nodular or linear) and bilateral hilar lymphadenopathy. Differential diagnosis from sarcoidosis is based on beryllium-specific lymphocyte transformation test performed on lymphocytes from BAL or blood.		
7) Chronic obstructive	COPD due to occupational	At risk are coal miners and hard rock miners	Initial symptoms are cough and sputum,	Smoking cessation is the most important	Generally not considered compensable

(*Continued*)

Table 3.   (*Continued*)

Disease	Definition	Causative Agents/ Occupations at Risk	Clinical Presentation/ Diagnosis	Management	Additional Comments
pulmonary disease (COPD)	exposures, i.e. occupational COPD, is clinically indistinguishable from COPD due to smoking. Persisting occupational asthma and reactive airways dysfunction syndrome may also be the cause.	exposed to silica, workers exposed to organic dust, e.g. cotton dust, grain dust and wood dust. Survivors of massive exposures to irritants, e.g. chlorine, ammonia and sulphur dioxide, are also at risk. Possible irritants include toluene diisocyanate, diesel exhaust, chromium, sodium hydroxide and aldehydes. Foundry workers with exposure to cadmium fumes are at higher risk of emphysema.	persisting or recurrent over time. Later exertional dyspnea can develop, possibly progressive. Crepitations or rhonchi may be present. Lung function tests indicate reduced FEV_1 and FEV_1/FVC ratio which are poorly-reversible with bronchodilators. CXR is usually normal or may show emphysematous changes, i.e. hyperlucent areas with flat and depressed diaphragms. Although the diagnosis of COPD is relatively straightforward, relation with occupational exposure may be difficult to establish, particularly in heavy smokers.	intervention. Avoid relevant occupational exposures.	

needed to screen out certain medical conditions that may increase the risk of pulmonary barotrauma, e.g. for divers, pilots and compressed air workers. Healthcare workers may be screened to exclude pulmonary tuberculosis (PTB) and other pre-existing infections prior to work as a baseline as well as for the protection of patients and other colleagues. Workers exposed to specific agents known to affect the respiratory system often require an examination of the respiratory system to determine fitness to work with the hazard and to establish their baseline function. Examples include workers exposed to silica, asbestos, cotton dust, respiratory allergens and irritants. Fitness to use respirators may also require an assessment of lung function, especially for the use of self-contained breathing apparatus (SCBA) or in workers with pre-existing respiratory disease.

Assessments following disease or injury

Assessments may be needed following a respiratory illness or injury for purposes of rehabilitation, return to work or job placement and work injury compensation. This could follow respiratory infections, e.g. SARS, TB, influenza, acute inhalational injury (smoke inhalation, chlorine, ammonia or other irritant gases) or chronic occupational lung diseases such as silicosis or asbestosis.

Assessment of the patient

Ideally, the assessment should be done when the patient is stable (i.e. not having an acute exacerbation or infection) and receiving optimum treatment. Unlike asthma, airflow limitation in chronic bronchitis and emphysema and pulmonary fibrosis is generally not improved greatly by treatment. Any acute episodes of bronchitis or infection should be adequately treated.

The degree of impairment of lung function can be assessed by properly conducted FEV_1, FVC and lung carbon monoxide diffusion capacity (DLCO) measurements. The values are compared with predicted normal values for the local population, corrected for race, sex, age and height. They can also be compared with baseline or previous values, if available. Values of 60–80% of the predicted have been classified as "mild impairment", those 40–60% as "moderate impairment", and those below 40–50% as "severe impairment". However, the degree of impairment of lung function is not the only factor affecting exercise capacity.

Other very important factors include the attitude and outlook of the patient, how he perceives his disease and his work. The subjective effort tolerance of the patient can be ascertained, for instance, by how far he can walk in a given time, how far he can walk on the level before getting breathless, how many flights of steps he can climb without getting breathless, etc. Assessments should be done periodically and the patient's subjective evaluation after a trial period at a particular job is always very useful.

Assessing the job demands and conditions

The physical demands of the job and its component tasks need to be assessed in relation to the individual's capacity to meet them. How much physical effort is required in terms of lifting, carrying or walking upstairs? What is the pace of his work? Can he take breaks or rest in between jobs? What about special or maintenance jobs? Does he need to use respirators? Breathing through a high-resistance filter may be demanding for a severely impaired worker.

The environment should also be assessed. Would the worker still be exposed to any known causative agent (e.g. for occupational asthma)? Is he exposed to dust, noxious and irritant fumes and gases? Is the environment hot or cold, high- or low-humidity? These factors may affect workers with asthma or chronic obstructive pulmonary disease (COPD).

Special considerations

Workers with specific allergies or hypersensitivities should ideally be transferred from any exposure to the specific causative agent, e.g. in the case of occupational asthma or hypersensitivity pneumonitis. Continued exposure could lead to further attacks which could be life-threatening or to chronic asthma and chronic obstructive airway disease.

For the chronic pneumoconiotic diseases, restrictions would depend on the risk of progression of the disease with continued exposure and on the adequacy of dust control at the place of work. Factors that favor a job transfer may include young patients, those who are symptomatic, those with complications such as active tuberculosis, those showing advanced disease (e.g. category 2 or 3 on chest X-ray), those with evidence of rapid progression and those with significant impairment of lung function. A transfer to a less dusty job would probably be helpful even if a dust-free job is not available.

Where the respiratory disease is progressive, lung function will deteriorate and the capacity for exercise will become increasingly limited. It is therefore important to periodically evaluate the patient in relation to his job demands. It is also important to reduce this progression wherever possible so that the worker can enjoy continued employment in his job as long as possible. Patients should be advised and encouraged to stop smoking. Exposures to environmental and occupational irritants or dust should be minimized wherever possible. The physician's attitude to the patient and his disease can also have a significant influence on the patient's perception of his fitness and well-being.

References

Akira M. (2008) Imaging of occupational and environmental lung disease. *Clin Chest Med* **29**: 117–131.

Bernstein IL, Chan-Yeung M, Malo J-L, Bernstein DI. (1993) *Asthma in the Workplace.* New York: Marcel Dekker.

Chia SE, Wang YT, Chan OY, Poh SC. (1993) Pulmonary function in healthy Chinese, Malay and Indian adults in Singapore. *Ann Acad Med Singapore* **22**: 878–884.

De Matteis S, Consonni D, Bertazzi PA. (2008) Exposure to occupational carcinogens and lung cancer risk: Evolution of epidemiological estimates of attributable fraction. *Acta Biomed* **79**(Suppl 1): 34–42.

Driscoll T, Nelson DI, Steenland K, *et al.* (2005) The global burden of non-malignant respiratory disease due to occupational airborne exposures. *Am J Ind Med* **48**: 432–445.

Driscoll T, Nelson DI, Steenland K, *et al.* (2005) The global burden of disease due to occupational carcinogens. *Am J Ind Med* **48**: 419–431.

Karjalainen A, Kurppa K, Martikainen R, *et al.* (2001) Work is related to a substantial portion of adult-onset asthma incidence in the Finnish population. *Am J Respir Crit Care Med* **164**: 565–568.

Le Moual N, Kauffmann F, Eisen EA, Kennedy SM. (2008) The healthy worker effect in asthma: Work may cause asthma, but asthma may also influence work. *Am J Respir Crit Care Med* **177**: 4–10.

Lin RT, Takahashi K, Karjalainen A, *et al.* (2007) Ecological association between asbestos-related diseases and historical asbestos consumption: An international analysis. *Lancet* **369**: 844–849.

Mannino DM, Buist AS. (2007) Global burden of COPD: Risk factors, prevalence, and future trends. *Lancet* **370**: 765–773.

Mapp CE, Boschetto P, Maestrelli P, Fabbri LM. (2005) Occupational asthma. *Am J Respir Crit Care Med* **172**: 280–305.

McCunney RJ. (2006) Should we screen for occupational lung cancer with low-dose computed tomography? *J Occup Environ Med* **48**: 1328–1333.

Pellegrino R, Viegi G, Brusasco V, *et al.* (2005) Interpretive strategies for lung function tests. *Eur Respir J* **26**: 720.

Poh SC, Chia M. (1969) Respiratory function tests in normal adult Chinese in Singapore. *Singapore Med J* **10**: 265–271.

Salvi SS, Barnes PJ. (2009) Chronic obstructive pulmonary disease in non-smokers. *Lancet* **374**: 733–743.

Schuitemaker A, van Berckel BN, Kropholler MA, *et al.* (2007) SPM analysis of parametric (R)-[11C]PK11195 binding images: Plasma input versus reference tissue parameteric methods. *Neuroimage* **35**: 1473–1479.

Tarlo SM, Balmes J, Balkissoon R, *et al.* (2008) Diagnosis and management of work-related asthma: American College of Chest Physicians Consensus Statement. *Chest* **134**(3 Suppl): 1S–41S.

Toren K, Blanc PD. (2009) Asthma caused by occupational exposures is common. *BMC Pulm Med* **9**: 7.

Chapter 5

Skin Disorders

David Koh[*,‡] *and Chee-Leok Goh*[†]

Introduction

Occupational dermatoses are defined as any pathological conditions of the skin for which job exposure can be shown to be a major direct or contributory factor. Although such disorders are rarely life-threatening, they can cause much morbidity and suffering to the workers. Occupational dermatoses are a significant cause of decreased productivity and sickness absence in industry.

Structure and Function of the Skin

The skin is the largest organ in the body, constituting about 10% of the normal body weight. It consists of an outer epidermis, the dermis and a subcutaneous layer (Fig. 1). The epidermis is about 0.1 mm in thickness. The outermost keratin layer and the stratum corneum provide the barrier functions of the skin. The rest of the epidermis consists of keratinocytes, some melanocytes and other cells, including

*Department of Epidemiology and Public Health, Yong Loo Lin School of Medicine, National University of Singapore.
†National Skin Centre, Singapore, Yong Loo Lin School of Medicine, National University of Singapore.
‡Corresponding author. E-mail: ephkohd@nus.edu.sg

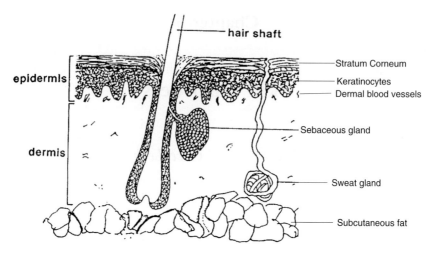

Fig. 1.   Structure of the skin.

Source: Reproduced with kind permission from Goh CL (1990), *Occupational Skin Diseases*, p. 4.

immunocompetent cells such as the Langerhans cells. The dermis is a supporting structure of connective tissue consisting of collagen and elastic bundles. It contains blood vessels and lymphatics in which immunocompetent cells such as macrophages, mast cells and lymphocytes are transported to the dermis. Cutaneous appendages such as hair follicles, sebaceous glands, eccrine and apocrine sweat glands, hair and erector pilorum muscles are found in the dermis. Beneath the dermis is a layer of subcutaneous fat, which acts as a cushion between the epidermis/dermis and the internal body structures.

The skin serves as an efficient protective layer of the body. Its high tensile strength and resilience provides defense against physical injury, especially shearing stress. The stratum corneum acts as a barrier against irritants and sensitizers, systemic poisons and microorganisms. The skin pigment, melanin, is believed to protect the skin against the damaging effects of ultraviolet light, and the continual renewal of the cellular epidermis discourages fungal and bacterial colonization. In addition, the skin's thermoregulation function is carried out by perspiration. Many other functions of the skin have been described, such as its role in Vitamin D metabolism and in the immune response.

Skin Barrier Functions

Skin barrier integrity plays an important role in contact dermatitis. As the body's skin surfaces are exposed to the environment, the skin's tough mechanical barrier serves as a first line of defense, sequestering the internal milieu from the harsh external environment. Keratinocytes are immunologically active cells. Traumatic barrier disruption alone, in the absence of signals from immune cells, stimulates both keratinocyte proliferation and cytokine production, which begin the process of wound repair and initiates features of skin inflammation.

The stratum corneum is a thin sheet of fully differentiated, enu-cleated corneocytes embedded in a lipid-rich matrix of sphingosine and ceramide. The stratum corneum has been referred to as the brick of the barrier and the lipid matrix as the mortar. Any derangement in the brick or mortar due to genetic or environmental factors may initiate the process of skin inflammation (Fig. 2).

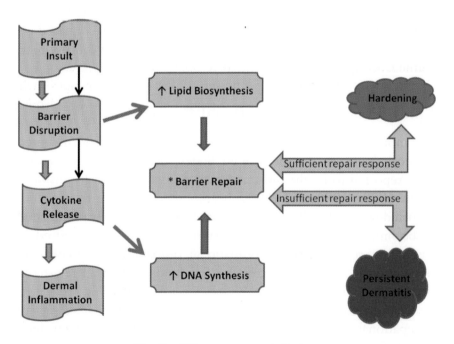

Fig. 2. Skin responses to irritation.

For example, the defective barrier function of patients with atopic dermatitis is relatively deficient in ceramide. This lack of hydrophobic "mortar" is believed to lead to an increase in transepidermal water loss, causing xerosis and probably susceptibility to contact irritants. Replacing ceramide through the application of ceramide-containing creams results in a restoration of the barrier function and significant clinical improvement. The understanding of these molecular derangements in the stratum corneum has important implications in the prevention and management of patients with contact dermatitis. Many genes encode for protein products integral to the proper assembly of the layers of the skin. The identification of these genes helps the occupational physician identify risk factors for contact dermatitis.

The impact of these important and dramatic new findings will compel investigators to search for environmental influences on the epithelial barrier. New investigations into understanding what makes a protein allergenic may begin to answer important further questions about barrier defense. For example, a recent animal study suggests that house dust mite allergen, which is a protease, can itself actively damage the epithelium *in vivo*. Recent attention has been placed on detergents and other environmental irritants which may contribute to epithelial damage in atopic dermatitis.

Epidemiology of Occupational Dermatoses

The morbidity from occupational dermatoses is not well-documented in most countries. In the United States, occupational dermatoses were reported to be the most common occupational health disorder in the 1970s, 1980s and 2000s. It accounted for more than 45% of reported work-related diseases, but this reported figure was estimated to be much lower than the true extent of the disease. In Sweden, where the registration of occupational diseases is comprehensive, occupational dermatoses accounted for about 50% of all registered occupational diseases.

Data from the US Bureau of Labor Statistics' annual surveys of occupational injuries and illnesses in the 1980s show that the incidence of occupational skin disease ranges from 16.2/10,000 per year to 6.3/10,000 per year in all industry divisions. In the manufacturing division, it ranged from 31.2/10,000 per year to 12.3/10,000 per year. In their Annual Survey in 2005, the Bureau reported that with an annual average employment of 109,127,000, there were 4 million injuries of which 242,500 were occupational. Skin disorders were among the commonest occupational disorders with 40,100 (16.5%) affected, followed by hearing loss (26,900 [11.1%]), respiratory conditions (20,200 [8.3%]) and poisonings (2800 [1.2%]).

Different occupational health systems and legislations in countries, reporting bias and selection bias would impact the reliability of estimates of prevalence and incidence of occupational skin diseases. An estimate of the incidence in Europe ranges from 0.7 to 1.5 cases per 1000 per year, with higher rates in specific high-risk occupational groups (Diepgen, 2003).

The UK has The Health and Occupation Reporting (THOR) network, a voluntary surveillance scheme. The average annual incidence rates of work-related skin disease reported from 2002 to 2005 were different for dermatologists and occupational physicians (Turner *et al.*, 2007). For dermatologists, the incidence rate was 91.3 (95% confidence interval [CI], 81.8–101.1) per million, while among occupational physicians, the incidence rate was 316.6 (95% CI, 251.8–381.3) per million. Most reports were of contact dermatitis.

In comparison, a voluntary surveillance scheme of occupational skin diseases in the Netherlands, started in 2001, showed a decline in the number of notifications from 2001 to 2005. The highest number of notifications, recorded in the first year of the scheme, was probably due to the reporting of a mixture of incident and prevalent cases. In the following years, the annual number of notifications declined. Hairdressers, nurses, metalworkers, mechanics and cleaners were those most commonly affected, with wet work and irritating substances the most frequently reported causative agents. Most patients with occupational contact dermatitis did not absent themselves from work (Pal *et al.*, 2009).

Under-reporting, under-recognition and misclassification of cases obscure the true magnitude of the problem. The true incidence has been estimated to be as much as 10 to 50 times higher than the reported figures. The reasons for the under-reported incidence include employees' fear of loss of job and limitation of future job prospects; and employer consternation over involvement in potential legal disputes and reimbursement. Other reasons include the limited disability caused by the skin condition, allowing affected persons to continue working; and the multi-factorial causes of occupational dermatoses, which may complicate diagnosis.

It has been estimated that about 20–25% of all reported occupational dermatoses resulted in time lost from work, averaging 10–12 lost working days per episode. The total economic losses as a consequence of occupational dermatoses can only be speculated at, but has been estimated (in the 1980s) to be in the region of US$222 million to US$1 billion annually in the United States. A more recent US report in 2004 on the Burden of Skin Disease Study indicated an impact of US$37 billion for 21 skin diseases (including physician visits, hospitalizations, missed work, medications). The estimated burden from contact dermatitis alone, reporting a prevalence of 72.29 million episodes that involve 9.2 million visits to offices and 1.6 million visits to emergency rooms, cost the nation about US$1.918 billion.

Throughout the world, there are relatively few reports on the epidemiology of occupational dermatoses in various specific occupations. The majority of published studies have been on hospital- or clinic-based populations, while the few reported field studies were limited by the use of unselected subjects and absent or unsuitable control groups for comparison.

In recent years, the impact of occupational skin disorders on quality of life has been increasingly studied (Rabin and Fraidlin, 2007; Nienhaus *et al.*, 2008; Lan *et al.*, 2008; Matterne *et al.*, 2009). In a study of over a thousand nurses in a university hospital, 22% of respondents reported the occurrence of hand eczema. The occurrence of hand eczema was significantly associated with nursing for >10 years (27% prevalence) and working in a special care unit (29% prevalence). Hand eczema was associated with suboptimal life quality. Among such persons, pruritus or burning sensations were associated with a lower quality of life (Lan *et al.*, 2008).

Another major area of ignorance is that of the risk factors for occupational dermatoses. Although it is known that the work environment plays a major role in the development of occupational dermatoses, genetic and other indirect factors (such as skin hygiene, age and work experience of workers and the presence of coexisting skin disease) may also contribute to the appearance of occupational dermatoses. There are very few epidemiological studies in the literature that have identified and quantified the various risk factors for occupational dermatoses.

Some genes may be associated with an increased risk of occupational dermatoses. For example, in a study of 153 workers frequently exposed to cement in southern Taiwan, 12% were found to be allergic to chromate. Sensitivity to chromate was significantly associated with TNF alpha promoter-308 heterozygous (GA) as compared with the GG genotype (OR 3.9, 95% CI, 1.1–13.2) or GST-T1 null genotype (OR 5.5, 95% CI, 1.4–36.2), but neither the GST-M1 nor the IL-4 genotypes (Wang *et al.*, 2007).

In a case-control study, subjects with intermediate or slow acetylators of NAT2 have a 2.01-fold (95% CI, 1.14–3.54) higher risk for hypersensitivity dermatitis induced by trichloroethylene (TCE) exposure, compared to the fast acetylators. When a non-fast NAT2 phenotype (intermediate and slow acetylators) and a slow NAT1 phenotype were combined, the risk for the disease was significantly increased (OR = 2.71, 95% CI, 1.29–5.70) to a level higher than that observed for the NAT2 non-fast acetylators phenotype alone (Dai *et al.*, 2009).

Types of Occupational Dermatoses

In a reported series of 1727 cases of occupational dermatoses which were confirmed by the Ministry of Labour in Singapore between 1983 and 1987, contact dermatitis was the most common presentation of occupational dermatoses. It accounted for 86% of all cases. About one fifth of the cases were from the construction industry, while the rapidly expanding electronics industry contributed to 15% of all cases. Many of these cases were assessed in a government skin hospital.

A published study of a series of 557 patients with occupational dermatoses seen at a Singapore government skin hospital between 1984 and 1985 reported that the majority of cases were of contact dermatitis. Irritant contact dermatitis was predominant (56%), followed by allergic contact dermatitis (39%). A small proportion (5%) of the cases were non-contact dermatitis, such as fiberglass dermatoses, miliaria and oil folliculitis. Most of the affected workers were from the construction (30%), metal and engineering (21%), electrical and electronic (16%), transport (6%) and food catering (4%) industries. Cutting fluids, oil, cement, solvents, detergents and soldering flux were among the most common occupational irritants. The common occupational allergens included chromates, rubber chemicals, resins, nickel and cobalt (Table 1). A few workers had contact urticaria to proteinaceous foods.

Table 1. Irritants and Allergens Causing Occupational Contact Dermatitis among Patients Seen at the National Skin Centre, Singapore

Year	2005/2009	2003/2004	1989–1998	1984/1985
Irritants				
No. of cases				
Wet work/detergents	79	25	133	37
Oil/grease	46	22	74	27
Solvents	18	14	133	53
Cement	43	11	NA	NA
Coolants/soluble oil	12	7	68	62
Food	1	4	NA	NA
Resins	9	3	NA	NA
Allergens				
No. of cases				
Chromate	5	28	132	106
Rubber Chemicals	9	7	65	35
Cobalt	1	6	41	28
Resins	9	6	44	13
Nickel	6	3	46	27
Colophony	2	2	11	3
Food	1	2	33	5

The above information relates to the types of occupational disorders seen in Singapore, a newly industrializing country. The pattern of occupational dermatoses will differ from country to country, depending on the types of industries present and the workforce characteristics. It should be remembered that most statistics from notification of occupational diseases are an underestimation of the true magnitude of the problem. Most of the cases reported also required tertiary assessment and management. The types of cases seen at the primary health care level would be different.

Prevalence Studies in Industry

Cross-sectional prevalence surveys provide a better reflection of the situation at the industry level. Some prevalence studies have been undertaken in different industries in Singapore (Table 2). However, the reported rates in all the studies were not strictly comparable, as they vary between point and period prevalence rates. The prevalence rates would differ for different industries, and also for different countries.

The Spectrum of Occupational Dermatoses

The most common presentation of occupational dermatosis is contact dermatitis. It accounts for over 90% of all cases seen at the secondary and tertiary levels of care. Other forms such as contact urticaria, disorders of pigmentation, skin cancers and others are uncommon.

Dermatitis

Dermatitis (or eczema) is an inflammation of the skin with characteristic morphology but varied causes. Dermatitis is characterized by redness, swelling, small fluid-filled blisters, and oozing in the acute state and scaly, lichenified, thickened, fissured appearance with pigmentary changes in the chronic stage.

Contact dermatitis, which is skin inflammation caused by direct skin contact with an environmental irritant or allergen, is the

Table 2.   Prevalence Rates of Occupational Dermatoses in Some Industries in Singapore

Industry	Prevalence Rate	n	%
Metal workers (Coenraads, 1985)	All dermatoses	50/751	6.7
Six-month period prevalence	Occupational dermatoses	42/751	5.6 (mainly dermatitis)
Prefabrication construction workers (Goh *et al.*, 1986)	All dermatoses	46/272	16.9
Unspecified period prevalence	Occupational dermatitis	38/272	14.0
Furniture sanders (Gan *et al.*, 1987)	All dermatoses	34/497	6.8
Unspecified period prevalence	Occupational dermatoses	19/497	3.8
Chrome platers (Lee and Goh, 1988)	Occupational dermatoses	14/37	37.8 (50% of cases were chrome ulcers)
Point prevalence			
Visual display unit workers (Koh *et al.*, 1990)	All skin complaints	82/672	12.2
One-year period prevalence	Work-related dermatoses	? 33/672	? 4.9
Electronics workers (Koh, 1993)	Occupational dermatoses	377/2567	14.7 (2/3 of all cases were solder burns and abrasions)
Point prevalence			

Note: ? indicates estimated figures, based on a history of improvement of the skin condition while off work.

most common presentation of occupational dermatosis. Most occupational dermatoses are eczematous reactions to an environmental contactant.

Endogenous dermatitis such as atopic, seborrhoeic, varicose and discoid dermatitis are dermatitis which are genetically inherent skin disorders. They are not caused by environmental agents. However, environmental factors or contactants often aggravate existing endogenous dermatitis.

Irritant contact dermatitis (ICD)

Irritants are substances which directly damage the skin at the site of contact or application. Skin inflammation caused by contact with irritants is called irritant contact dermatitis (ICD) (Figs. 3 and 4).

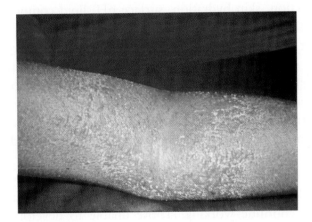

Fig. 3. Subacute contact dermatitis.

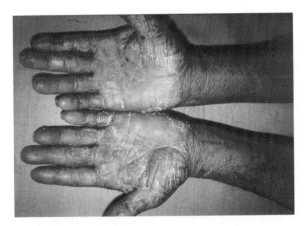

Fig. 4. Cumulative insult dermatitis.

Interaction between an irritant and the skin depends on several factors. These include the properties and nature of the irritant, specific individual factors and environment-related variables.

The pathological mechanisms in skin irritation involve skin barrier disruption, induction of a cytokine cascade and involvement of the oxidative stress network. This results in a subclinical, then visible inflammatory reaction. There are several non-invasive parameters for the evaluation of skin irritation and the irritant potential of compounds and their specific formulations. Among these are epidermal barrier function, skin hydration, surface pH, lipid composition, skin color and skin blood flow (Fluhr *et al.*, 2008).

Irritant contact dermatitis is more common than allergic contact dermatitis. It can present as acute, chronic and cumulative irritant dermatitis, delayed acute irritant dermatitis, irritant reaction, pustular irritant dermatitis, suberythematous irritation, sensory irritation, friction dermatitis and airborne dermatitis. Hand dermatitis is the most frequent manifestation of occupational ICD (Chew and Maibach, 2003).

In many instances, ICD resolves despite continued exposure. This process is known as "hardening", and this mechanism allows such patients to continue working. Those unable to develop hardening may progress to chronic ICD (Watkins and Maibach, 2009).

Acute irritant dermatitis

Strong irritants, for example, concentrated acids, alkalis or solvents, cause acute irritant contact dermatitis following a single exposure or repeated exposures. The skin structures are damaged directly by the irritant. The cause of acute irritant contact dermatitis is often obvious.

Strong irritants cause irritant contact dermatitis in almost all individuals. In contrast, weak irritants such as water and mild detergents tend to cause irritant contact dermatitis only in susceptible individuals (e.g. individuals with previous atopic dermatitis or hand eczema). Weak irritants tend to cause dermatitis only after repeated skin contact.

In the workplace, cases of acute irritant dermatitis often occur as accidents or as a result of workers' poor work habits, for example, failure to use gloves, boots or aprons when indicated, or from careless handling of acute irritants. It also results from workers' failure (usually due to ignorance) to recognize the hazards of corrosive work materials. Acute irritant dermatitis can very often be prevented and affected workers need not change their jobs. Health education is very important here. Where permissible, the use of impervious gloves, aprons and boots during work can prevent acute irritant contact dermatitis.

Cumulative insult irritant contact dermatitis

This type of irritant contact dermatitis is caused by repeated skin contact with weak irritants. Weak irritants cause irritant contact dermatitis in susceptible individuals only. The duration between the first exposure to the irritant and the appearance of dermatitis varies from weeks to years, depending on the nature of the irritant, frequency of contact and host susceptibility.

The clinical presentation is usually chronic dermatitis.

Cumulative insult dermatitis is exemplified by chronic hand dermatitis caused by water and detergents among dishwashers and housewives, and by cutting fluid dermatitis among metalworkers. Solvents such as thinners and kerosene, when used inappropriately as skin cleansers, often cause cumulative insult dermatitis.

Case Study 1

Five out of 15 newly employed persons in a metalworking factory complained of itchy rashes over the hands and forearms within two months of starting work. All five workers had a history of atopy, and an examination of the skin showed that the five had contact dermatitis of the dorsa of the hands and distal half of the forearms. Patch testing of the workers with the standard series of allergens and the metalworking fluid battery was negative. The provisional diagnosis was irritant contact dermatitis to metalworking fluid, and symptomatic treatment was initiated.

A workplace inspection showed that the hands and forearms of the workers were heavily contaminated with the machine cutting oils in the course of their work. The use of gloves was not feasible because of the risk of accidental entrapment by the moving parts of the machine and injury.

The workers were shown how to improve their work habits and how to minimize contact with the cutting oils by their supervisors. Advice was also given to improve personal hygiene, to avoid other irritants in domestic and other non-work situations, and to use emollient cream after work. The condition of four of the workers improved, and they could continue with their work. The fifth worker, who had hand eczema previously, continued to have problems and left the job.

Allergic contact dermatitis

Allergic contact dermatitis is an immunologic inflammatory reaction of the skin due to contact with an allergen. In contrast to irritant contact dermatitis, the inflammatory reaction is mediated through an immunological process. An individual does not develop any reaction to the allergen during his initial exposure to it. Often, repeat contacts are necessary before an individual becomes sensitized to an allergen. "I have been in contact with the substance for many months and never had any rash with it previously and therefore the substance cannot be the cause of my rash" is a misconception.

Different substances have different sensitizing potential, and these individuals have different susceptibility to sensitization by an allergen. Once an individual becomes sensitized to an allergen, further contact with it will trigger a type IV hypersensitivity reaction, during which chemical mediators are released from immunocompetent cells, leading to the manifestation of dermatitis. The dermatitis usually appears 36 to 48 hours after contact with the allergen. The dermatitis may be acute, subacute or chronic, depending on the sensitivity of the worker. Allergy to a substance is specific, and once developed, is usually lifelong.

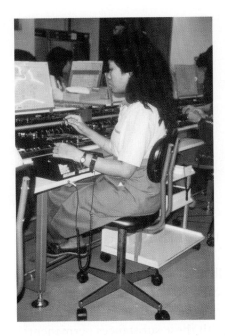

Fig. 5. Worker in an electronics company wearing an earthing wrist strap.

Case Study 2

About 5% of female electronics workers involved in microcomputer assembly work complained of rashes on their wrists. The workers were required to wear an anti-static earthing wrist strap while at work (Fig. 5).

All the affected workers gave a history of allergy to costume jewelry, and had dermatitis of varying severity at the site of contact with the wrist strap (Fig. 6). The metal stud of the wrist strap was examined, and a dimethylglyoxime test demonstrated the presence of nickel. The provisional diagnosis was that of allergic contact dermatitis to nickel. The problem was resolved by changing the wrist strap to another type that did not contain nickel.

Unlike a worker with irritant contact dermatitis, a worker who develops allergic contact dermatitis to a work substance may require a job change. Hence, it is important to differentiate irritant contact

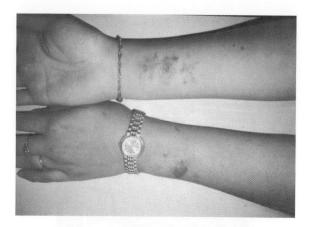

Fig. 6.   Allergic contact dermatitis due to nickel in wrist strap.

dermatitis from allergic contact dermatitis. Once an allergen has been identified as the cause of occupational dermatitis, it is necessary to inform the worker of the sources of the allergen and advise the patient to avoid contact with these substances permanently. One must also be aware that "automated processes" need maintenance. Workers maintaining such processes are exposed to chemicals used in the automated machines and may also develop contact allergy to the chemicals.

Patch testing

Patch testing is the definitive test for allergic contact dermatitis. The patch test procedure (Figs. 7 and 8) allows the dermatologist to identify the allergen that causes the dermatitis. The patch test procedure consists of applying a set of suspected allergens under occlusion on the skin of the upper back for 48 hours. The reaction to the test allergens is scored after the allergens are removed at 48 hours. A second scoring is made at 96 hours. Only patch test reactions which persist beyond 48 hours are considered positive allergic reactions. Patch testing must be carried out by an experienced dermatologist to avoid false positive and false negative test results. For example, a false positive reaction may result if the concentration of the test allergen applied on the skin is too high and a false negative patch test recording may result if the concentration of the test allergen is too low. In addition the relevance

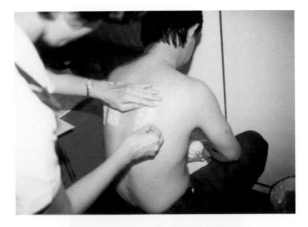

Fig. 7. Patch test being conducted.

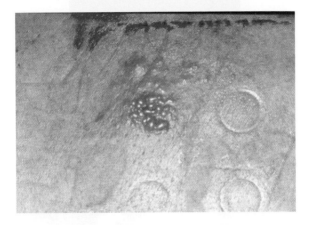

Fig. 8. Positive patch test result.

of a positive patch test reaction should be determined to ascertain if the existing dermatitis is due to the allergen.

Other types of environmentally induced skin disorders

Phototoxic and photoallergic contact dermatitis

A phototoxic substance is a substance which absorbs ultraviolet light and causes skin inflammation. Examples of phototoxic substances include medicaments (e.g. phenothiazines and tetracyclines), industrial

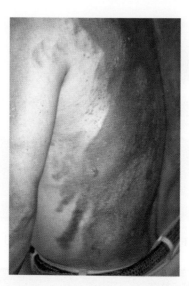

Fig. 9.   Phototoxic dermatitis due to application of lime juice from *Citrus hystrix* (as an insect repellent).

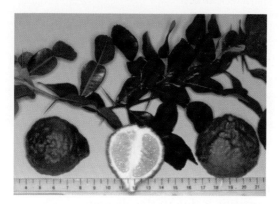

Fig. 10.   *Citrus hystrix* — the juice of this fruit contains psoralen, which causes photodermatitis.

chemicals (e.g. tars) and plant resins. Phototoxic contact dermatitis is not mediated through an immunologic mechanism. The reaction is dose-related. Phototoxic substances tend to cause reactions in almost all individuals who are exposed to it (Figs. 9 and 10).

Photoallergic contact dermatitis, like allergic contact dermatitis, is mediated through an immunological mechanism. The allergen becomes activated only in the presence of ultraviolet light. There is individual susceptibility to photoallergy. Examples of photoallergens include medicaments, fragrances, sunscreens and antiseptics. Photoallergic contact dermatitis can be confirmed by a photopatch test.

Contact urticaria

Contact urticaria (CU) is an immediate wheal and flare reaction of the skin to a contactant (an urticant). Unlike contact dermatitis, which tends to develop several days after skin contact, CU develops very soon after skin contact with the urticant. The clinical presentation is usually immediate urticarial eruption (within 30 minutes of contact), and in longstanding cases, dermatitis. CU is not uncommon.

CU may be immunologically mediated (type I hypersensitivity reaction = allergic CU) or non-immunologically mediated. The latter reaction is usually localized and not life-threatening, unlike allergic CU which can be generalized and life-threatening. Hence, there is a need to differentiate allergic from non-allergic CU. Allergic CU can be confirmed by a skin prick test (Fig. 11). The diagnosis should

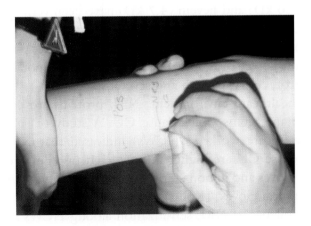

Fig. 11. Skin prick testing.

include an appropriate history, combined with specific skin tests, IgE determinations (e.g. radioallergosorbent test (RAST)) and occasionally provocation tests.

Causes of CU include foodstuff (e.g. meat, eggs, seafood, vegetables), animal dander and secretions (e.g. from caterpillars and other arthropods), plants and spices (e.g. seaweed, thyme and cayenne pepper), fragrances and flavorings such as Balsam of Peru and cinnamon oil, several types of medicaments (e.g. some antibiotics), metals (e.g. cobalt), some preservatives (e.g. formaldehyde and benzoic acids) and latex rubber (e.g. gloves).

In Finland, of 2759 workers with allergic contact reactions, 29.5% were due to CU (Kanerva *et al.*, 1996). It was much more common in women (70%) than in men (30%). The most common causes were cow dander (44.4%), natural latex rubber (23.7%), flour/grains (11.3%) and proteinaceous foodstuff. The occupations with the highest numbers of occupational CU were farmers, domestic animal attendants, bakers, nurses, chefs and dental assistants.

Contact urticaria (CU) to natural rubber latex (NRL) proteins

Hand eczema and atopy are the main risk factors for immunologic contact urticaria to NRL. Therefore, skin prick testing (SPT) with NRL allergen is recommended in all suspected to have CU to NRL. Prohevein (20 kD) and hevein (4.7 kD) have been verified to be the major NRL allergens in sensitized persons. Patients allergic to NRL may be cross-sensitized to birch, alder, hazel and oak pollen, hazelnut, almond, apple, pear, peach, kiwi fruit, plum, potato, tomato, paprika, carrot, celery, parsnip and several spices.

In the healthcare environment, NRL proteins are probably the most important agents which cause CU. A study of rubber gloves used by healthcare workers (HCWs) indicated that NRL proteins which can cause CU are higher in powdered (as compared to non-powdered) gloves and in non-sterile examination gloves (as compared to sterile surgical gloves) (Koh *et al.*, 2005).

The prevalence of NRL sensitization among HCWs ranges from 3% to 17% (Ahmed, Aw and Adisesh, 2004). Among sensitized persons, contact with NRL can cause itch, eczematous hand rash, urticaria, rhinitis, asthma or even anaphylaxis. There may be concurrent food allergy to bananas, avocados and kiwi fruit. Skin prick testing (SPT), using a commercial extract of NRL, can be performed to confirm the diagnosis. Blood tests can also be done for latex-specific IgE antibody detection.

Information on the prevalence of NRL sensitization is less readily available from developing Asian countries. In a study of 313 HCWs in Singapore, the point prevalence of NRL sensitization was 9.6%. In comparison, the point prevalence was 2.8% among 71 administrative staff. Glove-related symptoms were reported in 13.7% of all health-care workers, of whom 22.9% were sensitized to latex. Among the NRL-sensitized HCWs, 26.7% had glove-related symptoms, while the rest were asymptomatic. While the most common symptoms were itch and hand eczema, the most important discriminating symptom was CU. Only 1 out of 9 (11.2%) symptomatic NRL-sensitized subjects had sought previous medical attention for the problem (Tang *et al.*, 2005).

There is a need to increase the awareness of this condition among HCWs. Management of this condition includes health education and screening of workers with suspicious symptoms. Sensitized persons should be provided with latex-free alternatives at work, such as vinyl gloves. Measures should also be taken to minimize other sources of latex exposure.

Case Study 3

A restaurant chef complained of itch and rash over the fingers and hands whenever he prepared raw seafood. He noticed that the symptoms started within 15 minutes of handling the materials.

On examination, there was mild dermatitis of the hands. Patch testing with the standard series of allergens and the food handlers series did not produce any positive reactions. Prick testing was performed, using the materials that he believed were responsible for the symptoms. A strong wheal and flare reaction was noted for squid and shellfish. The diagnosis was contact urticaria. The chef was advised to avoid handling these contact urticants as far as possible, and to use gloves while at work.

Other types of occupational dermatoses

Other environmental agents, including physical agents (e.g. ionizing radiation, mechanical factors, ultraviolet light, heat and cold), can damage the skin. Some chemicals are absorbed percutaneously and can cause systemic toxicity (e.g. dioxins causing chloracne). Oil and grease can cause oil acne. Phenolic compounds such as para-tertiary butylphenol formaldehyde resins may cause skin depigmentation. Table 3 summarizes the causes of non-eczematous presentation of occupational dermatoses, while Figs. 12 to 15 illustrate some examples. Non-eczematous presentations of occupational dermatoses are uncommon. They account for less than 10% of all occupational dermatoses.

Table 3. Causes of Non-eczematous Occupational Dermatoses

Non-eczematous occupational dermatoses caused by physical agents

    Mechanical injury, e.g. frictional callosity, abrasions/lacerations
    Localized vibration (Raynaud's phenomenon)
    Temperature, e.g. miliaria from heat, frostbite from cold
    Ultraviolet light, e.g. photodermatitis, actinic damage
    Ionizing radiation, e.g. radiation burns, skin cancers

Skin infections and infestations

    Viral, e.g. herpetic whitlow
    Bacterial, e.g. pyoderma, pitted keratolysis
    Fungal, e.g. superficial and deep mycoses
    Parasitic, e.g. larva migrans, mite infestations

Others

    Acne and folliculitis, e.g. caused by oil and grease, aggravated by heat
    Skin ulceration — by chromic and other acids
    Pigmentary changes
    Hyperpigmentation — post-inflammatory, tar and pitch
    Hypopigmentation — phenolic compounds
    Generalized skin eruption — from trichloroethylene
    Lichen-planus-like eruptions — paraphenylenediamine dyes, photographic
      color developers
    Scleroderma — exposure to silica or vinyl chloride monomer
    Acquired porphyria cutanea tarda — hexachlorobenzene

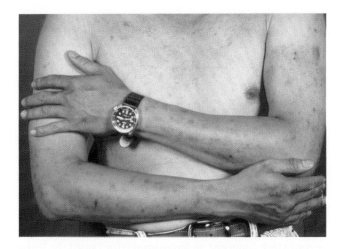

Fig. 12.   Grain mite infestation in a chef.

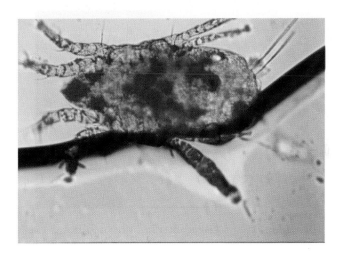

Fig. 13.   The mite was identified as *Pyemotes ventricosus.*

Skin cancers

Skin cancers from environmental carcinogens (such as ultraviolet light, polycyclic aromatic hydrocarbons and arsenic) are often induced after many years following exposure.

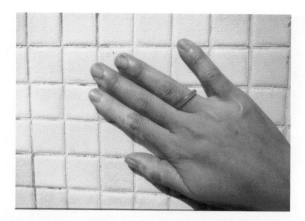

Fig. 14. Leukoderma in an electronics worker. The worker previously used a rubber finger cot (which contained an antioxidant) that caused the leukoderma.

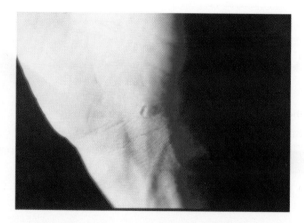

Fig. 15. Chrome ulcer in an electroplater.

Outdoor work is a well-recognized risk factor for skin cancer. In a study of data from a population-based cancer registry in Bavaria, outdoor workers were found to have a higher risk for basal cell carcinoma (BCC) (male [RR, 2.9; 95% CI, 2.2–3.9] and female [RR, 2.7; 95% CI, 1.8–4.1]) as well as squamous cell carcinoma (SCC) (male [RR, 2.5; 95% CI, 1.4–4.7] and female [RR, 3.6; 95%

CI, 1.6–8.1]) but not for cutaneous malignant melanoma (CMM) (Radespiel-Tröger *et al.*, 2009).

In some countries such as in Singapore, statutory regulations require designated workplace doctors to undertake special medical examinations of the skin to screen for skin cancers in workers exposed to potential skin carcinogens such as arsenic, tar, pitch, bitumen and creosote.

Industries and Occupations at Risk

Workers in some occupations are at a higher risk of developing occupational dermatoses than others. Table 4 lists some industries with

Table 4. Common Irritants and Allergens in Some Industries

Agriculture and Horticulture Industries

Allergens: Plants, gloves (rubber, chromates), animal feeds (antibiotics, preservatives, vegetables), antibiotics, pesticides, disinfectants, wood and its preservatives
Irritants: Animal feeds, fertilizers, solvents, plants, oils, disinfectants, pesticides

Chemical and Pharmaceutical Industries

Allergens: All chemicals and medicaments, gloves and masks (rubber chemicals)
Irritants: Chemicals, acids, alkalis, solvents, water, detergents, surfactants

Construction and Building Industries

Irritants: Cement (alkalis), wood dust, wood preservatives, fiberglass, solvents, oils, pitch, tar, paints
Allergens: Cement (chromates, cobalt), rubber gloves/boots, leather gloves/ boots (chromates), para-tertiary-butylphenol formaldehyde (PTBPF) resins, epoxy resins, woods, paints

Electronics and Electrical Industries

Irritants: Solvents, soldering fluxes, acids, alkalis, resins, fiberglass, metallic salts
Allergens: Resins (e.g. epoxy, acrylates, isocyanates, formaldehyde resins), soldering fluxes (amines and colophony), metals (nickel, chromates and cobalt), gloves/cots

(Continued)

Table 4.   (*Continued*)

Electroplating Industry

Irritants: Acids and alkalis (metal cleaners, pickling and plating solutions), chromic acid fumes, cleansers
Allergens: Metals and their salts, gloves, boots, aprons

Metal and Engineering Industries

Irritants: Cutting fluids, solvents, abrasives, metal slivers, grease, oils, hand cleansers
Allergens: Cutting fluids (metals, biocides, antioxidants, fragrances, resins), barrier creams, gloves

Food and Catering Industries

Irritants: Vegetables and fruit juices (enzymes, acids, alkalis), water and detergents, polishing agents
Allergens: Food (vegetables, seafood, salad dressings, meat, fruits, flavoring agents), gloves, antioxidants, preservatives, utensils (nickel)

Hairdressing Industry

Irritants: Shampoos, permanent wave solutions, water
Allergens: Nickel, formaldehyde, hair dyes, fragrances and preservatives, gloves

Healthcare Industry

Irritants: Water, soaps, detergents, solvents, resins, disinfectants, antiseptics, medicaments
Allergens: Gloves, medicaments, antiseptics, disinfectants, metals, formaldehyde, preservatives, resins

Transport and Shipbuilding Industries

Irritants: Cutting fluids, oils, grease, solvents, resins, metals, hand cleansers, fiberglass
Allergens: Cutting fluids and oils, gloves/boots, welding fumes, resins, metals, barrier creams, woods

Woodworking and Furniture Making Industries

Irritants: Wood dust, resins, soaps and detergents, solvents, oils, turpentine, lacquer, polishes
Allergens: Woods, plants, gloves, resins, formaldehyde, wood preservatives, turpentine

risks of occupational dermatoses and some of the commonly encountered occupational irritants and allergens.

An Approach to the Diagnosis of Occupational Dermatosis

The diagnosis of an occupational dermatosis requires not only a good knowledge of dermatology, but also a working knowledge of the patient's work process, materials, practice and habits. The clinical appearance of an occupational dermatosis (for example, dermatitis, acne, skin cancer) is exactly the same as a non-occupational skin disorder. The danger of overlooking an occupational dermatosis is that the patient's skin problem will recur when he returns to work. The failure to identify and avoid the causative agent of occupational dermatosis at a workplace may also result in failure to recognize similar skin problems in other workers.

It is essential that a detailed occupational history be obtained during any dermatological consultation. Occupational dermatosis should always be suspected when a worker presents with hand dermatitis and dermatitis on the exposed parts, as this is the most common presentation. Important elements to look out for in the occupational history and during clinical examination are listed in Box 1.

History Taking

Record of place of employment and job title

This includes particulars on the type of industry, the company address, contact telephone number and name of supervisor (in case there is a need to obtain more information). The job title will give an idea of the patient's work duties. It is often necessary to enquire about the worker's work tasks, and details of the patient's work exposure and contact to various work chemicals should be elicited. A simple way to go about doing this is to ask the worker to describe his daily work activities.

Box 1. Checklist of Important Considerations During History Taking and Clinical Examination

Occupational history

Place of employment
Job title
Typical workday activities
Material handling techniques
Protective clothing and equipment
Hygiene facilities and practice

Occupational factors in relation to the skin disorder

New job, materials, processes
Health and safety information on materials handled
Whether other workers affected
Improvement on weekends or holidays
Sick leave taken for skin disorder

Past occupational history

Past history of occupational dermatosis

Concurrent occupation(s)

Other general history

Atopic background (personal and familial)
Skin allergies
Other skin disorders
Treatment for skin disorder
Domestic exposure
Hobbies

Clinical examination

Is it dermatitis?
Is it contact (exogenous) dermatitis?
If it is contact dermatitis, is it irritant or allergic?
Are additional factors involved (e.g. sunlight)?
Is it a non-dermatitic occupational dermatosis?

Are there any predisposing and aggravating factors for the occupational dermatosis, and are these preventable?

Occupational factors in relation to the skin disorder

The history of the skin disorder, for example the duration of the rash, primary location, secondary spread (if any), should be correlated with the occupational history, such as the duration of employment. The relationship of the appearance of the skin disorders to any recent change in work duties, new processes or materials, or even to different batches of raw materials, may give a clue as to the occupational etiology of the skin disorder. Off days, weekends or vacations are usually associated with an improvement of the occupational dermatosis. A past history of the occurrence of similar skin disorders in other workers at the workplace may be another valuable piece of information which points to an occupational origin of the skin disorder.

Personal occupational factors

Incorrect material handling techniques may contribute to the cause of an occupational dermatosis. The worker should be asked about the way he handles work materials. Protective devices are often worn by workers. The type of protective equipment, the material it is made of, how it is used and maintained (to determine if this is improperly done) should be recorded. The availability of cleansing facilities, the types of skin cleansers used and the cleansing habits of the worker should be enquired about. Good personal hygiene reduces the risk of occupational dermatoses. However, extremely effective cleansers (e.g. solvents) are often skin irritants.

A personal history of similar skin problems should be obtained. A worker may have experienced a similar skin disorder in his previous employment. Exposure to the same work chemical or process in his present job may then cause a recurrence of the occupational dermatosis. The time off or sick leave taken by the patient for the skin disorder should also be recorded. Sick leave from occupational dermatoses may be compensable.

Seek the opinion of the worker regarding his skin problem. The worker can often help ascertain the cause of his skin disease.

Other general aspects of history taking

A history of treatment received (medicaments can cause or aggravate a skin disorder), skin allergies (the patient may have been exposed to the same allergen previously), a personal or family history of atopy (atopics are more susceptible to irritant contact dermatitis), and a history of other skin disorders or general illnesses should be recorded.

History of other occupational or environmental exposures

The cause of a skin disorder may not be apparent from the worker's work environment. It may be due to chemicals handled during his part-time job elsewhere. This information may be more difficult to obtain, especially if the patient is apprehensive that his main employer may disapprove of his part-time job. Skin disorders may also result from hobbies (e.g. from contact with solvents, resins and other materials used in do-it-yourself kits) or from domestic exposure (e.g. water/detergents during housework) and cosmetics.

The previous occupations of the worker should be obtained. Sensitization from exposure to chemicals in a previous job may have occurred. A record of past occupations may also be important for occupational dermatoses with long latent periods between work exposure to the chemicals and manifestation of disease, for example, skin cancers and ultraviolet light exposure and scleroderma and silica exposure.

*Overcoming common difficulties in obtaining
occupational history*

Often, difficulties are encountered during occupational history taking. The physician needs to understand various work processes. Workers performing similar work tasks in the same type of industry may work under different work conditions. A technical dictionary or reference book, such as the *ILO Encyclopaedia of Occupational Health and Safety*, may provide useful information. Alternatively, the help of an experienced occupational health colleague may be sought. The physician needs to have a knowledge of the common industries and their work processes in the country, and a knowledge of the common causes of occupational dermatoses in the various industries (see Table 4).

Additional information and follow up

Occasionally, further information on the nature of the chemicals which are handled by the worker may be required during investigation. The usual way of obtaining such information is to ask the worker for the Safety Data Sheets (SDS) which may be available for the work chemicals used. The SDS provides information on the nature of the substances and their possible health effects. Chemical safety and health databases (available either at the Poisons Centre, Occupational Health Centre or on the Internet) are other sources of information.

Where indicated, samples of the work materials handled by the worker should be obtained for patch testing or for chemical analysis. This may be necessary for the detection of impurities which may not be specified in the information sheet, or detection of decomposition products. The physician may need to arrange for a factory visit to better assess the worker's work conditions, to screen other workers for similar occupational dermatoses or to learn more about the work process.

Clinical Examination

A well-taken clinical and occupational history will often allow the physician to determine if the worker's skin disorder is work-related. Clinical examination, patch tests and laboratory tests will help the physician to confirm the diagnosis and ascertain the cause of the skin disorder. During the examination the following questions will help the physician in the management of occupational dermatoses.

Case Study 4

An outbreak of skin rashes occurred in a woodworking factory. 13 workers in two adjacent sections had the rashes, and the workers believed that their skin disorder was due to the wood dust and poor working conditions of the factory, such as poor ventilation and heat. The workers were concerned about the rashes because some of their family members were also affected.

A workplace investigation showed that the work environment was generally satisfactory. An examination of the affected workers showed popular rashes and excoriation marks with typical skin burrows at the finger webs and flexor surfaces of the wrists. The diagnosis was skin infestation by Sarcoptes scabiei.

The problem was resolved when the workers and their families were treated for scabies.

Is the skin disorder a dermatitis?

Most occupational dermatoses present as eczematous eruptions secondary to contact dermatitis. The ability to recognize the features of dermatitis is important.

Is the dermatitis a contact dermatitis?

Occupational contact dermatitis refers to dermatitis arising from contact with a work chemical. It should be distinguished from non-occupational contact dermatitis which are contact dermatitis arising from contact with non-occupational substances such as cosmetics, costume jewelry or medicaments. Contact dermatitis should also be distinguished from endogenous dermatitis (for example, atopic, seborrhoeic, discoid or hand and foot dermatitis), which is genetic in origin. It should be noted that workers with endogenous dermatitis are more susceptible to develop irritant contact dermatitis. It is not uncommon for contact dermatitis to coexist with endogenous dermatitis.

Is the contact dermatitis irritant or allergic in nature?

Irritant contact dermatitis results from direct skin injury from an irritant, for example, solvents or detergents. Allergic contact dermatitis is an immunological skin reaction and tends to be more severe. Unlike an irritant, an allergen tends to trigger a dermatitis readily, even if the allergen is present in minute quantities and in low concentrations.

Over three quarters of occupational contact dermatitis are irritant contact dermatitis. The remainder are allergic contact dermatitis or concomitant irritant and allergic contact dermatitis. Sometimes, more than one irritant or allergen may be the cause of the contact dermatitis. It is important to differentiate irritant from allergic contact dermatitis. The type of dermatitis a worker has affects his rehabilitation and future job placement. While patch testing is the definitive test for allergic contact dermatitis, there is no specific skin test to confirm irritant contact dermatitis. The diagnosis of irritant contact dermatitis is often based on clinical history, examination and after the exclusion of allergic contact dermatitis (by patch testing). All workers with contact dermatitis should be patch tested.

Are there aggravating factors (e.g. sunlight)?

If a photoallergic contact dermatitis is suspected, a photopatch test may be indicated. One should look for evidence of endogenous dermatitis.

Is there a non-eczematous occupational dermatosis?

About 5–10% of occupational dermatoses present as non-eczematous skin lesions. These include physical or mechanical injuries (e.g. heat, friction) and infections (see Table 3). When such disorders are suspected, relevant tests including skin scrapings for microscopy, prick tests, skin biopsy and serology may be necessary.

Are there any predisposing factors for the occupational dermatosis? Are these preventable?

Several factors are known to predispose an individual to developing occupational dermatoses. Individuals with constitutional predisposition, for example, atopy, are generally more susceptible to irritants.

Damaged skin, such as lacerated or abraded skin, may be predisposed to contact dermatitis.

Environmental conditions may also contribute to the development of occupational dermatoses. For example, a poorly ventilated and hot workplace induces workers to perspire excessively and aggravates heat-induced skin disorders and intertrigo. Sweat may also act as a solvent to enhance skin penetration of contact irritants and allergens. Workers who are ignorant of work hazards, and who do not observe good work habits and hygiene, are at higher risk of occupational skin disease.

Management of Occupational Dermatoses

The management of occupational dermatosis depends on its morphological presentation and cause. An accurate diagnosis is essential. The causative agent must be identified. A detailed history, thorough physical examination and, where indicated, relevant investigations including patch tests and laboratory tests, together with a factory visit, will often enable the physician to arrive at a correct diagnosis.

Specific Treatment

The worker should avoid the causative agent immediately if the dermatitis is severe. A temporary job change may be necessary. Severely affected workers should be given medical leave or hospitalized. Workers with mild dermatosis should be encouraged to resume work with proper protective garments and advised to observe good work habits.

Dermatitis is treated according to its severity. Acute dermatitis should be treated with wet compresses of normal saline or potassium permanganate (1:10,000) lotions until the dermatitis dries up. Chronic dermatitis should be treated with topical steroid creams or ointments of mild to moderate potency (e.g. hydrocortisone, betamethasone valerate, fluocinolone acetonide).

Potent steroids such as clobetasol dipropionate should be avoided or used for short periods only because of their potential side effects.

It is advisable to avoid combination steroid/antibiotic/antifungal preparations as they may pose problems of sensitization. Contact allergy to neomycin and quinolines present in such preparations is not uncommon. Oral antibiotics should be administered where secondary bacterial infection is suspected. Oral antihistamines should be given to relieve pruritus.

Other occupational dermatoses are treated according to diagnosis; for example, cutaneous larva migrans with cryotherapy and/or oral antihelmetics, and chromomycosis with oral antifungal agents.

Causes of chronicity of occupational dermatoses

Occasionally, a patient with an occupational dematosis may not respond to treatment.

Chronicity of an occupational dermatosis may be due to one or more of the following:

a. Continued exposure to the offending agent.
b. Severe longstanding dermatitis which generally takes longer to recover because the barrier functions of the skin are severely impaired.
c. Complications of treatment, such as superimposed contact allergy to medicaments.
d. Untreated complications, for example, secondary bacterial infection.
e. Underlying endogenous factors, e.g. atopic dermatitis.
f. Medico-legal problems: an avaricious worker may malinger or even inflict injury on himself in an attempt to seek compensation.

These conditions have to be considered and managed accordingly in a patient with chronic occupational dermatosis.

Rehabilitation

The primary consideration in the rehabilitation of a worker with occupational dermatosis is to get him back to work as soon as possible and, at the same time, prevent a relapse. The worker should be taken off work during the acute stage of the disease, but the physician should not encourage a long absence from work.

A permanent job change should be avoided wherever possible. A job change will require the worker to retrain for another job which may be expensive for the employee and the employer. It will also mean social adjustment for the worker: he has to adapt to a new working condition, colleagues and workplace. He may also suffer a salary reduction.

The physician should therefore consider the worker's age, skills, capability, intellect and available preventive measures before recommending a job change. Job change is usually recommended only for workers with allergic contact dermatitis and rarely for those with irritant contact dermatitis. This is because in allergic contact dermatitis, relapses tend to be more severe with each subsequent episode and even brief exposures to the allergen will trigger a reaction. However, when substitution of the allergen is possible, or contact with the allergen can be totally avoided by changing work procedures, a job change may not be necessary.

Studies have shown that allergic contact dermatitis from some occupational allergens (for example, chromate from cement, nickel and cobalt) has a poor prognosis. The dermatitis tends to persist even with the avoidance of the allergen. Therefore a job change may not benefit the worker significantly.

Another important factor to consider before recommending a job change is whether a personal history of atopy is present. Workers with an atopic background, especially those with a history of childhood atopic dermatitis or hand dermatitis, have a higher risk of developing irritant contact dermatitis when they are exposed to irritants. Job counseling is important for these workers, and they should be encouraged to do dry jobs.

The physician must distinguish between medical and social prognoses in workers with occupational dermatoses. Many workers with occupational dermatoses are able to continue working despite their dermatoses. Indeed, many do prefer to remain in their jobs despite their skin disorders, in order to avoid a salary reduction or a change to a less interesting or challenging job. Some who continue to be exposed to the work irritants or allergens may develop tolerance and hardening.

Prognosis of Occupational Contact Dermatitis

The prognosis of occupational contact dermatitis refers to the course of the dermatitis over a period of time with and without medical intervention. Understanding the prognosis of occupational contact dermatitis is important because it enables dermatologists and occupational physicians to (a) predict the course of the dermatitis of his patients; (b) implement risk management for patients who are exposed to contact irritants and allergens; (c) plan preventive measures against contact and occupational dermatitis; and (d) help the relevant authorities prioritize the implementation of preventive measures. The long-term outcome of occupational contact dermatitis has important medico-legal implications. It helps dermatologists and occupational physicians determine the amount of medico-legal compensation for patients with such skin disorders.

Epidemiology studies in the 1970s and 1980s generally reported the persistence of dermatitis among patients who developed occupational contact dermatitis. Recent reports appear to indicate that the prognosis is better than previously reported. The improvement in the prognosis can be attributed to the improvement in diagnostic test procedures; the ability of physicians to identify causative contact irritants and allergens; and the improvement in health education and effective preventive measures against occupational contact dermatitis.

Complete clearance of occupational contact dermatitis has been reported to range from 8% to 77% over follow-up periods ranging from one year to more than 10 years. Studies done between 1961 and 1989 indicated that total clearance of occupational contact dermatitis occurred in only 8% to 33% of patients. In a study of 555 patients who completed a follow-up questionnaire 2–3 years after initial consultation, 26% of women had complete healing, 22% had continual problems, and 52% had recurrence. Among the men, 31% had complete healing, 29% had continual problems, and 40% had recurrence

(Fregert, 1975). The prognosis was the same for those who changed their job or stopped working as it was for those who continued their eczema-inducing work.

In contrast, studies conducted after the 1990s appear to indicate that the total clearance rate is about 70%. 230 patients with occupational skin diseases were surveyed by a telephone interview at least two years after diagnosis. 78% of the workers were working, but 57% of those working had changed jobs, 67% because of their skin problem. Workers who changed their jobs tended to have a better outcome than those who did not (Holness and Nethercott, 1995). Wall and Gebauer (1991) reported that 61% of patients with occupational contact dermatitis lost time from work. 6% of these patients were off work for more than one year. The economic cost can thus be staggering.

In the most recent study on prognosis, a change in work and the presence of easily avoidable work-related allergies were associated with a good prognosis (Mälkönen *et al.*, 2009). Six months after diagnosis the skin disease had healed in 27% of the patients. The occupational skin disorder had cleared in 17% of those with no changes at work, compared to 34% among those who had changed their jobs/occupations. The best clearing occurred in patients with contact urticaria (35%), while the healing of allergic (27%) and irritant (23%) contact dermatitis was similar.

Long-term prognosis

In a 12-year Swedish follow-up study from 1987 to 1999, in a cohort of 2897 patients with occupational skin diseases, 70% had a persistence of skin symptoms (Meding *et al.*, 2005). Skin atopy was the strongest factor for poor prognosis, followed by contact allergy and female gender. 82% of the patients changed their work situation, and 44% changed their jobs. While the majority (62%) experienced no change in income, and 6% had better income, 32% had a reduced income. In the group with reduced income, 45% of persons had a reduction in income of greater than a quarter.

Prevention of Occupational Dermatoses

All occupational dermatoses are theoretically preventable. Standard principles of prevention include substitution or removal of the offending agent, isolation of the worker and enclosure of the work process. A well-ventilated workplace is desirable when volatile solvents and irritant dusts and fibers are used in the work process.

Pre-employment medical examinations and advice to workers and employers on job suitability (e.g. advising atopics to avoid wet work) and regular health education and training of workers (for hazard awareness, proper handling techniques and stressing the importance of good personal hygiene) play important roles in prevention.

The availability of conveniently sited washing and drying facilities in the workplace will encourage workers to utilize these facilities during breaks and after work. Proper skin cleansers should be provided, while abrasive detergents and solvents should be removed. The choice of cleanser will depend on the nature of the chemicals handled. A mild soap is usually adequate for office work. Non-aqueous cleansers may be needed to remove grease and oils. Unfortunately, strong cleansers tend to be corrosive and are more likely to cause irritant contact dermatitis.

The habit of using organic solvents and abrasive detergents as skin cleansers must be discouraged. The most effective prevention against occupational dermatitis is to avoid skin contamination during work. It may be better to have slightly dirty hands than to suffer from chronic dermatitis as a result of vigorous cleansing. Disposable towels should be provided for drying. Emollients or moisturizing creams applied after work may help to restore the barrier function of the skin.

Barrier Creams

The efficacy of barrier creams against occupational dermatitis is questionable. Most studies have found them to provide limited protection. Workers using barrier creams may have a false sense of security. However, the use of barrier creams has the advantage of increasing the worker's awareness of cleaning his skin during breaks and after work. It also facilitates skin cleansing.

Gloves

Personal protective equipment (e.g. gloves, sleeves, aprons and boots), if properly maintained and correctly used, can be a very effective means of preventing occupational dermatoses. One limitation of using gloves is the risk of accidents. The correct type of gloves should be used. The choice of the type of gloves is based on the type of chemical handled and the type of work process. They should cover the distal third of the forearm to be effective. Where dripping of liquid towards the elbow is inevitable, elbow-length gloves should be used. Alternatively, the dripping may be prevented by lowering the workbench or elevating the work platform.

Impervious gloves are occlusive, and may cause skin maceration. Gloves with a cotton lining may act as a wick and absorb sweat, enhancing a high-humidity microclimate adjacent to the skin. Workers should remember to remove gloves periodically and to change them when they become moist or when the inner lining is contaminated. Workers should be provided with several pairs of gloves to change. It should be remembered that workers can occasionally become sensitized to rubber chemicals in rubber gloves, or chromates and resins in leather gloves. Allergic contact dermatitis to gloves and boots is characteristic and should not be overlooked.

The use of clean work clothes is also advisable. Skin contact with clothing contaminated by irritants or allergens may cause dermatitis.

Surveillance

The company safety officers, nurses and physicians must maintain a vigilant surveillance on the occupational health of their workers so that prompt investigation and management of any outbreaks of occupational dermatoses can be undertaken.

Legislation

Different countries have different medico-legal legislation regulating occupational dermatoses. This may include regulatory laws on environmental standards for cutaneous hazards, provision of skin hygiene and washing facilities in the workplace, notification of occupational dermatoses, statutory medical examinations and workmen's compensation. Occupational health physicians and nurses, safety officers, general practitioners and anyone responsible for the healthcare of workers should be familiar with the occupational laws and regulations in their countries.

Percutaneous Absorption of Toxins

The skin is exposed to all environmental elements in the workplace. In addition to being a direct target organ for environmental chemicals, the skin is an important portal of entry for some environmental toxins into the body. The amount and rate of percutaneous absorption of contactants depend on several factors.

Different body sites have different skin permeability to chemicals. There is also individual variation. Besides, permeability depends on the state of the skin barrier. Absorption is enhanced through damaged skin or when substances are placed under occlusion. Another factor which affects the skin absorption rate is the physical and chemical nature of the chemical, for example, whether it is lipid or non-lipid soluble.

Skin notation in environmental standards

The skin notation is sometimes encountered in environmental standards for toxic agents. This notation serves to highlight the skin as an important portal of entry for the toxin. For example, in the American Conference of Governmental Industrial Hygienists (ACGIH) guidelines for threshold limit values (TLVs), this notation is described by the ACGIH to "refer to the potential contribution to the overall exposure by the cutaneous route including mucous membranes and eye — either by airborne, or more particularly, direct contact with the substance". It draws attention to the need for appropriate measures to prevent the cutaneous absorption of substances having a "skin notation" so that the TLV is not invalidated.

Thus for chemicals with skin notations (important examples include solvents and pesticides), respiratory protection alone may be inadequate, even for exposure levels within the prescribed TLVs. It should also be remembered that the skin notation of a chemical only refers to its potential for percutaneous absorption to be an important portal of entry into the systemic circulation, and not to the capacity of the substance to cause skin irritation or sensitization in workers.

Conclusion

The skin is an organ which is commonly affected by work-related disorders. As such, a good working knowledge of the epidemiology, etiology, diagnosis, management and rehabilitation of occupational dermatoses is required for practising occupational health professionals.

Occupational dermatoses are preventable. The principle of prevention, which is a major part of the ethos of occupational health practice, should be applied to safeguard the skin of workers wherever possible.

The study of dermatotoxicology has become increasingly important. For certain common workplace toxins such as solvents, it is known that the skin is an important route of entry into the systemic circulation. It is prudent to take note of "skin notations" when they appear in environmental standards, and to provide for appropriate cutaneous protection when indicated.

Further Reading

Frosch PJ, Menne T, Lepoittevin JP. (eds). (2006) *Contact Dermatitis*, 4th edn. Berlin: Springer-Verlag.

Kanerva L, Elsner P, Wahlberg JE, Maibach HI. (eds). (2004) *Condensed Handbook of Occupational Dermatology*. Berlin: Springer-Verlag.

Ng SK, Goh CL. (2002) *The Principles and Practice of Contact and Occupational Dermatology in the Asia-Pacific Region*. Singapore: World Scientific Publishing Co.

Zhai H, Wilhelm KP, Maibach HI. (2007) *Dermatotoxicology*, 7th edn. Boca Raton, FL: CRC Press, Taylor and Francis Group.

References

Ahmed SM, Aw TC, Adisesh A. (2004) Toxicological and immunological aspects of occupational latex allergy. *Toxicol Rev* **23**(2): 123–134.

Chew AL, Maibach HI. (2003) Occupational issues of irritant contact dermatitis. *Int Arch Occup Environ Health* **76**(5): 339–346.

Coenraads PJ, Foo SC, Phoon WO, Lun KC. (1985) Dermatitis in small scale metal industries. *Contact Dermatitis* **12**: 155–160.

Dai Y, Leng S, Li L, *et al.* (2009) Effects of genetic polymorphisms of N-Acetyltransferase on trichloroethylene-induced hypersensitivity dermatitis among exposed workers. *Ind Health* **47**(5): 479–486.

Diepgen TL. (2003) Occupational skin-disease data in Europe. *Int Arch Occup Environ Health* **76**(5): 331–338.

Fluhr JW, Darlenski R, Angelova-Fischer I, *et al.* (2008) Skin irritation and sensitization: Mechanisms and new approaches for risk assessment. 1. Skin irritation. *Skin Pharmacol Physiol* **21**(3): 124–135.

Fregert S. (1975) Occupational dermatitis in a 10-year material. *Contact Dermatitis* **1**: 96–107.

Gan SL, Goh CL, Lee CS, Hui KH. (1986) Occupational dermatoses among sanders in the furniture industry. *Contact Dermatitis* **17**: 237–240.

Goh CL, Gan SL, Ngui SJ. (1986) Occupational dermatitis in a prefabrication construction industry. *Contact Dermatitis* **15**: 235–240.

Goh CL. (1990) *Occupational Skin Diseases*. Singapore: PG Publishing.

Holness DL, Nethercott JR. (1995) Work outcome in workers with occupational skin disease. *Am J Ind Med* **27**: 807–815.

Kanerva L, Toikkanen J, Jolanki R, Estlander T. (1996) Statistical data on occupational contact urticaria. *Contact Dermatitis* **35**(4): 229–233.

Koh D, Goh CL, Jeyaratnam J, Kee WC, Ong CN. (1990) Dermatological symptoms among Visual Display Unit operators using Plasma Display and Cathode Ray Tube screens. *Ann Acad Med S'pore* **19**: 617–620.

Koh D, Ng V, Leow YH, Goh CL. (2005) A study of natural rubber latex allergens in gloves used by health care workers in Singapore. *Br J Dermatol* **153**: 954–959.

Koh D. (1993) A study of occupational dermatoses in the electronics industry. *J Occup Med S'pore* **5**: 1–76.

Lan CC, Feng WW, Lu YW, *et al.* (2008) Hand eczema among University Hospital nursing staff: Identification of high-risk sector and impact on quality of life. *Contact Dermatitis* **59**(5): 301–306.

Lee KS and Goh CL. (1988) Occupational dermatosis among chrome platers. *Contact Dermatitis* **118**: 89–93.

Mälkönen T, Jolanki R, Alanko K, *et al.* (2009) A 6-month follow-up study of 1048 patients diagnosed with an occupational skin disease. *Contact Dermatitis* **61**(5): 261–268.

Matterne U, Apfelbacher CJ, Soder S, *et al.* (2009) Health-related quality of life in health care workers with work-related skin diseases. *Contact Dermatitis* **61**(3): 145–151.

Meding B, Lantto R, Lindahl G, *et al.* (2005) Occupational skin disease in Sweden — a 12 year follow up. *Contact Dermatitis* **53**: 308–313.

Nienhaus A, Kromark K, Raulf-Heimsoth M, *et al.* (2008) Outcome of occupational latex allergy — work ability and quality of life. *PLoS One* **3**(10): e3459.

Pal TM, de Wilde NS, van Beurden MM, *et al.* (2009) Notification of occupational skin diseases by dermatologists in The Netherlands. *Occup Med* (*Lond*) **59**(1): 38–43.

Rabin B, Fraidlin N. (2007) Patients with occupational contact dermatitis in Israel: Quality of life and social implications. *Soc Work Health Care* **45**(2): 97–111.

Radespiel-Tröger M, Meyer M, Pfahlberg A, *et al.* (2009) Outdoor work and skin cancer incidence: A registry-based study in Bavaria. *Int Arch Occup Environ Health* **82**(3): 357–363.

Tang MBY, Leow YH, Ngm V, *et al.* (2005) Latex sensitization in health-care workers in Singapore. *Ann Acad Med Singapore* **34**: 376–382.

Turner S, Carder M, van Tongeren M, *et al.* (2007) The incidence of occupational skin disease as reported to The Health and Occupation Reporting (THOR) network between 2002 and 2005. *Br J Dermatol* **157**(4): 713–722.

Wall LM, Gebauer KA. (1991) A follow up study of occupational skin disease in Western Australia. *Contact Dermatitis* **24**: 241–243.

Wang BJ, Shiao JS, Chen CJ, *et al.* (2007) Tumour necrotizing factor-alpha promoter and GST-T1 genotype predict skin allergy to chromate in cement workers in Taiwan. *Contact Dermatitis* **57**(5): 309–315.

Watkins SA, Maibach HI. (2009) The hardening phenomenon in irritant contact dermatitis: An interpretative update. *Contact Dermatitis* **60**(3): 123–130.

Chapter 6

Hematological Disorders

Wee-Tong Ng[*,‡] *and Kee-Seng Chia*[†]

Physiology of the Hematological System

All blood cells are derived from a multipotent hemopoietic stem cell. These cells may self-replicate or differentiate to form committed progenitor cells of the various blood cells lines: erythrocytes, monocytes, neutrophils, eosinophils, basophils, lymphocytes and platelets.

Erythropoiesis is controlled both by growth factors within the marrow as well as the hormone erythropoietin. Progenitor cells committed to erythropoiesis divide and differentiate in the presence of growth factors like interleukin 3 (IL-3). Erythropoietin is produced by the peritubular cells of the kidneys in response to hypoxia. It further modulates the maturation of the erythroblasts into erythrocytes. Erythrocytes have a life span of 120 days and the senescent cells are removed by the phagocytic action of reticuloendothelial cells in the spleen and liver. In males, the normal red cell count is between 4.5 to $6.5 \times 10^{12}/1$ with a hemoglobin (Hb) of 13.5 to 18.0 g/dl. In females, the red cell count is between 4.0 to $5.5 \times 10^{12}/1$ and a hemoglobin of 11.5 to 16.5 g/dl.

*Department of Geriatric Medicine, Singapore Aeromedical Centre.
†Department of Epidemiology and Public Health, Yong Loo Lin School of Medicine, National University of Singapore.
‡Corresponding author. E-mail: wtng@pacific.net.sg

White cells are formed in the bone marrow and its regulation is less well-understood compared to erythrocytes. Granulocytes can be rapidly mobilized from the bone marrow in response to inflammatory stimulus. Various growth factors in the bone marrow (including GM-CSF) promote marrow turnover and its release.

Lymphocytes, on the other hand, mature mainly in the lymphoid tissues, some in the thymus (T-cells) and others (B-cells) in other lymphoid tissues (probably in the Peyer's patches). The prime function of the B-cells is to divide in response to contact with antigens to produce plasma cells which in turn produce antibodies. The T-cells assist the B-cells in the primary immune response and are also responsible for cell-mediated immunity.

There is little difference in normal white cell values between males and females. The total number of white cells is 4 to 11×10^9/l. This is made up of 2.0 to 7.5×10^9/l neutrophils (40–75%), 1.5 to 4.0×10^9/l lymphocytes (20–50%), 0.2 to 0.8×10^9/l monocytes (2–10%), 0.04 to 0.4×10^9/l eosinophils (1–6%) and 0.01 to 0.1×10^9/l basophils (<1%).

Anemia Due to Inorganic Lead

Mechanism of Anemia Due to Inorganic Lead

Lead-induced anemia can be attributed to the combined effects of

1. inhibition of heme synthesis;
2. promotion of heme breakdown;
3. decreased lifespan of erythrocytes; and
4. interference with globin chain synthesis.

Of these, the inhibition of heme synthesis is probably the most important mechanism in causing anemia. Lead inhibits the activities of δ-aminolevulinic dehydratase (δ-ALAD), ferrochelatase and coproporphyrinogen decarboxylase (Chisolm, 1971; Hernberg, 1980). This inhibition and the resultant negative feedback leads to increased δ-aminolevulinic acid (δ-ALA) and coproporphyrin III in the urine and accumulation of protoporphyrins in the erythrocytes (Fig. 1).

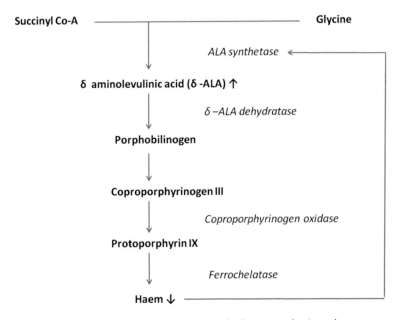

Fig. 1. Effect of inorganic lead on the heme synthesis pathway.

The breakdown of heme is catalyzed by the enzyme heme oxygenase. The synthesis of this enzyme is regulated by a repressor protein. Lead binds to the -SH group of this protein, leading to an increase in heme oxygenase.

Lead also causes structural and functional changes in the erythrocytic membranes, which lead to increased osmotic and mechanical fragility and a shortened erythrocyte lifespan. The mechanism of action is complex and probably involves P5′N (pyrimidine 5′-nucleotidase), inhibition of the Na^+ and K^+ pump as well as reduction in cytochrome oxidative phosphorylation (Sakai, Araki and Ushio, 1990). There is also some evidence that a decrease in the activity of the P5′N pathway has an effect on Hb levels in workers without manifest hemolytic anemia (Kim *et al.*, 2002).

Lead also inhibits the production of the α- and β-globin chains, although the effect on the α-chain is greater. This may also be a factor in the pathogenesis of lead-induced anemia (White and Harvey, 1972).

Lead is also known to induce constipation. This is often associated with bleeding piles which aggravates the anemia induced by lead on the hematological system. Diarrhea has also been described as one of the gastrointestinal effects of inorganic lead. This is probably via the stimulation of intestinal smooth muscle by inorganic lead. However, in clinical practice and where blood lead levels are below 1000 $\mu g/l$, constipation is the more common symptom encountered.

Sources of Exposure to Inorganic Lead

Lead is the most commonly used non-ferrous metal. Its ductility, high resistance to corrosion and other properties make it one of the most useful metals. An exact estimation of the amount consumed globally is difficult because of the lack of reliable statistics and reporting systems. It is estimated that the present world production is about 8.9 million metric tons and about 3 million tons are recycled annually. In 1985, production in the United States was about 488,000 metric tons, and the amount recovered from scrap was 594,000 metric tons (US Department of the Interior, 1991). The largest single use of lead is in the manufacture of lead-acid storage batteries. About 80% of the lead used in batteries is re-smelted as scrap. The next largest use of lead is in the form of organic lead (tetraethyl and tetramethyl lead) as an anti-knock additive in petroleum. With the introduction of unleaded petrol and the environmental concern of inorganic lead pollution from vehicle exhaust, this use has decreased in recent years. Lead is also widely used in the construction and shipbuilding industries for cathodic protection of the superstructures of ships and bridges. It is also widely used as a component in lead alloys, paint pigments as well as in the production of polyvinyl chloride (PVC) stabilizers.

It is unlikely that general environmental exposure to inorganic lead from the use of leaded petrol will give rise to significant anemia. However, in communities where significant industrial pollution exists, anemia can be a common feature of excessive lead exposure. Furthermore, in many developing countries where secondary lead smelting in small-scale enterprises are common, there can be excessive lead exposure. Family members including children are often at risk since they either participate in the smelting or live in close proximity as these are usually household enterprises.

Diagnosis and Management of Inorganic Lead Poisoning

Pre-employment and periodic medical examinations

In many countries, workers exposed to inorganic lead are required to have pre-employment and periodic medical examinations. At pre-employment examinations, workers with underlying anemia will require further investigations. Nutritional anemias and anemia due to blood loss can be treated. Once treated, these workers can proceed to work in lead environments. However, workers with congenital anemias like thalassemia should not work in lead environments.

During pre-employment examinations, the hemoglobin and blood lead (PbB) measurements should be monitored. PbB is an indicator of recent exposure to lead. Among non-exposed subjects in communities without industrial lead pollution and using unleaded petrol, the PbB should be less than 100 μg/l. Among moderately exposed workers, the level is between 100 and 250 μg/l. Exposed workers tend to have levels above 250 μg/l. The World Health Organization recommends a health-based exposure limit of 400 μg/l (WHO, 1980) but several countries have adopted other limits: 300 μg/l by the American Conference of Governmental Industrial Hygienists (ACGIH, 2009) and 700 μg/l by the European Communities (EC Council Directive, 1982).

Where possible, the erythrocyte activity of δ-ALAD should be measured. There is a good negative correlation between the erythrocyte activity of δ-ALAD and PbB (Alessio and Foa, 1983). Even at PbB levels of below 400 μg/l, the enzyme activity is depressed. There is suggestive evidence that the no-effect level is around 100 μg/l. It has also been shown that the *in vitro* measurement of δ-ALAD in the erythrocyte is a good indicator of δ-ALAD inhibition *in vitro*.

Among workers with a past history of high exposure to lead, the erythrocyte activity of δ-ALAD continues to be inhibited out of proportion to the current PbB even after removal from exposure. This is partly due to the high affinity of inorganic lead to the bones. In a steady state, about 90% of the total body burden of lead is present in the bones and teeth. Even with cessation of exposure, bone lead decreases very gradually (Nilsson *et al.*, 1991). Bone lead is therefore an important source of "endogenous exposure" because of its slow turnover and the large storage capacity of the bones.

However, the routine measurement of erythrocyte activity of δ-ALAD is limited by technical problems. The blood sample has to be stored at below 4°C and preferably be measured within 24 hours. For this reason, the measurement of delta-aminolevulinic acid in the urine (ALA-U) is a useful alternative. Due to the inhibition of δ-ALAD of the maturing erythrocytes by lead, the transformation of ALA into porphobilinogen is obstructed. Furthermore, the lowered heme level stimulates the action of ALA synthetase, resulting in an increase in ALA in the serum and urine (Fig. 1). However, the correlation between ALA-U and PbB is weaker than that of erythrocyte activity of δ-ALAD.

As a practical guideline, male workers with a hemoglobin of less than 11 g/dl or a PbB of more than 500 μg/l should be removed from further lead exposure until there is significant improvement in the biological parameters as well as work practice and environmental control. If the PbB is less than 500 μg/l but the Hb is between 11 and 13 g/dl, the worker should also be suspended and the anemia investigated. Females with a Hb of less than 10 g/dl and a PbB of 400 μg/l should be suspended. Similarly, if their Hb is between 10 and 12 g/dl, they should be suspended. Pregnant and lactating females should not be exposed to lead work.

One of the major roles of periodic medical examinations is to control the environmental exposure. Where group data shows an increasing trend in average PbB levels, environmental control measures need to be evaluated and further enforced. There is often a breakdown of exhaust ventilation and poor housekeeping, resulting in a higher environmental concentration in the workplace. Poor work practices among workers and improper use of personal protective equipment are further contributing factors to the increase in PbB levels.

Health education

During medical examinations, the personal health education of the workers is crucial in preventing lead-induced anemia. The workers should be educated on the following:

1. health effects of lead exposure;
2. the long half-life (20–30 years) of lead and the ineffectiveness and dangers of chelating agents;
3. proper use and maintenance of respirators;
4. importance of good personal hygiene to reduce oral ingestion of lead;
5. avoiding eating with hands and smoking at the workplace;
6. importance of a proper diet to control constipation and avoid bleeding piles; and
7. separate washing of workplace clothing to avoid exposing family members, especially children.

Case Study 1

A young Malay worker complained of lethargy and was found to be clinically pale. There were no other significant clinical findings. He had been working as a production operator in a factory that manufactured polyvinyl chloride (PVC) stabilizers for the past three years. This was his first job. There are several types of PVC stabilizers, the most common being inorganic lead stabilizers. The work process begins with the smelting of lead ingots and oxidation of the lead into lead oxide (litharge). The litharge is then combined with sulphuric acid into lead sulphate or with stearic acid into lead stearate. These salts are then packed or mixed before packing. Workers are exposed to lead fumes in the smelting process and lead dust in the packing and mixing area.

Investigations revealed he had a hemoglobin level of 10 g/dl. He was also found to have occult bleeding in the stool examination. Further examination revealed bleeding internal piles. It was assumed that the anemia was a result of the bleeding piles. However, after treatment of the piles, the patient continued to be anemic and was subsequently referred to an occupational health physician. After confirming the occupational history of inorganic lead exposure, laboratory investigation revealed a blood lead level of 400 μg/l. The urinary level of aminolevulinic acid (ALA-U) was also high.

He was diagnosed to have anemia due to lead overexposure and bleeding piles. The bleeding piles were also aggravated by constipation due to inorganic lead exposure. He was removed from further exposure to inorganic lead and given oral iron, folate and vitamin B. Three months later, the blood lead was down to 200 μg/l. The ALA-U was normal and the hemoglobin rose to 13.7 g/dl.

There is a traditional belief that milk is an effective antidote for lead toxicity because of the high calcium content. Calcium is effective in decreasing the gastrointestinal absorption of lead, probably because of the competition for the same intestinal binding sites. However, when the blood calcium is high, it can compete with free lead in the blood for skeletal binding sites as well as displacing the lead that is bound to the bones. The net result is an increase in the free blood lead level.

Suspension from exposure

As lead is a cumulative poison, suspension from exposure is not an effective means of preventing the health effects. It has to be borne in mind that after a period of suspension, the lowered PbB does not indicate that the body burden of lead is now lower. Returning the worker to exposure will in fact result in a further increase in the body burden, even if the PbB is below the exposure limit. Therefore, suspension merely decreases the rate of increase in the body lead burden.

With X-ray fluorescence techniques, it is now possible to measure the level of bone lead (Ahlgren *et al.*, 1980). This can be taken as a measure of the body burden of lead. Unfortunately, it is still not possible to use the bone lead as a predictor of long-term adverse health effects. Hence, retired workers should continue to be monitored periodically for early adverse health effects (especially on the neurological and renal systems).

Use of chelators

Chelating agents are organic compounds capable of binding to metal ions to form a ring structure, or a chelate. The common chelators used for lead poisoning include calcium disodium ethylenediaminetetraacetic acid ($CaNa_2$ EDTA), d-penicillamine (Cuprimine) and 2,3-dimercaptosuccinic acid (DMSA). Dimercaprol (British anti-Lewisite or BAL) has also been recommended.

$CaNa_2$ EDTA is not metabolized by the body, and following an intravenous injection, 50% of it is excreted in an hour and 90% in seven hours. Oral EDTA has also been shown to decrease the gastrointestinal absorption of lead. Its role in acute lead poisoning is controversial especially in those with lead encephalopathy. Among patients with EDTA therapy, the encephalopathy symptoms increased due to the liberation of bone lead into the blood.

Penicillamine is effective for chelating copper in Wilson's disease. However, its effectiveness for other metals is not well-established. It has the advantage of oral administration but it interferes with vitamin B6 metabolism and has the same side effects as penicillin. DMSA is very promising and is effective when given orally. Its side effect profile is much better than the other chelators and its efficiency in chelating heavy metals is very much higher. In a recent animal study, DMSA improved the glomerular filtration rate in lead-poisoned rats but not the tubulointerstitial scarring seen. It is therefore postulated that DMSA may also induce hemodynamic changes (Khalil-Manesh *et al.*, 1992).

Chelators should be used only in severe lead poisoning with clinical signs and symptoms. "Prophylactic chelation", that is, the use of chelating agents or related drugs to prevent elevated blood lead or the use of drugs to routinely lower blood lead to predetermined concentrations, is strongly discouraged. It is, in fact, prohibited by the US Occupational Safety and Health Administration (OSHA). Chelation is recommended only when the blood lead level exceeds 800 μg/l with severe clinical manifestations of lead poisoning. In children, there is little justification to use chelators when the blood lead is below 400 μg/l. The main reason for the cautious use of chelators

154 Textbook of Occupational Medicine Practice, 3rd Edition

is their high nephrotoxicity and the depletion of other essential metals like zinc and iron.

Chelators are also used to aid in the diagnosis of lead poisoning. Following a standard dose of a chelator, all the urine excreted over a time period (usually 24 hours) is collected and the lead content estimated. This "mobilizable" lead content is also a good indicator of the body burden of lead.

Toxic Hemolysis

Oxidant Hemolysis

Work-related methemoglobinemia and oxidative hemolysis are caused by several aromatic nitro and amino compounds (Halsted, 1960). Examples include aniline, nitroaniline, toluidine, naphthalene and trinitrotoluene (Kearney, Manoguerra and Dunford, 1984). These are common in the manufacture of aniline dyestuffs, pesticides, antioxidants in rubber production and explosives. Urea herbicides are also metabolized to aniline-derived products (Watt *et al.*, 2005).

In order for the hemoglobin molecule to carry oxygen effectively, the iron molecule must be in the reduced state (ferrohemoglobin). When the oxygen is released, the iron molecule is oxidized into the ferric state (ferric hemoglobin or methemoglobin). The normal individual has less than 1% of methemoglobin because of the effective reduction of methemoglobin into ferrohemoglobin via NADH cytochrome b_5 reductase.

Methemoglobin also increases the oxygen affinity to the remaining heme groups of the hemoglobin tetramer, resulting in decreasing oxygen delivery to the tissues. Furthermore, the hemoglobin can be denatured and precipitated as Heinz bodies. The presence of Heinz bodies alters the membrane stability of the red blood cells, resulting in hemolysis.

Apart from exposure to exogenous oxidative chemicals, inborn structural abnormalities of the hemoglobin as well as a decrease in the reduction capabilities due to metabolic abnormalities like glucose-6-phosphate dehydrogenase (G6PD) deficiency cause workers to be more susceptible to oxidative damage. During an acute hemolytic episode, older erythrocytes tend to be destroyed and are replaced by young red cells and reticulocytes. These reticulocytes will have normal G6PD levels and any screening for G6PD activity immeaditely after an acute hemolytic episode is useless. Workers should therefore be screened for G6PD deficiency at the pre-employment examination if its prevalence is high in the community.

Acute exposure to agents causing methemoglobinemia and hemolytic anemia is usually associated with spills and improper usage. With mild exposure, the worker presents with asymptomatic peripheral cyanosis (i.e. blueness of the nail beds). With more severe exposure, central cyanosis may be present and the patient may complain of breathlessness, headache and fatigue. Freshly drawn blood appears to be dark maroon-brown and does not become red with exposure to air. When the methemoglobin level is more than 50%, the patient may be disorientated or comatose. Laboratory investigations will reveal hypoxia and subsequently anemia and hemolysis.

The effects of naphthalene exposure can also cross the placenta, resulting in the newborn infant having symptoms identical to the mother's (Molloy *et al.*, 2004). Therefore, extra care must be taken to prevent pregnant women from exposure to oxidative chemicals.

The treatment of acute exposure includes rapid recognition and removal of the offending agent. If the methemoglobin level is more than 30%, 100% oxygen should be given by mask. Methylene blue should be administered with care. Methylene blue acts as a co-factor with NADPH to reduce the methemoglobin to ferrohemoglobin. NADPH is derived from the hexose monophosphate shunt and requires G6PD. Methylene blue in itself has oxidative potential and may precipitate a hemolytic crisis in patients with G6PD deficiency. Hence, methylene blue should only be administered in patients without G6PD deficiency.

Methylene blue is given intravenously as a 1% solution (dose: 1–2 mg/kg) over 10 minutes. The effect should be seen within an hour. If the patient responds, the dose could be repeated at hourly intervals. If the patient does not respond, methylene blue administration should be stopped, as the patient may be G6PD deficient. Supportive therapy should be used instead. These patients should be screened for G6PD deficiency 1–2 months after the poisoning episode because during a hemolytic episode, older red blood cells are destroyed and replaced by immature cells. Among patients with G6PD deficiency, the level of the enzyme is normal in such cells.

Ascorbic acid has been recommended as it is also able to reduce methemoglobin into ferrohemoglobin. However, the rate of reduction is very slow and is of doubtful value. Furthermore, it may potentiate renal toxicity.

Workers exposed to oxidative agents should be screened for G6PD deficiency. Biological monitoring would include end-of-shift measurements of methemoglobin levels (to be kept below 5%), reticulocyte count and appropriate metabolites (e.g. urinary *p*-aminophenol for aniline; *p*-nitrophenol and *p*-aminophenol for nitrobenzene).

Hemolysis from Heavy Metals

Arsenic and arsine

Arsenic is often present as a contaminant in metal ores or products. In the presence of hydrogen ions, it reacts to form a volatile, colorless and non-irritating gas, arsine (AsH_3). The gas is much heavier than air and has a garlicky smell. It is easily inhaled and absorbed, as it does not irritate the respiratory tract. Exposure situations include the smelting of metals like zinc and the cleaning of acid storage tanks. Antimony is also present with arsenic and, under the same conditions, stibine is also produced. The toxicity of stibine is similar to that of arsine. Arsine gas is also used extensively today in the growth and preparation of crystals and conducting devices in the semiconductor industry.

The mechanism responsible for arsine-induced hemolysis is not well-understood. However, it is recognized that the presence of oxyhemoglobin is a necessary component of the overall mechanism as the conversion of oxyhemoglobin to carboxyhemoglobin prevents the hemolysis of erythrocytes (Rael, Ayala-Fierro and Carter, 2000).

About 20% of all acute arsine poisoning is fatal. Exposure to 250 ppm is instantly fatal. At levels of 25–50 ppm, exposure for more than 30 minutes is also fatal. At lower concentrations, hemolysis develops after a latent period of a length inversely proportional to the extent of exposure. Patients are often alarmed by the painless hemoglobinuria and seek medical attention for it. Associated signs and symptoms include nausea and vomiting, abdominal cramps, headache, malaise, tachycardia, tachypnea and hypotension. Subsequently, acute renal failure may follow.

Case Study 2

Two workers were clearing up a clogged floor drain in a chemical manufacturing plant (Parish, Glass and Kimbrough, 1979). The workers used a drain cleaner containing sodium hydroxide, sodium nitrate and aluminium chips. Unknown to the workers, the plant used to be involved in the manufacture of arsenical herbicides more than five years ago. The nascent hydrogen produced from the drain cleaner reacted with the arsenic residues in the clogged drain. The workers spent 2–3 hours clearing the drain and noticed the drain bubbling when the cleaner was used. The next morning, both workers were admitted for acute hemolytic anemia.

Anemia is not present initially. The plasma-free hemoglobin is high and the blood appears brownish-red from the presence of methemalbumin (oxidized hemoglobin bound to albumin). The peripheral blood film will show schistocytosis (red cell fragmentation), poikilocytosis, basophilic stippling and polychromasia. When the hematocrit starts to fall, reticulocytosis increases. The level of unconjugated bilirubin is also raised. Renal function is affected by the obstruction by renal tubular hemoglobin casts as well as the direct toxicity of arsine on the renal tubular and interstitial cells. Levels of arsenic in the blood and urine are useful indicators of exposure rather than guidelines for therapy.

Initial therapy includes the management of shock and adequate renal perfusion. Exchange transfusion is required if the free hemoglobin level exceeds 500 μg/dl. Repeated exchange transfusion may be necessary. If renal failure develops, hemodialysis may be necessary. All patients must be monitored closely for further hemolysis and deterioration of renal function. The use of chelators is of doubtful value, and may even potentiate the renal dysfunction. Survivors of acute arsine poisoning should be followed up yearly for residual renal impairment.

Lead-induced hemolysis

The main effect of inorganic lead is the inhibition of heme synthesis. However, in very high exposure situations, as in the use of a blow-torch on leaded materials, severe acute intravascular hemolysis may occur. It is believed that the inhibition of pyrimidine-5′ nucleotidase by lead is similar to the hereditary deficiency of the enzyme. In the hereditary condition, there is accumulation of pyrimidine containing nucleotides within the red blood cells. These nucleotides are believed to compete with adenine nucleotides in binding to active sites of kinases in the glycolytic pathways and affect the membrane stability of the red blood cells.

Aplastic Anemia due to Occupational Exposure

Bone marrow damage is uncommon in industry and only a small percentage of aplastic anemias are due to environmental and occupational causes. The most common occupational causes are benzene and irradiation.

Benzene

In the early years, benzene exposure was high and was the most common cause of toxic aplastic anemia. There were even cases of fatal aplastic anemia from exposures exceeding 100 ppm.

At lower levels of exposure, the changes depend on which cell line(s) suffer the brunt of the injury. There is however great variation in susceptibility and the evidence of toxicity may appear weeks or years later. There have been reports of cases developing several years after exposure has ceased.

Anemia is often the first effect to be noted, followed by leukopenia, thrombocytopenia and finally pancytopenia. The bone marrow may show evidence of acellularity, with replacement of fatty tissue to islands of hypercellularity, without evidence of new cells in the peripheral blood.

Aplastic anemia due to acute benzene exposure has a better prognosis than idiopathic aplastic anemia. When the patients are removed from exposure, as many as 40% of them may recover completely. However, if hypocellularity persists for more than 4 to 6 months, recovery is not likely. Those who develop aplastic anemia after exposure has ceased are also unlikely to recover and it may form part of a preleukemic syndrome. Bone marrow transplantation and immunosuppressive therapy are the current mainstays of treatment. The successful use of *ex vivo* activated mononuclear cells (immunotherapy) in the treatment of benzene-induced aplastic anemia has also been reported (Chen *et al.*, 2003).

Petrochemical industries and petroleum refineries are the main sources of benzene exposure. Benzene is also used in the manufacture of plastics, synthetic fibers and synthetic rubber. In laboratories, benzene is often used for the extraction of organic substances. Though the concentration of benzene in industrial solvents (like toluene and xylene) is low, exposure to benzene may be high because of the large volume of industrial solvents used and if the work is carried out in confined spaces.

Biological monitoring of benzene-exposed workers include the hemoglobin level, full blood count and peripheral blood film. The end-of-shift urinary phenol level is useful for estimating the benzene exposure if the environmental concentration is above 5 ppm. For exposures below 5 ppm, urinary trans, trans-muconic acid (ttma) and urinary S-phenylmercapturic acid (SPMA) are better biomarkers. Pregnant and nursing mothers as well as young persons (below 18 years) should not be occupationally exposed to benzene. Ex-workers should be followed up periodically for delayed onset of toxicity.

Ionizing Radiation

Hemopoietic cells are highly radiosensitive. An acute, high-dose, total-body exposure (200–300 rem) will cause a high percentage of these cells to be killed so that normal replacement of aging leukocytes, platelets and erythrocytes will be significantly impaired. Platelets and leukocyte levels will be maximally depressed in 3 to 5 weeks. Aplasia of lymphoid tissues is also common with the depression of the immune response. At doses above 500 rem, death from fatal hemorrhage and infection may occur. The most important long-term effect is leukemia.

Exposure situations can be either from acute, high-dose exposure in nuclear accidents or long-term, low-level exposure as in the practice of radiology. Radiology is also used in various industrial settings, in particular to evaluate the quality of welded joints.

Work-related Hematological Malignancies

Leukemia

Ionizing radiation, benzene, ethylene oxide and antineoplastic drugs have been shown definitively to cause leukemia. Other causal associations not conclusively established include employment in agricultural work, exposure to formaldehyde and exposure to low-frequency electromagnetic radiation. A further description of occupational leukemia can be found in the chapter on occupational cancers.

Multiple Myeloma

Multiple myeloma is a clonal differentiated B-cell neoplasm. Its incidence appears to be on the rise and this has aroused a concern that it may be associated with environmental or occupational factors. Many epidemiological studies have shown an association with agriculture work, benzene exposure, high-dose radiation, pesticides and petroleum products. These are however inconclusive.

References

Ahlgren L, Haeger-Aronson B, Mattsson S, Schutz A. (1980) *In vivo* determination of lead in the skeleton following occupational exposure. *Br J Ind Med* 37: 109–113.

Alessio L, Foa V. (1983) Lead. In: Alessio L, Berlin A, Roi R, Boni M (eds). *Human Biological Monitoring of Industrial Chemicals Series*, pp. 105–132. Luxembourg: Commission of the European Communities, Luxembourg.

American Congress of Governmental Industrial Hygienists. (2009) Threshold limit values for chemical substances and physical agents and biological exposure indices. Cincinnati: ACGIH.

Chen J, Liu W, Wang X, *et al.* (2003) *Ex vivo* immunotherapy for patients with benzene-induced aplastic anemia. *J Hematother Stem Cell Res* **12**(5): 505–514.

Chisolm JJ Jr. (1971) Lead poisoning. *Sc American* **224**: 15–23.

EC Council Directive of 28 July 1982 (82/605/EEC) on the protection of workers from the risks related to exposure to metallic lead and its ionic compounds at work. *Official Journal of the European Community* **25**: 12–21.

Halsted HC. (1960) Industrial methaemoglobinaemia. *J Occup Med* **2**: 591.

Hernberg S. (1980) Biochemical and clinical effects and responses as indicated by blood lead concentration. In: Singhal RL, Thomas JA (eds). *Lead Toxicity*, pp. 367–399. Baltimore: Urban and Schwarzenberg.

Kearney TE, Manoguerra AS, Dunford JV Jr. (1984) Chemically induced methaemoglobinaemia from aniline poisoning. *West J Med* **140**: 282.

Khalil-Manesh F, Gonick CH, Cohen A, *et al.* (1992) Experimental model of lead nephropathy: II. Effect of removal from lead exposure and chelation treatment with dimercaptosuccinic acid (DMSA). *Env Res* **58**: 35–54.

Kim Y, Yoo CI, Lee CR, *et al.* (2002) Evaluation of activity of erythrocyte pyrimidine 5′-nucleotidase (P5N) in lead exposed workers: With focus on the effect on hemoglobin. *Ind Health* **40**(1): 23–27.

Molloy EJ, Doctor BA, Reed MD, Walsh MC. (2004) Perinatal toxicity of domestic naphthalene exposure. *J Perinatol* **24**(12): 792–793.

Nilsson U, Attewell R, Christoffersson JO, *et al.* (1991) Kinetics of lead in bone and blood after end of occupational exposure. *Pharm Toxicol* **69**: 477–484.

Parish GG, Glass R, Kimbrough R. (1979) Acute arsine poisoning in two workers cleaning a clogged drain. *Arch Env Health* **34**: 224–227.

Rael LT, Ayala-Fierro F, Carter DE. (2000) The effects of sulfur, thiol, and thiol inhibitor compounds on arsine-induced toxicity in the human erythrocyte membrane. *Toxicol Sci* **55**: 468–477.

Sakai T, Araki T, Ushio K. (1990) Accumulation of erythrocyte nucleotides and their pattern in lead workers. *Arch Env Health* **45**: 273–277.

US Department of the Interior. (1991) *Minerals Yearbook for 1990*, Vol. 1. Washington DC: Government Printing Office.

Watt BE, Proudfoot AT, Bradberry SM, Vale JA. (2005) Poisoning due to urea herbicides. *Toxicol Rev* **24**(3): 161–166.

WHO. (1980) Recommended health-based limits in occupational exposure to heavy metals. WHO Technical Report Series 647, WHO, Geneva.

White JM, Harvey DR. (1972) Defective synthesis of α and β globin chains in lead poisoning. *Nature* **236**: 71–73.

Chapter 7

Neurological Disorders

Roberto Lucchini* and Sin-Eng Chia[†,‡]

Introduction

About 40% of chemicals in the workplace are known to affect the nervous system and about 30% of occupational standards are based on behavioral or neurological endpoints (Lucchini *et al.*, 2005). Much of our knowledge of the effects of neurotoxicants on workers' health comes from epidemiological studies. These studies are important because they provide evidence of the effects of long-term exposure to many neurotoxicants.

Metals have been poisoning man almost since the day he first learned to use them. The neurotoxic effects of lead, mercury, arsenic and manganese were known since the 19th century (Raffle *et al.*, 1987). The first description of "manganism", the clinical manifestation deriving from manganese intoxication, was published by Couper (1837) only 20 years after the first description of the "shaking palsy" by Sir James Parkinson (Parkinson, 2002).

Roberto Lucchini* and Sin-Eng Chia[†,‡]

*Department of Experimental and Applied Medicine, Section of Occupational Health and Industrial Hygiene, University of Brescia, Brescia, Italy.
†Department of Epidemiology and Public Health, Yong Loo Lin School of Medicine, National University of Singapore.
‡Corresponding author. E-mail: ephcse@nus.edu.sg

163

But it was only in the late 20th century that experimental, clinical and epidemiological experiences have confirmed that exposure to organic solvents can result in neurobehavioral effects besides its known effect of peripheral neuropathy (Hänninen, 1985; Johnson, 1987).

Etiologic Agents

Metals

Arsenic

Peripheral neuropathy is not a common feature of acute arsenic poisoning. In chronic arsenic exposure, the typical neurological manifestation is a combined sensory and motor polyneuropathy (Heyman *et al.*, 1956; Feldman *et al.*, 1979). Paresthesias and painful hyperesthesias may be the initial presenting symptoms. Sensory deficits are prominent. Motor defects appear initially in the distal parts of the lower limbs with wasting of the extensor muscles of the feet and toes. Involvement of the upper limbs is less common. Effects on the central nervous system are rare. Exposure to arsenic is associated with mucosal irritation, desquamating rash, myalgias, peripheral neuropathy, and white transverse (Mees) lines on the fingernails (Ropper and Samuels, 2009). Chronic occupational exposure at levels above the air concentration of 10 $\mu g/m^3$ can cause increased neurological symptoms and dose-related abnormalities of visual evoked potential, electroneurography and electroencephalography (Halatek *et al.*, 2009).

Lead

Lead can damage both the central and peripheral nervous systems, e.g. acute encephalopathy and radial palsy. Acute encephalopathy, characterized by delusion, delirium and hallucination, is rare. When present, it is associated with very high exposure, usually to organic lead (e.g. alkyl lead compounds). Radial palsy, or "wrist drop" as it is commonly known, is now an uncommon complication of lead poisoning.

Neurobehavioral changes, consistent with mild toxic encephalopathy, have been reported in lead workers. These consist of sleep difficulties, headaches, fatigue, difficulty in learning new material and adjusting to new situations. Neurobehavioral testing will show elevated mood disorders, deficits in memory and impairment of visuomotor performance. Chia *et al.* (1997) reported that cumulative exposure to lead affects performance on neurobehavioral tests in adults, especially perceptual and motor skills. Cumulative lead exposure may also cause long-term cognitive effects that can be visualized by MRI in smaller amounts in specific brain regions (Schwartz *et al.*, 2007). The calculation of the benchmark dose in studies on occupational lead exposure has showed that neurotoxic effects are initiated at blood lead levels of around 18 μg/dl (Murata *et al.*, 2009).

Severe neurological defects have been reported for blood lead (BPb) concentrations of 100 to 200 μg/dl (Hernberg, 1976). Radial palsy can develop if BPb levels exceed 120 μg/dl. There is no evidence in adults of peripheral neuropathy below BPb levels of 40 μg/dl (Jeyaratnam *et al.*, 1985; Chia *et al.*, 1996).

Manganese

Manganese is especially known for its acute behavioral manifestations ("manganese madness"). Manganese miners were reported to develop irritability, nervousness and emotional liability. Some experienced visual and auditory hallucinations, and compulsive, repetitive and uncontrolled actions.

Chronic manganese exposure may lead to poisoning of the central nervous system, called "manganism". Exposure of at least 2–3 years to airborne manganese of concentrations above 1 mg/m^3 (WHO, 1981) is believed to be sufficient for the development of neurologic abnormalities; but there is marked individual susceptibility (Emara *et al.*, 1971).

Manganism involves a degenerative change of the basal ganglia, producing an extrapyramidal symptomatology of the Parkinsonian type. At the early stages, it presents with asthenia, somnolence, muscular tenderness and behavioral changes (irritability and apathy). Later, it involves disorders of gait, dysarthria, mask-like facies, tremor and adiadochokinesis (Chandra, Seth and Mankeshwar, 1974). After chronic exposure to air levels below 200 μg/m^3, early signs of motor function impairment can be revealed by neurobehavioral (Lucchini *et al.*, 1999) and brain MRI testing (Chang *et al.*, 2009). Prolonged exposure to lower levels may be responsible for increased Parkinsonism, as shown in manganese-exposed welders (Racette, 2001; 2005). This may be due to a different toxicity of manganese in the basal ganglia, that could be limited to the globus pallidus at high-exposure doses, but may extend to the substantia nigra pars compacta with low-level, long-term exposure (Lucchini *et al.*, 2009).

Case Study 1

A 50-year-old woman who had been occupationally exposed to manganese for 21 years (1963–1984). The patient had suffered from palpitations and had tremor since 1968 and had been misdiagnosed as having hyperthyroidism. In 1980, she showed symptoms such as headache, giddiness, palpitation, salivation, failing memory, lower limb myalgia, myasthenia, and tetany and numbness in arms and legs. Physical examination at that time showed her hands, tongue and eyelids to be tremulous, rigidity or hypertonicity of muscles, and a positive finger-nose test. The patient was subsequently (in 1982) diagnosed to have chronic mild manganese poisoning by an occupational diseases diagnosis group (Ky et al., 1992).

Mercury

Tremor is the characteristic sign of inorganic mercury poisoning. A fine tremor involving the eyelids, lips, tongue and fingers may progress to a very coarse tremor. Handwriting may become irregular, shaky and illegible. Mixed peripheral neuropathy can occur, though it is not common (Vroom and Greer, 1972).

Inorganic mercury can also cause the behavioral changes referred to as "erethism". It is characterized by nervousness, insomnia, loss of memory, irritability and excessive shyness. Erethism is not common today as it is usually associated with high levels of mercury exposure. However, low-level exposure to mercury vapors could induce symptoms of difficulties in concentration and mild impairment of cognitive functions (Piikivi and Hänninen, 1977). Alterations in visual field threshold, contrast sensitivity and color discrimination have been detected in workers exposed to low levels of mercury vapor (average urinary mercury of 22.3 μg/g creatinine) (Barboni *et al.*, 2009). Neuroendocrine changes (increased serum prolactin) and motor coordination imbalance were observed in those working in chlor-alkali plants and the production of thermometers and neon lamps, with average urinary mercury levels of 8.3 μg/g creatinine (Lucchini *et al.*, 2003).

Solvents

Case Study 2

A 55-year-old man was seen at a medical clinic on many occasions for the last few months for complaints of giddiness. He was well before going to work and only developed giddiness after beginning work. Physical examinations by the attending doctors were normal on all these occasions. Since he insisted on asking for a medical certificate to stay home from work, he was diagnosed as "malingering" by the doctors at the clinic and referred to the Occupational Health Clinic. His occupational history showed that this patient had been working as a fitter in a shipyard for the last 15 years. Each day he had to use considerable amounts of organic solvents to clean the ship engine. Over the last few months, he developed giddiness after the degreasing job — this was the reason why he did not want to go back to work! Further investigations were conducted for the patient that showed his symptoms were suggestive of early chronic toxic encephalopathy due to exposure to the organic solvents.

Solvents are widely used in industry and agriculture and they have been studied for neurotoxic effects both on the central (CNS) and peripheral nervous system (PNS). Behavioral methods have frequently been used in the study on effects of exposure to organic solvents for some three decades. There is an ever-increasing number of publications in this area of research. Today, the prenarcotic effects of acute solvent exposures are widely accepted, as well as the CNS effects of long-term, low-level exposures (Iregren, 1996). Exposure to a mixture of solvents can cause deficits in attention and cognitive processing speed (Meyer-Baron *et al.*, 2008). Long-term exposure leads in some workers to the development of chronic solvent-induced encephalopathy (CSE), a non-progressive disease in which no severe deterioration of functioning occurs after diagnosis and exposure cessation (van Valen *et al.*, 2009). Cerebral impairment has been demonstrated in the fronto-striato-thalamic circuitry (Visser *et al.*, 2008).

In general, acute exposure to a high concentration of organic solvents causes confusion, dizziness, headache, poor concentration, motor incoordination and other related symptoms. Most of these symptoms are reversible if the exposure concentrations are not too high, but residual deficits may persist. The behavioral effects of solvents associated with chronic exposure can be divided into three levels of increasing severity (Johnson, 1987). The first involves mood changes: easy fatiguability, decreased reactivity to environmental stimuli and some degree of mental confusion. Neurobehavioral tests are usually normal but symptoms of depression, irritability, fatiguability and confusion are present. The second is represented by a mild toxic encephalopathy that includes features of mood disorder together with impaired cognitive function. Sleep disorders and memory impairments are also common. The third level is chronic dementia, and represents the least common and most advanced form of CNS effects. The prognosis of phase 1 is benign. Workers can fully recover if they are quickly removed from the excessive solvent exposure. The prognosis of phase 2 depends on its severity. At the early stages of phase 2, recovery can be complete. However, if removal from exposure does not happen early in phase 2, recovery may not be complete. The third stage of the disease is not reversible. One would still recommend removal from solvent exposure as this will prevent further deterioration (Chia, 1998).

Long- and medium-term exposure to organic solvents containing carbon disulphide, *n*-hexane and methyl *n*-butyl ketone are well-known for causing mixed peripheral neuropathies (Baker, Smith and Landrigan, 1985).

Case Study 3

A 40-year-old female production worker from an electronic factory complained of numbness in her hands. She has been a diabetic for the last 10 years. Her blood sugar was always well controlled with oral hypoglycemic agents. She was diagnosed by her physician with peripheral neuropathy secondary to diabetes mellitus.

In a follow-up for the diabetes, it was found that she used solvents to clean the electronic components, and the solvent was found to contain n-hexane as a contaminant. Therefore, she was suspected to have solvent-induced peripheral neuropathy caused by n-hexane exposure. After the contaminated solvent was replaced, she recovered completely and did not experience any numbness in her hands.

Pesticides

The Food and Agriculture Organization (FAO, 1986) defines a pesticide as any substance or mixture of substances intended to prevent, destroy or control any pest, including vectors of human or animal disease, unwanted species of plants or animals causing harm during or otherwise interfering with the production, processing, storage, transport or marketing of food, agricultural commodities, wood and wood products, or animal feedstuffs, or which may be administered to animals for the control of insects, arachnids or other pests in or on their bodies. Pesticides can be classified according to their use into three main categories: insecticides, fungicides and herbicides. The effects of pesticides on the nervous system may be due to their acute toxicity, as in the case of most insecticides, or may contribute to chronic neurodegenerative disorders, most notably Parkinson's disease.

This family of chemicals comprises the organophosphates, the carbamates, the pyrethroids, the organochlorines and other compounds.

Some of the more common pesticides which pose occupational hazards could be listed in the following groups:

Organochlorine compounds

Acute or subacute intoxication from organochlorines produces a picture of generalized nervous system excitability: apprehension, excitability, dizziness, headache, disorientation, confusion, weakness, paresthesia, muscle twitching, tremor, convulsions and coma. Examples of these compounds are dichlorodiphenyl-trichloroethane (DDT) and chlordecone (Kepone).

Organophosphorus compounds

Organophosphorus (OP) insecticides are used most commonly in agriculture and are probably the most frequent causative agents of neurologic disease among agricultural workers, especially those in the developing countries. Dithiocarbamates like maneb and mancozeb are also widely used fungicides which have been shown to cause neurotoxic effects in workers. Acute poisoning caused by OP originates from its inhibition of acetylcholinesterase action. Symptoms and signs seen: muscarinic effects (miosis, salivation, vomiting, diarrhea, bronchial hypersecretion), nicotinic effects (muscular fasciculation, tremor, muscular cramps) and central nervous effects (impaired consciousness, convulsions, coma). Polyneuropathies are not a common effect, although some OP compounds can induce a delayed motor polyneuropathy affecting mainly the lower limbs (Davis and Richardson, 1980). In contrast, evidence of long-term CNS alterations in humans from low, chronic exposure to OPs is contradictory, and current evidence does not fully support the existence of clinically significant neuropsychological effects, neuropsychiatric abnormalities or peripheral nerve dysfunction in workers chronically exposed to low levels of OPs (Costa *et al.*, 2008).

Neurodegenerative effects are also reported, leading to Parkinsonian disturbances in agricultural workers exposed to organochlorine pesticides (Elbaz *et al.*, 2009). Use of organochlorine

2,4-dichlorophenoxyacetic acid, the herbicide paraquat and the insecticide and acaricide permethrin has been shown to be associated with Parkinsonism in farmers (Tanner *et al.*, 2009).

Common Work Situations which Give Rise to These Occupational Diseases

Metals

Arsenic

In Singapore, the commonest exposures to arsenic are from the electronic component manufacturing and wood preservation industries (Chia *et al.*, 1993a). Although the electronics industry has the highest number of workers, their exposure is usually very low. The exposure is confined to the manufacture of electronic wafers where arsenic is used to enhance electrical conductivity. This process is enclosed although exposure is possible during maintenance (LaDou, 1990).

Arsenic exposure could be high in wood preservation plants. Dust is generated during the pouring and mixing of dry wood preservatives that contain arsenic. Although no dust is generated when wood preservatives are used in paste form, skin contact is unavoidable during the release of treated wood from the pressurized tanks (Fig. 1) (Ho *et al.*, 1982).

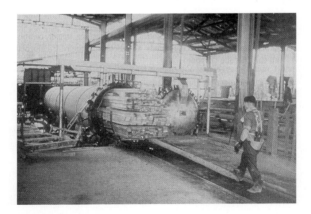

Fig. 1. Wood being placed into a pressurized tank for treatment with preservatives containing arsenic.

High levels of arsenic can be found in drinking water from both natural and anthropogenic sources. Workers occupationally exposed to arsenic and residents in areas with high arsenic content in drinking water can be at a higher risk for the development of adverse effects.

Other exposures to arsenic occur in the manufacture of glass (where arsenic is used to remove bubbles from molten glass), alloy manufacturing, manufacture and use of antifouling paints, taxidermy (arsenic trioxide) and pottery (arsenic trichloride).

Lead

Some common industries where workers can be exposed to lead include telecommunication, manufacture and recycling of electronic parts and components, manufacture of plastic materials, and manufacture, storage and recycling of primary batteries (Fig. 2). The iron industry, plastics industry (stabilizers in PVC compounding) and industries working with fabricated metal products are additional sites for occupational lead exposure. Other sources include the printing industry (typesetting), manufacture and use of antifouling paints, manufacture and use of glazes for China porcelain, enamels and glazed tiles, and lead soldering.

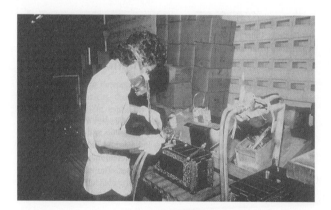

Fig. 2.   Burning of lead ingot to join the connectors in the assembly of storage batteries.

Organic lead exposure is usually confined to the refining and use of gasoline (organic lead is used as an anti-knock agent) and the production and transportation of anti-knock agents.

Manganese

Manganese is used in the manufacture of dry cell batteries, animal feed, matches and fireworks, and in the iron and steel industry. Exposure typically occurs in mining, ferroalloy production, smelting, welding, refining and milling of manganese compounds. A study conducted by Gan, Tan and Kwok (1988) reported that the highest manganese exposure was in manganese mills. Other studies indicate that the highest levels are in mining and ferroalloy production (IEH/IOM, 2004).

Mercury

The chlor-alkali plant produces chlorine, hydrogen and sodium hydroxide by brine electrolysis, using elemental mercury as a flowing cathode. The mercury is kept in brine or water during normal operations. Mercury exposure can occur during "rebuilding" when the electrolyzing chambers are drained, exposing the mercury (Chan *et al.*, 1982). Mercury is used to recover gold by amalgamation, with an extraction process that can cause occupational exposure and contamination of air, soil, rivers and lakes.

Workers in the artisanal and small-scale gold-mining sector are thought to use mercury more than in any other single sector, and the number of poor miners has grown considerably in many regions across Africa, Asia and South America (Swain *et al.*, 2007). In the laboratory, elemental mercury is used as a pressure medium in various pressure gauges for carrying out pressure, volume, and temperature measurements.

Other possible sources of exposure to mercury include amalgam preparation in dentistry, production of thermometers and neon lights, paint and pigment manufacture, and the pharmaceutical industry (preparation of drugs and disinfectants).

Solvents

Solvents are used in industries for a variety of purposes. Different forms of surface coatings are made possible by solvents, e.g. printing inks and paints, dilutants for paints, spreading preparations for papers and fabrics, and fiberglass production. They are also used for extracting oils, fats and other substances from different materials. Some solvents are used for degreasing, gluing and dry cleaning purposes. The extent and amount of solvent usage varies from industry to industry.

Toluene is probably the most extensively reported organic solvent for causing toxic encephalopathy, especially among toluene abusers (King, 1983). It is widely used as a paint, lacquer and ink dilutant.

The shoemaking, leather and glove industries were among the most frequently reported sources of peripheral neuropathy from organic solvents (Spencer *et al.*, 1980). The main solvents responsible were *n*-hexane, methyl *n*-butyl ketone and carbon disulphide. Most of the cases occurred in subjects who worked in small, poorly ventilated rooms where good work hygiene conditions were absent (Gilioli, Cassitto and Foà, 1983).

Pesticides

Approximately 90% of all pesticides are used for commercial purposes and the remainder for structural pest control, horticulture, and home and garden purposes.

Common work exposure situations usually involve agricultural workers. Horticultural workers may also be exposed to significant levels of pesticides. In horticulture, occupational exposure to the pesticides occurs mainly during the mixing of the compound with water and in the spraying of the mixture (Tan, 1982).

Workers involved in the formulation and manufacture of pesticides are also exposed to its hazards. Those who repack pesticides (most of whom do not know the nature of what they are packing) are also at risk. These operations are done in warehouses or cottage industries with little or no preventive measures adopted.

Clinical Presentation

There are many problems in trying to establish a direct cause–effect relationship when examining workers exposed to potentially neurotoxic agents who manifest signs and symptoms of neurotoxicity (especially those relating to central nervous system effects).

The nervous system responds to neurotoxic substances in many ways. The actual mechanism responsible for neurotoxic effects is still unclear for many substances. Furthermore, little information is generally available about the possible neurotoxic properties of many chemicals. Only a small number of the estimated 60,000 chemicals in the workplace have been evaluated for neurotoxic effects. However, 1000–1500 new chemicals are being introduced into the industries each year (Anger, 1990). For chemicals with known neurotoxic properties, there is generally uncertainty about the level and duration of exposure required to produce neurotoxic effects.

In addition, workers are generally exposed to a mixture of chemicals, like in the cases of solvents and of pesticides. Therefore, in practice, it is very difficult to isolate the effect of a single chemical. On the other hand, according to the "multi-hit" theory, the CNS is particularly suceptible to cumulative exposure to multiple agents compared to a single exposure (Lucchini and Zimmerman, 2009).

Very few symptoms or signs of neurologic impairments are specific to neurotoxicity caused by chemicals. It may be difficult at times to differentiate from other (non-occupational) causes of neurological dysfunction. Symptom reporting may not be very useful in the diagnostic process of CSE, which needs objective evaluation with neuropsychological testing (Bast-Pettersen, 2009).

In order to establish that the presenting problem is related to or caused by work exposure, a detailed occupational history is important. This should be followed by environmental assessment (where feasible) to determine the types of agents and level of exposure. Biological monitoring (if available) of the patient and other workers would give a better picture of the body burden of the exposed substance.

How to Distinguish between an Occupational and a Non-occupational Disease

Occupational history

In general, the symptomatology of a non-occupational neurological disorder cannot be differentiated from that of a occupational disease, apart from a suggestive exposure history. This is where taking a comprehensive occupational history becomes very important in helping to distinguish an occupational disease from one that is not work-related.

The following is a suggested checklist for taking an occupational history:

Present illness

Are the symptoms associated with work? In other words, do the symptoms improve during vacations or weekends?

Identify patterns suggesting either improvement or exacerbation on withdrawal from exposure. This is true for stage one of behavioral effects.

Do other workers have similar symptoms?

Identifying others who may have been affected may lead to further inquiries that clarify the individual patient's problem.

Are you currently exposed to any metals, solvents or pesticides?

Think of the possible neurotoxic agents; remember that there are many substances with possible effects on the nervous system that we may not be aware of.

Who else did you see regarding the problems?

This is a valuable way of getting further information from others who may have seen the patient at an earlier phase of the disease, e.g. behavioral changes.

Work history

List in chronological order all the jobs. Describe a typical workday and job duties.

Ascertain the degree and duration of exposure to possible neurotoxic substances.

Was protective equipment issued? And if so, do you use it? How frequently do you use it?

Consider if protection was given to workers and whether the protection was adequate. One should also check if respirators (masks) used are the appropriate types.

Is ventilation in your workplace adequate?

Obtain a general impression of adequacy of ventilation by air movement and odors.

Was a pre-employment examination done? What about periodic medical examinations?

Important information could be obtained regarding baseline results and trends of investigation results if these examinations were conducted.

Besides your regular work, do you have another job? List additional jobs.

Some significant exposures may not be due to the regular job but occur during a part-time job outside normal working hours.

Ask about abnormal circumstances in the workplace. Has there been any increase in workload recently? Was there a breakdown/shutdown? Have there been any changes to the production line or introduction of new chemicals?

Identify possible outbreaks or clusters of a neurological condition in the workplace.

Subjective symptoms questionnaire

The recording of subjective complaints using a standardized questionnaire is of importance to provide a consistent information base for all patients with neurotoxic exposure. Symptom reports are usually the first manifestation of the disease before any detectable neurological or psychological testing. Subtle changes could be detected, especially if the standardized questionnaire is used periodically for workers.

Table 1 shows a sample of one such questionnaire (Johnson, 1987).

Table 1.   Symptoms Questionnaire

A. Chronic Symptoms

Below is a list of questions concerning symptoms you may have had.

Check the appropriate box if you have been experiencing the symptoms in the past month.

If you have experienced the symptom, please indicate in the space provided.

1. Are you tired more easily than expected for the amount of activity you do?

    (1) not at all __   (2) a little __   (3) moderately __   (4) quite a bit __   (5) extremely __

2. Have you felt lightheaded or dizzy?

    (1) not at all __   (2) a little __   (3) moderately __   (4) quite a bit __   (5) extremely __

3. Have you had difficulty concentrating?

    (1) not at all __   (2) a little __   (3) moderately __   (4) quite a bit __   (5) extremely __

4. Have you been confused or disoriented?

    (1) not at all __   (2) a little __   (3) moderately __   (4) quite a bit __   (5) extremely __

5. Have you had trouble remembering things?

    (1) not at all __   (2) a little __   (3) moderately __   (4) quite a bit __   (5) extremely __

6. Have your relatives noticed that you have trouble remembering things?

    (1) not at all __   (2) a little __   (3) moderately __   (4) quite a bit __   (5) extremely __

7. Have you had to make notes to remember things?

    (1) not at all __   (2) a little __   (3) moderately __   (4) quite a bit __   (5) extremely __

8. Have you found it hard to understand the meaning of newspapers, magazines and books you have read?

    (1) not at all __   (2) a little __   (3) moderately __   (4) quite a bit __   (5) extremely __

(*Continued*)

Table 1. (*Continued*)

9. Have you felt irritable?
   (1) not at all __   (2) a little __   (3) moderately __   (4) quite a bit __   (5) extremely __

10. Have you felt depressed?
   (1) not at all __   (2) a little __   (3) moderately __   (4) quite a bit __   (5) extremely __

11. Have you had heart palpitations even when not exerting yourself?
   (1) not at all __   (2) a little __   (3) moderately __   (4) quite a bit __   (5) extremely __

12. Have you had a seizure?
   (1) not at all __   (2) a little __   (3) moderately __   (4) quite a bit __   (5) extremely __

13. Have you been sleeping more often than is usual for you?
   (1) not at all __   (2) a little __   (3) moderately __   (4) quite a bit __   (5) extremely __

14. Have you had difficulty falling asleep?
   (1) not at all __   (2) a little __   (3) moderately __   (4) quite a bit __   (5) extremely __

15. Have you been bothered by incoordination or loss of balance?
   (1) not at all __   (2) a little __   (3) moderately __   (4) quite a bit __   (5) extremely __

16. Have you had any loss of muscle strength in your legs or feet?
   (1) not at all __   (2) a little __   (3) moderately __   (4) quite a bit __   (5) extremely __

17. Have you had any loss of muscle strength in your arms or hands?
   (1) not at all __   (2) a little __   (3) moderately __   (4) quite a bit __   (5) extremely __

18. Have you had difficulty moving your fingers or grasping things?
   (1) not at all __   (2) a little __   (3) moderately __   (4) quite a bit __   (5) extremely __

(*Continued*)

Table 1. (*Continued*)

19. Have you had numbness or tingling in your fingers lasting more than a day?

    (1) not at all ___   (2) a little ___   (3) moderately ___   (4) quite a bit ___   (5) extremely ___

20. Have you had numbness or tingling in your toes lasting more than a day?

    (1) not at all ___   (2) a little ___   (3) moderately ___   (4) quite a bit ___   (5) extremely ___

21. Have you had headaches at least once a week?

    (1) not at all ___   (2) a little ___   (3) moderately ___   (4) quite a bit ___   (5) extremely ___

22. Have you had difficulty driving home from work because you felt dizzy or tired, even though you'd slept enough?

    (1) not at all ___   (2) a little ___   (3) moderately ___   (4) quite a bit ___   (5) extremely ___

23. Have you felt "high" from the chemical you smell at work?

    (1) not at all ___   (2) a little ___   (3) moderately ___   (4) quite a bit ___   (5) extremely ___

24. Have you had a lower tolerance for alcohol (takes less to get drunk)?

    (1) not at all ___   (2) a little ___   (3) moderately ___   (4) quite a bit ___   (5) extremely ___

B. Acute Symptoms during the Workday

During the last month that you have worked, have you noticed that you felt or experienced any of the following symptoms during the workday?

1. Headaches

    (1) not at all ___   (2) a little ___   (3) moderately ___   (4) quite a bit ___   (5) extremely ___

2. Tired

    (1) not at all ___   (2) a little ___   (3) moderately ___   (4) quite a bit ___   (5) extremely ___

3. Lightheaded or "high"

    (1) not at all ___   (2) a little ___   (3) moderately ___   (4) quite a bit ___   (5) extremely ___

(*Continued*)

Table 1.   (*Continued*)

4. Difficulty concentrating
   (1) not at all __ (2) a little __ (3) moderately __ (4) quite a bit __ (5) extremely __
5. Confusion
   (1) not at all __ (2) a little __ (3) moderately __ (4) quite a bit __ (5) extremely __
6. Difficulty remembering things
   (1) not at all __ (2) a little __ (3) moderately __ (4) quite a bit __ (5) extremely __
7. Irritable
   (1) not at all __ (2) a little __ (3) moderately __ (4) quite a bit __ (5) extremely __
8. Incoordination
   (1) not at all __ (2) a little __ (3) moderately __ (4) quite a bit __ (5) extremely __
9. Loss of muscle strength
   (1) not at all __ (2) a little __ (3) moderately __ (4) quite a bit __ (5) extremely __

If you have answered yes to any of the symptoms above, do these symptoms come on when you are using a specific substance? Please explain.

Source: Johnson (1987).

Clinical History and Examination

Other than a general examination of the various systems, specific emphasis should be placed on the nervous system. The neurological examination should include an examination of the cranial nerves, coordination, sensation, strength, gait and tendon reflexes (Baker and Seppalainen, 1987). Particular emphasis should be placed on a careful mental status examination, as suggested above.

Peripheral Nerve Function

Early symptoms of peripheral nerve dysfunction is numbness or tingling in the extremities, starting usually in the lower limbs, then moving to the upper limbs. If exposure persists, weakness (distal more than proximal) may follow with sensory symptoms (diminished vibration or pain sensation, bilateral reduced or absent ankle reflexes). Atrophy and muscular fasciculation may develop later.

Central Nervous System

Acute exposure to high concentrations of a neurotoxic substance generally results in a non-specific narcotic effect. The toxic substance is easy to identify because of the acute onset of symptoms when exposure occurs.

Chronic low-level exposure is much more difficult to relate to central nervous system dysfunction because of the lack of specific symptoms, the lack (in many instances) of objective methods for assessment, biases introduced by compensation and a possible "healthy worker effect". The most common complaints are difficulties with concentration and memory. Verbal reasoning, remote and recent memory, complex concept formation, and dexterity may also be affected. In addition, patients may report headache, light-headedness, vertigo, blurred vision, poor coordination, tremor and weakness of the extremities. The more severely affected patients may complain of difficulties with attention and organization together with general depression, irritability and fatigue.

It must be stressed that patients who have been exposed to a central neurotoxin (e.g. solvents) may complain of cognitive dysfunction without any other physical signs. A standard neurobehavioral test battery is therefore an important adjunct investigative tool.

Diagnostic and Laboratory Tests

Tests for Exposure

Environmental monitoring

Environmental monitoring is used to assess the types of chemical and exposure levels at the work site. Wherever possible, personal monitoring of the workers should be carried out rather than collecting static area samples. This is especially so for workers who have to move around the workplace and are not stationed at a particular work process. It is best to consult an industrial hygienist for the environmental monitoring. However, in certain factories, the safety officer or engineer may be able to do the monitoring if they have been trained.

Knowledge of the types of chemicals that the workers are exposed to and the exposure levels are very useful information and need to be obtained by the physician.

Biological monitoring

Biological monitoring is complementary to environmental monitoring. Where biological monitoring techniques are available, they provide information on body burden (internal exposure) which reflects the balance between uptake, biotransformation and excretion, in contrast to environmental monitoring which measures the airborne concentration in the workplace or breathing zone.

Biological monitoring is especially useful where skin absorption or inadvertent ingestion could be a significant route of exposure.

Skin exposure to solvents is especially common among painters, degreasers and printers (Chia *et al.*, 1993a). It is common practice for these workers to use solvents to clean paint/ink or oil stains from their skin (Chia, Tan and Kwok, 1987).

Oral ingestion of metal dust can also be a significant factor, especially in some cultural practices. Chia, Chia and Ong (1991) reported that oral ingestion of lead, through eating of food with hands contaminated by lead compounds, among the Malay workers could be a possible cause for the higher mean blood levels compared to that of the Chinese workers. Other possible confounders like age, exposure duration, cigarette smoking and lead-in-air concentration were adjusted for the analysis.

The important point to note for chronic effects is that current biological monitoring results may not be reflective of past exposure. It would, therefore, be more useful to look at serial results of biological markers rather than just a single result.

Biological monitoring for some of the heavy metals are quite well-established. Blood lead and manganese are useful measures of body burden. Similarly, this is true for the urinary level of mercury, arsenic and manganese. Measures of red blood cell or plasma cholinesterase activity would be useful in determining the acute effect of organophosphate.

There are, however, a limited number of biological monitoring techniques applicable to solvents. Examples of solvents that have biological exposure indices (BEI) include carbon disulphide, dimethylformamide (DMF), *n*-hexane, methanol, methyl chloroform, methyl ethyl ketone (MEK), perchloroethylene, styrene, toluene, trichloroethylene and xylene (ACGIH, 2009). Even for the limited solvents with BEI the techniques for analysis of these substances or their metabolites are only available in certain laboratories in the world.

Table 2 shows a summary of biomarkers that monitor exposure to some known neurotoxic chemicals.

Tests to Confirm Clinical Findings or to Detect Subclinical Effects

Neurophysiological tests

Electroencephalography

Electroencephalography (EEG) records the surface (cortical) electrical activity of the brain. In recent years, imaging studies have

Table 2. Biomarkers for Monitoring Exposure to Some Neurotoxic Chemicals (ACGIH, 2009)

Chemical Agents	Biological Fluid	Tentative Maximum Permissible Values	Remarks/ Sampling Time
Metals			
Arsenic, elemental and soluble inorganic compounds	Urine	35 μg/g creatinine	End of workweek
Inorganic lead	Blood	30 μg/dl	Not critical
Total inorganic mercury	Blood	15 μg/L	End of shift at end of workweek
Total inorganic mercury	Urine	35 μg/g creatinine	Prior to shift
Solvents			
Carbon disulphide	Urine (2-thiothiazolidine-4-carboxylic acid)	0.5 mg/g creatinine	End of shift
Methanol	Urine	15 mg/L	End of shift
Methyl ethyl ketone	Urine	2 mg/L	End of shift
Toluene	Urine (hippuric acid)	1.6 g/g creatinine	End of shift
	Blood	0.05 mg/L	Prior to last shift of workweek

supplanted it as a method for localizing anatomic pathology. It is more useful as a pathophysiologic tool, detecting abnormal cerebral function that cannot be visualized radiographically or magnetically. Thus, the use of EEG is more appropriate in the evaluation of transient states (e.g. seizures), evolving conditions (e.g. encephalitis) and global disorders (e.g. dementia).

Studies of significant EEG findings among workers exposed to solvents are equivocal. Seppalainen, Lindstrom and Martelin (1980) reported that abnormalities were more frequent among patients with mild solvent poisoning. The abnormalities were usually slow wave abnormalities, one-third local and about two-thirds diffuse or generalized. However, no increase in frequency of abnormal EEGs was found among industrial or car painters exposed to solvents of about 30% of the hygienic limits in comparison to reference groups of manual workers without solvent exposure (Seppalainen, 1973; Elofsson *et al.*, 1980).

EEGs of patients who are intoxicated by toluene may show diffuse or focal slow or sharp wave complexes (King *et al.*, 1981). In general, EEG may be useful in detecting encephalopathic processes, but the findings are non-specific and it cannot confirm that an abnormality is due to a work-related disease.

Electroneuromyography

Electroneuromyography (EMG), which consists of motor and sensory nerve conduction studies and needle electrode examination of muscles, is a valuable and sensitive test. It can recognize and distinguish abnormalities of the anterior horn cell, dorsal sensory ganglion cell, nerve root, peripheral nerve, neuromuscular junction, muscle membrane or muscle fiber.

EMG is a sensitive and useful method of identifying and diagnosing patients with mild toxic neuropathy. The prominent feature of neuropathy caused by various solvents has been the distal slowing of both motor and/or sensory conduction velocities (depending on the causative agent) (Allen *et al.*, 1975; Cianchetti *et al.*, 1976). EMG has also showed neurogenic abnormalities in patients with *n*-hexane polyneuropathy (Sobue *et al.*, 1978).

Because of its sensitivity, the examiner must be cautious of over-interpretating the results. A study at the Mayo Clinic found that up to a third of unselected patients with an EMG diagnosis of polyneuropathy had minor or subclinical disease thought not to warrant intervention by the clinician (Thomas and Dale, 1981). To avoid problems of over-interpretation, EMG should be a focused and restricted examination with specific questions asked: Does the worker have polyneuropathy detectable by EMG? Is this polyneuropathy due to agent exposure or is it due to some concomitant disease?

Neuroradiological tests

Computed tomography and magnetic resonance imaging

Computed tomography (CT) is not very useful as a diagnostic tool for toxic encephalopathy. Orbaek *et al.* (1987) studied 32 patients with chronic toxic encephalopathy due to occupational exposure to organic solvents. They concluded that chronic toxic encephalopathy induced by solvents shows no evidence of brain atrophy in CT, despite poor psychometric test performance.

Magnetic resonance imaging (MRI) is one of several technological advances that have occurred in recent years. MRI uses a magnetic field and radio frequency waves (not radiation). It is non-invasive and is based on the principle of imaging the hydrogen proton (Gilman, 1992). The intensity of images in a certain region of the CNS is given by the "proton spin-lattice relaxation time" (T_1), a measure of the rate at which the protons (hydrogen nuclei) return to thermal equilibrium after being perturbed in a magnetic field. The T_1 rate, and consequently the contrast in brain MRI, is influenced by the water and fat content and by the presence of paramagnetic ions such as manganese (Mn), iron (Fe) and copper. Manganese accumulates selectively in the globus pallidus of the basal ganglia and can be visualized by brain MRI. A semi-quantitative method to compute a pallidal index can be used to assess Mn deposition in the brain and has been found to be predictive of neurobehavioral alterations in welders (Chang *et al.*, 2009).

Neurobehavioral tests

A variety of neurobehavioral methods are available for evaluating nervous system effects in working populations exposed to chemical and physical agents. However, these methods have important limitations. The standardization of techniques has often been variable. Various factors can influence test performance and mask the impact of exposure or job-related factors. In addition, specific abnormal neurobehavioral tasks cannot be related to specific neuropathological processes or disease conditions.

The selection of neurobehavioral tests will depend on the settings and purposes under which the testing is performed, and the kind of person suitable to perform the tests in different situations.

World Health Organization neurobehavioral core test battery

At the clinic level, prospective surveillance programs could be developed for monitoring workers exposed to neurotoxic agents. A short standardized neurobehavioral test would be useful. A suggested test battery is the World Health Organization (WHO) neurobehavioral core test battery (NCTB). The complete set of tests is given in Table 3. The details of this test battery are described in Johnson (1987).

Factors influencing test performance

Test scores are influenced by many factors other than exposure to toxicants. These factors can confound the interpretation of the results if the factors are not recognized and controlled for in the test. Generally, the factors could be classified as subject factors, examiner factors and environmental factors.

Table 3.   WHO Neurobehavioral Core Test Battery

Test	Functional Domain Tested
Profile of mood states	Affect
Simple reaction time	Attention/Response speed
Digit span	Auditory memory
Santa Ana dexterity test	Manual dexterity
Digit symbol	Perceptual-motor speed
Benton visual retention	Visual perception/memory
Aiming (pursuit aiming II)	Motor steadiness

Subject factors to be considered include age, sex, education, socioeconomic status, health and drug history, circadian rhythm and fatigue, and motivation. Examiners should preferably be from the same culture and be able to speak fluently in the subject's native language. Examiners must interact with all subjects in a consistent and standardized manner. Environmental factors which could affect the test include lighting, noise, temperature and humidity.

Interpretation of the results

One major problem in the interpretation of test results is the lack of baseline data for the worker's performance prior to exposure to toxicants. The non-specific nature of the toxicant in question and the variability of the worker's performance create problems in interpretation. Efforts should be made to obtain the baseline data wherever possible. As with neurophysiological tests, serial results of the workers are often more meaningful and important than a single reading for an individual diagnosis.

Other tests

A worker with a neurological disorder with an appropriate history may not definitely be suffering from a work-related disease. To further clarify pathological processes, hematological and biochemical tests may be necessary.

Assessment of Clinical Status

Pre-employment Examination

As in any pre-employment examination, the general principles apply: Is the worker fit for this particular job in which he is seeking employment? What are the baseline examinations and investigations that should be conducted?

To answer the above questions with sufficient confidence and a clear conscience, the attending physician must know the job requirements and the possible hazards. What is the working environment? What is the work process? What are the work tools? Does the job expose the worker to any substances that may cause the worker to be more susceptible to developing ill-health?

The physician would need to know also the likely agents the worker may be exposed to. What are the likely target organ systems? Based on this knowledge, the appropriate tests (as discussed earlier) may be conducted to obtain the baseline results. Wherever possible, the relevant and available biological monitoring markers (Table 2) should be done to determine the pre-exposure levels.

In addition, workers who are exposed to organic solvents could be given a subjective symptoms questionnaire (Table 1) and a standard neurobehavioral test (Table 3). These questionnaires and tests become very useful during the periodic medical examination to evaluate early cases of toxic encephalopathy.

Workers with certain medical conditions or complications may be more susceptible to neurotoxic substances in the workplace. Extra caution must be taken in deciding if such workers are fit for employment. When in doubt, it is always good practice to consult and discuss the worker's medical condition with specialists in that particular field.

Periodic Examinations

The objective of periodic examinations is the detection of early cases of subclinical effects or excessive absorption of the exposed substances. The frequency of the examination is dependent on the degree of exposure to the hazards.

History taking and clinical examination should be specific to the hazard concerned. Serial results of the workers are more important than a single result. It is good practice to study the relationship of the results over different medical examination periods. Rising trends in the results should alert the physician to the likelihood of pending excessive absorption or early effects of the agent. The appropriate interventions should then be carried out.

If the workers' biological monitoring results exceed the permissible values, they should be transferred to another section where there is no exposure to the hazard. Similarly, this would apply to workers who develop symptoms and or signs of neurological or behavioral dysfunction.

Fitness to Return to Work

Whether a worker is fit to return to work (exposure to neurotoxic agent) will depend on the cause of his unfitness in the first instance. If it is due to excessive absorption, e.g. high blood lead levels, he could return to his former job when his blood lead levels return to the permissible level, and there are no other contraindications.

In a situation where a worker develops peripheral neuropathy due to a neurotoxic substance, following which he recovers completely, re-exposure to the causative agent should be prohibited.

References

Allen N, Mendell JR, Billmaier DJ, *et al.* (1975) Toxic polyneuropathy due to methyl *n*-butyl ketone: An industrial outbreak. *Arch Neurol* **32**: 209–218.

American Conference of Governmental Industrial Hygienists. (2009) *Threshold Limit Values for Chemical Substances and Physical Agents Biological Exposure Indices.* ACGIH, Cincinnati.

Anger WK. (1990) Worksite behavioral research: Results, sensitive methods, test batteries and the transition from laboratory data to human health. *Neurotoxicology* **11**: 629–720.

Baker EL, Seppalainen AM. (1987) Human aspect of solvent neurobehavioral effects. *Neurotoxicology* **7**(4): 43–56.

Baker EL, Smith TJ, Landrigan PJ. (1985) The neurotoxicity of industrial solvents: A review of the literature. *Am J Ind Med* **8**: 207–217.

Barboni MT, Feitosa-Santana C, Zachi EC, *et al.* (2009) Preliminary findings on the effects of occupational exposure to mercury vapor below safety levels on visual and neuropsychological functions. *J Occup Environ Med* **51**(12): 1403–1412.

Bast-Pettersen R. (2009) The neuropsychological diagnosis of chronic solvent induced encephalopathy (CSE) — A reanalysis of neuropsychological test results in a group of CSE patients diagnosed 20 years ago, based on comparisons with matched controls. *Neurotoxicology* **30**(6): 1195–1201.

Chan OY, Kwok SF, Tan KT, Chio LF. (1982) A study of mercury exposure in laboratories and chlorine manufacturing, including beta-2 microglobulin excretion. *Proc 10th Asian Conf Occup Health* **2**: 557–562.

Chandra SV, Seth PK, Mankeshwar JK. (1974) Manganese poisoning: Clinical and biochemical observation. *Environ Res* **7**: 374–380.

Chang Y, Kim Y, Woo ST, *et al.* (2009) High signal intensity on magnetic resonance imaging is a better predictor of neurobehavioral performances than blood manganese in asymptomatic welders. *Neurotoxicology* **30**(4): 555–563.

Chia SE, Phoon WH, Lee HS, *et al.* (1993a) Exposure to neurotoxic metals among workers in Singapore: An overview. *Occup Med (Lond)* **43**(1): 18–22.

Chia SE, Ong CN, Phoon WH, *et al.* (1993) Neurobehavioural effects on workers in a video-tape manufacturing factory in Singapore. *Neurotoxicology* **14**(1): 51–56.

Chia SE, Tan KT, Kwok SF. (1987) A study on the health hazard of toluene in the polythene printing industry in Singapore. *Ann Acad Med Singapore* **16**(2): 294–299.

Chia SE, Chia KS, Ong CN. (1991) Ethnic differences in blood lead concentration among workers in a battery manufacturing factory. *Ann Acad Med Singapore* **20**(6): 758–761.

Chia SE, Chia KS, Chia HP, *et al.* (1996) Three-year follow-up of serial nerve conduction among lead-exposed workers. *Scand J Work Environ Health* **22**: 374–380.

Chia SE, Chia HP, Ong CN, Jeyaratnam J. (1997) Cumulative blood lead levels and neurobehavioral test performance. *Neurotoxicology* **18**: 793–804.

Chia SE. (1998) Exposure to solvents and behavioural effects (Editorial). *Singapore Med J* **39**: 191–192.

Costa LG, Giordano G, Guizzetti M, Vitalone A. (2008) Neurotoxicity of pesticides: A brief review. *Front Biosci* **13**: 1240–1249.

Couper J. (1837) On the effects of black oxide of manganese when inhaled into the lungs. *Br Ann Med Pharmacol* **1**: 41–42.

Cianchetti G, Abbritti G, Perticoni G, *et al.* (1976) Toxic polyneuropathy of shoe-industry workers: A study of 122 cases. *J Neurol, Neurosurg and Psychiatry* **39**: 1151.

Davis CS, Richardson RJ. (1980) Organophosphorus compounds. In: Spencer PS, Schaumburg HH (eds). *Experimental and Clinical Neurotoxicology*, pp. 527–545. Baltimore: Williams and Wilkins.

Elbaz A, Clavel J, Rathouz PJ, *et al.* (2009) Professional exposure to pesticides and Parkinson's disease. *Ann Neurol* **66**(4): 494–504.

Elofsson SA, Gamborale F, Hindmarsh A, *et al.* (1980) Exposure to organic solvents: A cross-sectional epidemiologic investigation on occupationally exposed car and industrial spray painters with special reference to the nervous system. *Scand J Work Environ Health* **6**: 239–273.

Emara AM, El-Ghawabi SH, Madkour OI, El-Samra GH. (1971) Chronic manganese poisoning in the dry battery industry. *Br J Ind Med* **28**: 78–82.

FAO (Food and Agriculture Organization). (1986) International code of conduct on the distribution and use of pesticides. FAO, Rome.

Feldman RG, Niles CA, Kelly-Hayes M, *et al.* (1979) Peripheral neuropathy in arsenic smelter workers. *Neurology* **29**: 939.

Gan SL, Tan KT, Kwok SF. (1988) Biological threshold limit values for manganese dust exposure. *Singapore Med J* **29**: 563–568.

Gilioli R, Cassitto MG, Foà V. (eds). (1983) *Neurobehavioral Methods in Occupational Health*. Oxford: Pergamon Press.

Gilman S. (1992) Advances in neurology. New Engl J Med 326(24): 1608–1616.

Halatek T, Sinczuk-Walczak H, Rabieh S, Wasowicz W. (2009) Association between occupational exposure to arsenic and neurological, respiratory and renal effects. *Toxicol Appl Pharmacol* **239**(2): 193–199.

Hänninen H. (1985) Twenty-five years of behavioral toxicology within occupational medicine: A personal account. *Am J Ind Med* 7(1): 19–30.

Hernberg S. (1976) *Effects and Dose-Response Relationship of Toxic Metals*. Amsterdam: Elsevier Scientific.

Heyman A, Pfeiffer JB, Willet RW, Taylor HM. (1956) Peripheral neuropathy caused by arsenical intoxication. *New Engl J Med* **254**: 401.

Ho SF, Phoon WH, Tan KT, Kwok SF. (1982) Study on the usage and health hazards of arsenic in wood prservation plants. *Proc 10th Asian Conf Occup Health* **2**: 563–568.

Institute for Environment and Health/Institute of Occupational Medicine (IEH/IOM). (2004) *Occupational Exposure Limits: Criteria Document for Manganese and Inorganic Manganese Compounds* (Web Report W17). MRC Institute for Environment and Health, Leicester, UK. http://www.le.ac.uk/ieh.

Iregren A. (1996) Behavioural methods and organic solvents: Questions and consequences. *Environ Health Perspect* **104**(Suppl. 2): 361–366.

Jeyaratnam J, Devathasan G, Ong CN, *et al.* (1985) Neurophysiological studies on workers exposed to lead. *Br J Ind Med* **42**: 173–177.

Johnson BL. (1987) *Prevention of Neurotoxic Illness in Working Populations.* New York: John Wiley & Sons, p. 27.

King M. (1983) Long-term neuropsychological effects of solvent abuse. In: Cherry N, Waldron HA (eds). *The Neuropsychological Effects of Solvent Exposure.* Havant, Hampshire: Colt Foundation, pp. 75–84.

King MD, Day RE, Oliver JS, *et al.* (1981) Solvent encephalopathy. *BMJ* **283**: 663–665.

Ky S, Deng HS, Xie PY, Hu W. (1992) A report of two cases of chronic serious manganese poisoning treated with sodium para-aminosalicylic acid. *Br J Ind Med* **49**: 66–69.

LaDou J. (1990) Health issues in the micro-electronics industry. *J Occup Med Singapore* **2**: 9–22.

Lucchini R, Apostoli P, Perrone C, *et al.* (1999) Long-term exposure to "low levels" of manganese oxides and neurofunctional changes in ferroalloy workers. *Neurotoxicology* **20**(2–3): 287–297.

Lucchini R, Calza S, Camerino D, *et al.* (2003) Application of a latent variable model for a multicenter study on early effects due to mercury exposure. *Neurotoxicology* **24**(4–5): 605–616.

Lucchini R, Benedetti L, Albini E, Alessio L. (2005) Neurobehavioral science in hazard identification and risk assessment of neurotoxic agents — What are the needs for further development? *Int Arch Occup Environ Health* **78**: 427–437.

Lucchini R, Zimmerman N. (2009) Lifetime cumulative exposure as a threat for neurodegeneration: Need for prevention strategies on a global scale. *Neurotoxicology* **30**: 1144–1148.

Lucchini RG, Martin CJ, Doney BC. (2009) From manganism to manganese-induced Parkinsonism: A conceptual model based on the evolution of exposure. *Neuro Mol Med* **11**(4): 311–321.

Meyer-Baron M, Blaszkewicz M, Henke H, *et al.* (2008) The impact of solvent mixtures on neurobehavioral performance: Conclusions from epidemiological data. *Neurotoxicology* **29**(3): 349–360.

Murata K, Iwata T, Dakeishi M, Karita K. (2009) Lead toxicity: Does the critical level of lead resulting in adverse effects differ between adults and children? *J Occup Health* **51**(1): 1–12.

Orbaek P, Lindgren M, Olivecrona H, Haeger-Aronsen B. (1987) Computed tomography and psychometric test performance in patients with solvent induced chronic toxic encephalopathy and healthy controls. *Br J Ind Med* **44**(3): 175–179.

Piikivi LT, Hanninen H. (1977) Psychological performance and long-term exposure to mercury vapors. In: Hernberg S, Kahn H (eds). *Proceedings from Effects of Early Action of Toxic Substances on the Organism*, pp. 165–169. Helsinki: Tallinn.

Parkinson J. (2002) An essay on the shaking palsy. *J Neuropsych Clin Neurosc* **14**: 223–236.

Raffle PAB, Lee WR, McCallum RI, *et al.* (1987) *Hunter's Diseases of Occupations*, 7th edn. London: Hodder and Stoughton, pp. 239–296.

Ropper AH, Samuels MA. (2009) *Adams and Victor's Principles of Neurology* 9th edn. New York: McGraw-Hill Medical.

Racette BA, McGee-Minnich L, Moerlein SM, Mink JW. (2001) Welding-related parkinsonism: Clinical features, treatment, and pathophysiology. *Neurology* **56**(1): 8–13.

Racette BA, Antenor JA, McGee-Minnich L, Moerlein SM. (2005) [18F]FDOPA PET and clinical features in parkinsonism due to manganism. *Mov Disord* **20**(4): 492–496.

Schwartz BS, Chen S, Caffo B, Stewart WF. (2007) Relations of brain volumes with cognitive function in males 45 years and older with past lead exposure. *Neuroimage* **37**(2): 633–641.

Seppalainen AM, Lindstrom K, Martelin T. (1980) Neurophysiological and psychological picture of solvent poisoning. *Am J Ind Med* **1**: 31–42.

Seppalainen AM. (1973) Neurotoxic effects of industrial solvents. *Electroencephalogr Clin Neurophysiol* **34**: 702–703.

Spencer PS, Schaumburg HH, Sabri MI, *et al.* (1980) The enlarging view of hexacarbon neurotoxicity. *CRC Crit Rev Toxicol* **7**(4): 279–356.

Sobue I, Iida M, Yamamura Y, Takayanagui T. (1978) *n*-Hexane polyneuropathy. *Int J Neurology* **11**: 317.

Swain EB, Jakus PM, Rice G, *et al.* (2007) Socioeconomic consequences of mercury use and pollution. *Ambio* **36**: 45–61.

Tan KJ. (1982). Occupational exposure to organophosphorous insecticides in Singapore. *Proc 10th Asian Conf Occup Health* **1**: 208–211.

Tanner CM, Ross GW, Jewell SA, *et al.* (2009) Occupation and risk of Parkinsonism: A multicenter case-control study. *Arch Neurol* **66**(9): 1106–1113.

Thomas JE, Dale AJD. (eds). (1981) *Clinical Examinations in Neurology.* Philadelphia: WB Saunders.

van Valen E, Wekking E, van der Laan G, Sprangers M. (2009) The course of chronic solvent induced encephalopathy: A systematic review. *Neurotoxicology* **30**(6): 1172–1186.

Visser I, Lavini C, Booij J, *et al.* (2008) Cerebral impairment in chronic solvent-induced encephalopathy. *Ann Neurol* **63**(5): 572–580.

Vroom FQ, Greer M. (1972) Mercury vapour intoxication. *Brain* **95**: 305–318.

WHO. (1981) *Manganese, Environmental Health Criteria 17.* World Health Organization, Geneva, Switzerland.

Chapter 8

Mental Health Disorders

Ee-Heok Kua^{*,‡} *and Ken Ung*[†]

Ee-Heok Kua*,‡ *and Ken Ung*†

Introduction

The importance of mental health in the workplace is often under recognized. There has been an inordinately high focus on work stress, which often serves as a catch-all phrase for every mental health problem which occurs in the workplace. Mental health problems in the workplace can be broadly categorized into mental disorders, work stress and difficulties stemming from a lack of emotional competence.

The Global Burden of Disease Study sought to estimate the burden of different illnesses, using a standard unit called the disability-adjusted life year (DALY) to aid comparisons (Table 1) (Murray and Lopez, 1997). For established market economies, neuropsychiatric disorders accounted for 25.1% of disability — the highest for any single category.

*Yong Loo Lin School of Medicine, National University of Singapore, National University Health System, Singapore.
†Adam Road Hospital, Singapore.
‡Corresponding author. E-mail: pcmkeh@nus.edu.sg

Table 1. Disability-adjusted Life Years of Various Medical Disorders in the Established Market Economies

Neuropsychiatric Disorders	25.1%
Cardiovascular disorders	18.6%
Cancers	15.0%
Injuries	11.9%
Respiratory disorders	4.80%
Digestive disorders	4.40%
Musculoskeletal disorders	4.20%
Others	16.0%

Source: Global Burden of Disease Study.

Mental Health Issues in the Workplace

Mental Disorders

In 1998, Norwegian Prime Minister Kjell Bondevik went public with the admission that his 3.5-week sick leave was for a "depressive reaction" partly attributable to stress from work. Since the landmark case of Carter vs. General Motors in 1960, American courts have allowed for worker compensation for mental stress that causes a mental disorder. This move has been followed by courts in the United Kingdom, Europe and Australia. These cases merely represent the tip of the iceberg of mental illness in the work setting.

The impact of psychiatric disorders on work has been well accepted but not systematically studied. In an important study, Kessler and Frank (1997) attempted to estimate the lost and reduced work days due to various psychiatric illnesses using 4091 respondents from the US National Comorbidity Study (NCS) (Fig. 1). Depression was the single most important diagnosis in terms of work days lost or reduced. Importantly, having more than one disorder substantially increased disability. Employees are usually fearful of disclosing a history of any mental disorder as it may jeopardize their job.

Mild mental disorders are prevalent in the community and local estimates suggest a 12-month prevalence of 8–10% in the community (Fones *et al.*, 1998) (Fig. 2). Such illnesses often arise in early or mid-adulthood — the period of maximum economic productivity.

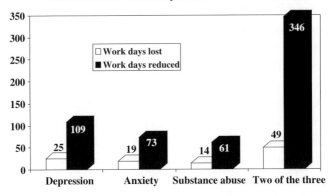

Fig. 1. Lost/reduced work days due to psychiatric illnesses (adapted from Kessler and Frank, 1997).

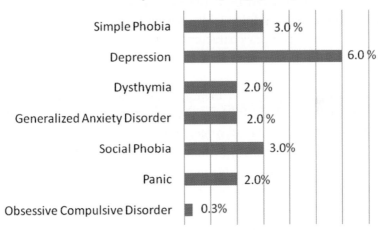

Fig. 2. Prevalence of mild mental disorders in the community.

Depression

The burden of depression has been the best studied of all the mental disorders. Depression imposes an enormous burden on society as it tends to afflict those in early and mid-adulthood — the time of maximum economic productivity. It is common, often recurrent, often underdiagnosed and often undertreated. A recent study

(Finkelstein, Berndt and Greenberg, 1996) estimated that depression cost the US economy $23 billion due to absenteeism and lost productivity and $8 billion due to premature death (in addition to the $12 billion in direct healthcare costs). In 1995, the estimated annual economic cost was $6000 per depressed worker (with employers directly bearing a cost of more than $4200 per depressed worker) (Greenberg *et al.*, 1996). A comparison of records of a large health maintenance organization (HMO) showed that depressed patients incurred an extra $1975 ($4246 vs. $2371) in health costs per year compared to non-depressed patients (Gregory, von Korff and Barlow, 1995).

Depressive illness differs from feeling depressed (which is an everyday phenomenon) by virtue of being more prolonged, severe and incapacitating (Box 1). Depression responds well to drug treatments, electroconvulsive therapy (ECT) and psychotherapy. The hopelessness engendered by depression may lead to attempts at suicide or even to successful suicide. A small proportion of depressives also have manic episodes characterized by elated mood and disinhibited and inappropriate behavior.

Case Study 1: A Sad Story — Michael

Michael was 30 years old when he got depressed. Although a worrier by nature, he was never depressed before. He complained of being depressed for 2–3 months. He was unable to work and slept poorly, waking up at 4 a.m. and not able to sleep again. He lost 4–5 kg in weight. He also complained of regularly feeling anxious and uptight. During these periods his heart would pound quickly and he felt sweaty, shaky and giddy. He admitted being very scared about these feelings. His wife said he had lost interest in sexual activities over the last few months.

Neither he nor his wife could identify a trigger for his depression. Their marriage was happy and although there was some stress at work, it was mild. Michael went on a course of antidepressants but was no better after a month. As he was not improving, hospital admission was advised. He came to the ward but became panicky and unfortunately refused to

Box 1.   Depression

Depression: How sad is sad?

How long?   At least two weeks
How bad?   Bad enough to:
            Have thoughts about death/suicide
            Have difficulties with sleeping
            Have changes in appetite or weight
            Have little interest in usual pleasures
            Have no energy
            Be markedly slowed down or agitated
            Be unable to concentrate or focus
            Feel worthless or guilty

Depression and suicide

90% of those who commit suicide suffer from some mental disorder at the time of suicide.

The commonest disorder is depression.

~5–10% of severely depressed patients will eventually commit suicide.

Physical illnesses, social isolation and male sex are risk factors.

stay and stopped taking his medications. Michael never made his next appointment and I learnt later that he had jumped to his death not long after he was last seen.

Comment: Depression often arises in early or mid-adulthood. Those who are vulnerable may develop depression even in the absence of a severe stressor. The stigma of mental illness unfortunately often results in a reluctance to be admitted to a psychiatric facility for appropriate treatment. As is often the case, the patient had become unable to work productively because of his depression. Over 90% of those dying through suicide have been shown to be mentally ill at the time of their suicide, with depression being the single most common diagnosis.

Anxiety

Anxiety disorders refer to any of these five related disorders: (1) generalized anxiety disorder, which is characterized by pervasive and incapacitating worry over normal everyday matters; (2) panic disorder, characterized by repeated episodes of panic accompanied by uncomfortable and frightening bodily sensations; (3) phobias, characterized by strong, unreasonable and incapacitating fears of objects or situations; (4) obsessive-compulsive disorder, characterized by recurrent intrusive, senseless thoughts and the accompanying rituals which are performed to reduce the anxiety level; and (5) post-traumatic stress disorder (PTSD), characterized by frightening re-experiences, bodily over-arousal and avoidance related to a traumatic event.

Phobias related to social and performance situations can lead to a significant reduction in efficiency. Avoidance is often associated with it. Panic disorders often lead to agoraphobia, a fear of situations where getting help or escape is difficult. This may lead the sufferer to avoid traveling alone. Those in certain occupations may be more prone to suffering from PTSD by virtue of their proximity to traumatic events, for example, those in the armed forces, policemen and firefighters. Anxiety disorders respond well to medications and psychotherapy.

Case Study 2: The Frequent Flyer — James

James, an executive in his late thirties, works for a company specializing in technical equipment. Part of his job description is to fly to other parts of the region to coordinate the sales of such equipment. He likes his job but intensely dislikes flying. His fear is extreme, and on a recent occasion he stopped a plane from taking off by rushing for the door and demanding to be let off just before the plane was due to take off. His regular airline had been fully booked and he was uncomfortable with the alternative carrier. To make matters worse, the recent Silk Air crash had intensified his fears.

He was able to persuade his wife to accompany him on some trips. This allayed his anxieties but was not practical on a regular basis. He tried a variety of medications with partial success and eventually found that practicing a relaxation exercise to the taped voice of his psychologist worked well.

Comment: Flying phobia is much more of a problem for someone who has to fly regularly. Not uncommonly, avoidance in the form of giving up the job for one which does not require any flying takes place. In this example, the patient has rightly chosen to work to overcome his fear.

Case Study 3: The Fearful Driver — Susan

Susan, an insurance agent in her mid-twenties, had her first panic attack whilst driving on the highway. She described experiencing a sudden, intense fear and thoughts of "choking and suffocating to death" whilst in the tunnel. It was accompanied by markedly distressing bodily sensations such as palpitations, breathlessness and dizziness. She went to the emergency department of a nearby hospital immediately but all the results were normal. After a few subsequent attacks, she began to dread traveling alone. She feared that she would lose control of the car and crash during an attack. She was however able to travel quite comfortably if she was accompanied. She presented for treatment as her traveling restrictions were interfering severely with her work as an insurance agent. She responded well to a combination of medications and cognitive behavioral psychotherapy.

Comment: Panic disorder and agoraphobia respond particularly well to cognitive behavioral psychotherapy, which seeks to help the sufferer identify and overcome inappropriate and dysfunctional thoughts and behaviors.

Alcohol and substance abuse

Alcohol abuse and dependence was the driving force behind the employee assistance movement in the US in the post-war years. Part of the motivation was the recognition of the costs alcohol abuse and dependence was having on industry. Reporting cases of opiate abuse is mandatory under Singapore law. Most companies lack any coherent protocol for dealing with a suspected abuser, though many will usually give the worker one chance at treatment before terminating employment. It is imperative to assess readiness for change in the abuser (pre-contemplation; contemplation; action; maintenance; resolution or relapse). Treatment involves an initial stage of weaning a person off the substance (detoxification) and subsequent stages of maintenance and relapse prevention. Support from groups such as Alcoholics Anonymous may help in the maintenance and relapse prevention stages.

The one-year treatment outcome of alcohol dependence at the National University Hospital, Singapore, had an encouraging result with about 60% in abstinence. One significant factor was that all the patients after discharge were cared for at home by their families (Kua *et al.*, 1990; Kua, 2004).

Case Study 4: A Sobering Tale — Raj

Raj, a self-employed businessman in his forties operating shipping services, presented for treatment somewhat reluctantly at the instigation of his wife and brother. He downplayed his drinking problem and consistently denied that he was an "alcoholic". He admitted to drinking two bottles of beer (his wife and brother said it was 2–3 times this amount) every day after work. He had started drinking whilst in the Navy but this had increased significantly over the last two years after he left to start his own business. His wife reported that he would come back drunk every night and that recently he had missed several important contracts as he could not get up in time. He admitted to feeling tremulous and irritable if he did not consume a small amount of alcohol in the morning. Unfortunately, Raj checked out of treatment after a few days and a pattern of readmissions and premature discharges occurred. Eventually, further admissions were blocked by the psychiatrist as he showed little change and continued to deny the severity of his drinking. He eventually lost his business and his wife through divorce.

Comment: It is common for those dependent on alcohol and other substances to underestimate their consumption and to deny the problem until a late stage. Unfortunately at this stage significant and sometimes irreversible health, occupational and familial dysfunction may have occurred.

Schizophrenia and other psychotic illnesses

The hallmark of schizophrenia and other related psychotic illnesses is the loss of touch with reality manifesting as psychotic symptoms — hallucinations (false perceptions), delusions (false beliefs) and bizarre behavior. These disorders may also be accompanied by disorganization of thought, leading to severe occupational impairment. A significant proportion of patients respond well to medications. In the presence of paranoid persecutory beliefs, the potential risks to others in the workplace have to be carefully considered, as illustrated by the case below. Contrary to popular opinion, violence and aggression is very much the exception rather than the rule and is limited to only a small minority of such cases.

Case Study 5: The Mentally Ill Worker — The Human Resource Manager's Dilemma

Mr Lee is in his late thirties and has been suffering from paranoid schizophrenia for the last two years. His job in a chemical company involves the use of potentially hazardous chemical agents. He has given good service to his present company for the last 15 years and has even received a long service certificate of commendation. Over the last two years, however, he has become withdrawn and suspicious. Things came to a head recently when he accused two fellow co-workers of being involved in a conspiracy with the police to spy on him. He complained that his computer terminal was wired to a central one in the organization and that his moves and communications were being monitored. He was seen by a psychiatrist and prescribed medications but was never compliant with medications or his appointments. His job performance had steadily declined. According to his HR manager, he was only performing at about 10% of what was expected for his job seniority. In addition, his colleagues felt that they had to constantly monitor and "babysit" him. His HR manager was also worried about the possibility of an unpleasant and dangerous situation involving toxic chemicals in view of his paranoid beliefs about his colleagues. On the occasions when his HR manager attempted to talk to him about his job performance, he reacted

206 Textbook of Occupational Medicine Practice, 3rd Edition

angrily, saying that his Union would resist any move to retire him prematurely. The company doctor felt unable to make a decision about him and requested that the hospital convene a "medical board" to decide on his ability to work.

Comment: Mr Lee's case is not uncommon and his lack of compliance is likely to work against him significantly. Unfortunately, psychiatrists are often hesitant to say anything which may be construed as detrimental to their patient and consequently little if any practical significance may be communicated. His poor performance, lack of compliance and the potential for harm to others make his retirement on health grounds reasonable. If possible, alternative, less demanding, safer jobs can be offered (preferably at the same pay) but not uncommonly this is unacceptable to the patient (or the company). Hospitals do not convene medical boards on behalf of private companies and the psychiatrist's role here is to provide a medical opinion on fitness to work. The final decision remains the responsibility of the company.

Psychosomatic Problems

Psychosomatic problems are those where psychological factors are felt to be the predominant driving force behind physical symptoms or loss of function. The mind and body are intricately connected and in such cases, the body may "speak" on behalf of the mind via physical symptoms. Studies of those going to see their family physician have found that over half have little or no physical abnormality that can be detected, suggesting that reassurance and biopsychosocial factors may be behind the majority of consultations. Psychosomatic problems are a major contributor to absenteeism and health utilization.

Case Study 6: The Painful Issue of Pain — Albert

Albert, a supervisor at a construction firm in his forties, first presented to the emergency services with left chest pain. He was admitted for further investigations which proved to be normal. A musculoskeletal cause of his pain was entertained and analgesics were prescribed. Further history taking also revealed that his wife was suffering from chronic renal failure and having regular dialysis, that he was having to look after his 12-year-old son as well, and that he was having difficulties with his superior at work whom he felt was victimizing him. He felt like shouting back at his superior but controlled himself and felt trapped as he did not wish to impose more work on the workers he was supervising. He improved rapidly and after three days was well enough to be discharged. He was given a medical certificate for a further two days which he felt was insufficient. He requested an additional two days but his doctor refused. He angrily retorted that this being the case, he would come back with chest pain again at night. True to his word, he presented to the emergency department with the same pain and was readmitted much to the chagrin of his doctor. A request was made for the psychiatrist to assist in his management. Before he could be seen again, he had presented himself for readmission for giddiness and headache.

Comment: Psychosomatic problems require close collaboration between the physician and the psychiatrist. Albert was assessed and an attempt was made to help him see a link between his stress, feelings, bodily symptoms and behavior, which was partially successful. He was seen regularly as an outpatient and a problem-solving orientation was outlined. Over 60% of private companies employing 25 or more employees in Singapore implement measures to control sickness absence (usually counseling, disciplinary procedures and attendance allowance or bonus). Over 13% use computerized records to monitor sickness absence (Chan, Gan and Sia, 1997).

Sleep Problems

Inadequate sleep resulting in fatigue, reduced alertness and increased error and accidents is the primary sleep problem in the workplace. Major disasters such as the Three Mile Island accident, the Chernobyl accident, the tragedy of the space shuttle *Challenger* and the accident of the supertanker *Exxon Valdez* have all been partly attributed to inadequate sleep. Estimates of the costs range from US$300 billion in the Chernobyl disaster to US$52 billion in the *Exxon Valdez* accident (US$1 billion to clean up the oil spill, US$1 billion in fines and an outstanding US$50 billion in civil suits) (Moore-Ede, 1993). Signs of inadequate sleep include feeling sleepy in the day; irritability and poor concentration; and difficulty keeping awake in boring or mundane situations (watching TV or listening to boring or mundane talks/ lectures). A study of 3087 subjects in the community in Singapore found 15.5% complaining of insomnia (male 12.9%, female 17.5%) (Yeo *et al.*, 1996).

Personality Disorders

Everyone has weaknesses and faults within their personality. When these are particularly severe, causing significant impairment and/or distress to the sufferer or others, a diagnosis of a personality disorder (Box 2) is entertained. As the term "personality" denotes, such attributes are enduring and longstanding, evident from late childhood or early adolescence onwards. Such painful (for others) and pain-full (full of pain themselves) people can cause severe dysfunction within a company.

Box 2.   Personality Disorder, Behavior and Thoughts

Personality Disorder and Behavior
Based on DSM-IV personality disorders

Paranoid	Suspicious and hypervigilant
Schizotypal	Eccentric non-conformity
Schizoid	Solitary and self-reliant
Dependent	Over-dependence on others
Obsessive	Perfectionist, rigid and meticulous
Avoidant	Timid and poor conflict tolerance
Histrionic	Overdramatic and needy for attention
Antisocial	Opportunist and predatory
Narcissistic	Morbid self-love and self-interest
Borderline	Impulsive, chaotic and hypersensitive

(Continued)

(*Continued*)

Personality Disorder and Thoughts

Dependent clinger	"I'm helpless, weak and needy. Don't abandon me!"
Fearful avoider	"I may get hurt or rejected. I can't stand being hurt."
Obsessed perfectionist	"I must not err. I must always be in complete control."
Antisocial troublemaker	"People are there to be taken advantage of."
Detached loner	"Don't violate my personal space."
Suspicious paranoid	"All people are potential enemies."
Dramatic attention seeker	"I need to impress all the time."
Narcissistic egotist	"I am very special."

Work Stress

There is a myth that stress at work is bad. As stress is ubiquitous in our environment and day-to-day life, the only form of "stress-free" life would be no life at all — death. A distinction has to made between stress and distress. Indeed, one should expect work to be stressful in that it brings challenges and improves performance but it should not be distressing. Where stress becomes distress depends on the type, duration and intensity of the stress as well as the person the stress acts on. Depending on this stress–person interaction, three outcomes are possible: "break down", "break even" and "break through". It must be remembered that work has positive effects too. Job loss has been shown to have a significant effect on the health and well-being of many unemployed people and their families.

In our local context, actual figures relating to the costs and consequences of work stress are hard to come by, but a recent cover story in *Asian Business* suggests from anecdotal data and observations that work and executive stress is on the rise in Asia (Asian Business, 1995). Because of the complexity involved in stress research, available figures are not precise and merely represent "guesstimates". What they do show, however, and there is little disagreement here, is that work stress contributes significantly to serious mental and physical ill-health and that it is costly — to individuals, families and organizations.

Effects of work stress

Some possible effects of having too much stress at work are listed in Table 2.

Sources of work stress

Work environment and ergonomics

Stress occurs when environmental factors are extreme; fluctuate greatly or are unexpected and/or unpredictable; or are poorly matched for the job concerned (e.g. lighting).

Ergonomic factors relate to the poor equipment or workplace design and to poor techniques relating to the usage of equipment. A local study of 363 civil servants found that minor illnesses not resulting in sickness absence were more strongly correlated with work stress than minor

Table 2.   Possible Effects of Work Stress

Physical	Psychological	Behavioral	Occupational
Aches and pains	Depression	Smoking	Absenteeism
Tense feeling	Anxiety/worry	Drinking	Decreased productivity
Headaches	Fear	Recklessness	Low morale
Stomach pain	Hysterical overreaction	Absent-mindedness	Increased accidents and errors
More infections	Irritability	Overeating	Increased turnover
Poor sleep	Distrust	Aggression	Sabotage and violence
Tiredness	Poor concentration	Compulsions	Dissatisfaction
Hair loss	Loss of balance	Social withdrawal	More sick leave

illnesses resulting in sickness absence. Improving the physical work environment appeared to alleviate absenteeism more (Woo *et al.*, 1999).

Type of work

Examples of these factors include shift work, long hours and risky occupations. Studies have found that shift work may lead to poor health in various occupations. A longer work shift (though this helps workers re-adapt to their sleep patterns) and being married with children adds to the stress.

Experts are increasingly concerned about the ill-effects of working hours that are too long. The irony is that working beyond 40 hours a week is now thought to lead to decreasing productivity.

Certain occupations have a potential for harm or death (for example, in policemen, armed forces personnel and firefighters) and this may lead to stress. The constant presence of or potential for risk and danger can lead to a constant state of arousal, which may wear down the body and mind.

Demands and control/resources

Work overload may be due to either having too much or too difficult work (or both). Overload may also be the result of inadequate resources or support available within the organization. One aspect of overload is the requirement to keep up with information or technology. Although new technology can be a great help in reducing our workload, in certain circumstances, coping with new technology and information can be stressful — particularly if there is inadequate support and training. Some corporations now have chief information officers (CIOs) to help manage the vast flows of information. Work overload is consistently found to be the most important source of stress (Boey *et al.*, 1997).

Work underload results from too little work or work which is unchallenging, unstimulating, routine or boring. Repetitive, dehumanizing work (Cooper and Smith, 1985) has been described as a form of work stress (especially short-cycle, monotonous, repetitive, machine-type work). Having no meaningful work is very stressful — unemployment increases the risks of mental and physical ill health (Fryer and Payne, 1986).

Role factors

Role factors encompass the roles, expectations and responsibilities associated with work.

Role ambiguity or uncertainty occurs when individuals are uncertain about just what exactly their job entails, for example, its objectives, their superior's expectations, what is and is not part of the job. Any change to the job or one's position may bring uncertainty.

Role conflict occurs when the person finds a mismatch between what the job demands and what the person feels is right, is part of the job or is what he actually wants to do.

Responsibilities can be either for people or for things. Responsibility for people (and especially if one has to make unpleasant decisions about them) appears to be the more stressful of the two. The opposite, of having little influence in decisions, can also be stressful.

Non-participation may be associated with role ambiguity and perceptions of lack of control within the organization.

Career development, termination, transition, expectation and entitlement

Examples of transition include job entry, job loss (Kates, Greiff and Hagan, 1990), relocation, retrenchment, retirement and corporate merger. In relocation, those most stressed appear to be married couples with young children, while those least stressed are married without children (Cooper, 1981).

Examples of career blockage include non-promotion, demotion, lack of progress and career blockage in women. Poor pay or remuneration and lack of appreciation can be potent sources of work stress.

Uncertainties about one's continued ability to remain in work can be highly stressful, such as a lack of job stability and/or fear of dismissal or retrenchment. The knowledge that one's performance is being monitored can be stressful, especially if the feedback/findings are not used wisely and tactfully.

Interpersonal factors

Poor interpersonal relationships and unhealthy attachments account for a great deal of stress at work. The quality of employer/executive–employee relationships is one of the most (if not the most) important non-technological factors which affects productivity (Rizzo and Mendez, 1990). Certain qualities such as self-centredness, abrasiveness (driven, over-demanding perfectionists bordering on the tyrannical — often highly ambitious, impatient, insensitive, overly negative and aggressive) (Levinson, 1978) and shyness may cause problems with relating in the workplace. Stress arises in relationships with superiors when there is a perception of unfairness, inconsideration or victimization.

Stress from peer relationships usually arises from competition, communication difficulties and personality conflicts. A study on work stress and mental distress in Singapore found that the main work problem in managers was conflict with employers or directors (superiors) and not their workers. Their scores on the Work Environment Scale indicated that they had little support from their superiors and perceived the work pressure to be overwhelming. Workers however cited difficulty with fellow workers as their main problem and complained of poor peer cohesion (Kua *et al.*, 1989).

There is a myth that equates success with the "strong", hard-driving, tough, independent boss. What matters more is whether an executive can comfortably depend on the support of others and trust them. A successful executive is confident of himself and confident on relying on others. Confidence, trust and mutual respect are important qualities here.

Home–work interface

A healthy family life protects people from stress, whereas an unhealthy one merely adds to the stress at work. Stresses include marital conflicts, children, in-laws, maids and grandparents. Repeated separations and absences due to work-related travel appear to be stressful for some families (Land, 1988).

Dual-career stress refers to women having to work as well as looking after the family. Problems which may arise are overload, money issues, jealousy, postponing having children, etc. A study of 500 consecutive admissions to the psychiatric unit at the National University Hospital, Singapore, found that married working women were most vulnerable to mental illness. The most often cited stressor was their husbands. Married women had higher work stress (58.5% vs. 46.2%) and family stress (37.7% vs. 32.3%) than singles (Kua *et al.*, 1996).

Self–work interface

With increasingly competitive and materialistic attitudes, money is often a major source of stress. Studies suggest that so long as a person is not in poverty, having more does not necessarily bring happiness. In a report on policemen who commit suicide, financial stresses were listed as the commonest major stress factor.

Any significant life event or change is stressful — even changes which we may see as positive, i.e. promotion, pregnancy, going on vacation, though changes which are perceived as negative are even more stressful. There is some evidence to support the notion that too many life changes in a particular time span will increase stress and therefore the likelihood of falling ill physically or mentally.

Organization structure, culture and climate

Organizational factors and "office politics" can be a substantial stress factor. Like any family, an organization has a particular structure, culture and climate. Management researchers Kets de Vries and Danny Miller describe five types of maladaptive organization functioning:

(1) The dramatic organization: Headed by dramatic, power-hungry, megalomaniacal individuals. An example of such an individual would be Robert Maxwell who was described by his workers as tyrannical and megalomaniacal.
(2) The paranoid organization: Characterized by suspicion and insecurity, tracking and fighting enemies (real and imaginary) to such an extent as to neglect its business and customers' needs and desires.
(3) The compulsive organization: Characterized by constant striving for total control, completeness and thoroughness.
(4) The depressive organization: Characterized by defeatist attitudes, inactivity, lack of confidence and passivity. Examples include Ford and General Motors in the 1980s.
(5) The schizoid organization: The CEO becomes a recluse and is unavailable, withdrawing from contact and leaving a leadership vacuum. One such example is Howard Hughes and the Hughes Aircraft Company (de Vries and Miller, 1990).

Box 3. What the Worker Can Do

Acknowledge
↓
Appraise
↓
Act
↓
Adjust

four steps to personal stress management

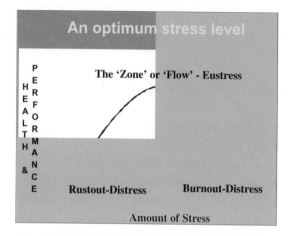

Fig. 3. Stress levels and performance and health.

Stress management

Stress management requires first the acknowledgment that one may be suffering from undesirable effects of stress (Box 3); followed by an appraisal of the sources of stress (for example, by means of a checklist as shown in Box 4), its effects and possible resources, changes and interventions for that individual. Interventions are acted upon with the goal of behavior and cognitive change. A review to adjust and improve one's coping strategies is the final step (Fig 3).

Box 4.   Work Stress Checklist

Work Stress Checklist

Rate how the following sources of work stress apply to you over the **last month**.
Stress ratings: 1 = None   2 = Slight   3 = Moderate   4 = High
                5 = Intense

(Continued)

(*Continued*)

1.	My work environment	1	2	3	4	5
2.	Poor equipment or office design (ergonomic factors)	1	2	3	4	5
3.	Shift work	1	2	3	4	5
4.	Long working hours	1	2	3	4	5
5.	Risky/Dangerous work	1	2	3	4	5
6.	Too much work/ demands (overload)	1	2	3	4	5
7.	Too difficult work (overload)	1	2	3	4	5
8.	Time pressures and deadlines (overload)	1	2	3	4	5
9.	Lack of resources/ personnel (overload)	1	2	3	4	5
10.	Too little work (underload)	1	2	3	4	5
11.	Too easy or unstimulating work (underload)	1	2	3	4	5
12.	Keeping up with new developments and technology	1	2	3	4	5
13.	Traveling related to work	1	2	3	4	5
14.	Traveling to and from work	1	2	3	4	5
15.	Uncertainty about what job is all about	1	2	3	4	5
16.	Conflict between my own beliefs/values and my organization's	1	2	3	4	5
17.	Difficulty in managing/ making decisions about people	1	2	3	4	5

(*Continued*)

(*Continued*)

18.	Lack of power and influence	1	2	3	4	5
19.	Major job transition (i.e. relocation, job entry)	1	2	3	4	5
20.	Job insecurity/Major organization transition	1	2	3	4	5
21.	Poor pay or rewards	1	2	3	4	5
22.	Feeling undervalued or unappreciated	1	2	3	4	5
23.	Lack of or difficulty with promotion	1	2	3	4	5
24.	My relationship with my superior(s)/ boss(es)	1	2	3	4	5
25.	My relationship with my peers/colleagues	1	2	3	4	5
26.	My relationship with my subordinates	1	2	3	4	5
27.	Interference of work with my private and social life	1	2	3	4	5
28.	Interference of work with my family life	1	2	3	4	5
29.	Lack of communication in my organization	1	2	3	4	5
30.	Office "politics"	1	2	3	4	5
31.	Poor corporate culture, structure and climate	1	2	3	4	5
32.	Other: _____	1	2	3	4	5

What organizations can do

The traditional approach to work stress has been to make the employee responsible for managing his stress and that the employee should be thankful if the organization provides some resources to help "stress-proof" the employee (Table 3). Thankfully this view is slowly changing and some enlightened organizations are acknowledging that an important source of stress may be the organization itself. The result has been healthier employees and organizations with the added benefits of improved morale, performance, absenteeism rates, turnover rates and productivity (Zaccaro and Riley, 1987).

Table 3.   What Organizations Can Do

1. **Environmental and Ergonomics**
   Environmental factors
      Improve design of working environment; assess and reduce stressful environments
      Facilitate task accomplishments
      Soothing ambience, colors, sounds, scents, visuals, temperature
      Remove noxious agents, dangerous conditions
      Improve air quality to reduce sick building syndrome
   Ergonomic factors
      Improve design of work tools/equipment
      Education on lifting, back care, repetitive strain, VDU strain, etc.

2. **Type of Work**
   Shift work
      Allow for consistent/fixed vs. rotating shifts
      Select shifts which minimize body clock disruption
   Long hours
      Limit work hours; flexible work schedules
      Allow employee to manage time to fit needs
   Dangerous work
      Maximize safety; adequate training and support

3. **Demands and Control/Resources**
   Work overload
      Set more reasonable quotas; establish reasonable performance goals
      Make resources, training and support adequate and accessible

(*Continued*)

Table 3.   (*Continued*)

Work underload
Provide quotas/targets; job/task redesign

4. **Role Factors**
   Ambiguity/Uncertainty
   Define job requirement(s) and areas(s) of responsibility clearly
   Make rewards contingent upon performance; frequent feedback on performance
   Allow for feedback of worker's perception of problems; access to supervisors.
   Role conflict
   Eliminate conflicting expectations; improve person–work match or fit
   Non-participation
   Participative management

5. **Career Development, Termination, Transition, Expectation and Entitlement Transitions**
   Provide transition stage counseling, i.e. retirement, relocation (Siegel, 1988; Sherwood and DeSimone, 1983), retrenchment, etc.
   Career development
   Self and organizational assessment
   Clarification of career paths; provision of career counseling

6. **Interpersonal Factors**
   Relationship factors
   Encourage constructive relationships; provide group/unit goals and rewards; encourage collectivism vs. individualism (where appropriate); encourage access to supervisors; provide accessible counseling; provide adequate training in communication, assertiveness and team building; provide opportunity to address and resolve conflicts; provide methods for integrating new employees; create support groups

7. **Home–Work Interface**
   Home–work interface
   Recognize and provide for work–family interface
   Enhance fit between work and home responsibilities; allow for "home-based" work
   Engage service providers to help with errands, shopping, etc. for employee
   Dual-career stress
   Provide options for childcare; on-site childcare
   Flexible schedules; adequate maternity (and paternity) leave without penalty
   Provision of education/skills on parenthood, marital enhancement, etc.

(*Continued*)

Table 3. (*Continued*)

8. **Self–Work Interface**
   Self–work interface
   Support of employees to engage in areas of personal interest

9. **Organization Structure, Culture and Climate**
   Climate
   Allow regular feedback of worker's suggestions, perceptions of problems and the organization
   Structure
   Reduce authoritarianism and increase employee control and responsibility; increase co-worker support; allow for semi-autonomous work groups; assess task demands Institute restructuring to provide more satisfying, less stressful work
   Culture
   "Learning" organization; social and charitable focus

Emotional Competence(s)

Emotional factors relating to work performance have become one of the fastest growing fields in organizational psychology. Howard Gardner's concept of "multiple intelligences", Robert Sternberg's "successful intelligence" and Daniel Goleman's popularization of the concept of emotional intelligence (Goleman, 1995; 1988) has helped to heighten awareness of the importance of emotional competency in the work setting. Unfortunately, popular science has accelerated far beyond proper scientific evaluation of many of these concepts (Box 5).

The three most highly sought-after skills in new employees in the mid-nineties in the United States were good communication, interpersonal and teamwork skills. Such emotional competency can be thought of as specific "life skills" which determine one's success at work. IQ scores have been found to correlate poorly with career success, with figures ranging from 25% (Hunter and Schmidt, 1984) to 4% (Sternberg, 1996). This is especially so for so-called "professional" careers (i.e. medicine, law, engineering) (Spencer and Spencer, 1993).

Box 5.   Emotional Competencies and Training

Emotional Competencies

Self-awareness

Self-confidence

Self-control

Self-esteem

Creativity and flexibility

Optimism and realism

Commitment, challenge
and change

Learning and self-mastery
focus

Strong core values

Wisdom and common sense

Getting along

Listening and communicating

Anger control

Conflict control

Problem solving

Collaboration

Teamwork

Helping others

Service orientation

Emotional Competencies Training

Adapted from Goleman D, *Working with Emotional Intelligence*
(1998)

Assess

The work

The individual

The resources

Readiness to change

Motivation

Feedback

Set specific realistic goals

Individualize

Arrange Support

Provide models

Encourage practice

Encourage learning

Prevent relapse

Reward change

Reward effort

Evaluate and improve

Provide help

Developing a corporate mental health program

The level of organizational input into corporate mental health can
vary from non-existent to comprehensive, with the provision of full
leisure, sport and recreation facilities, complete medical cover that
includes mental illnesses, and employee assistance programs (EAPs)

which identify and assist troubled employees (often with the provision of counseling services). EAPs evolved in the United States out of industrial alcoholism programs in the post-war years. EAPs are more likely to be offered by larger corporations, especially those in the communications, transportation, utilities, finance, realty and insurance industries. 81% of corporations engaged an external provider compared to 17% which utilized internal providers. In the local context, corporate mental health programs vary from non-existent to partial. Most organizations offer medical and dental benefits, and some may have their own doctors, but it is unlikely any will go so far as providing an EAP.

The care of mentally ill workers is usually through a private or public health provider. Such healthcare providers are likely to feel that their first obligation is to their client and consequently are reluctant to offer any significant findings that may be damaging to their client. Corporations should understand this and always seek the consent of the employee to liaise with their healthcare provider. Asking specific questions relating to medical facts requiring "yes", "no" or factual answers will usually facilitate a useful response. External healthcare providers will usually leave the final decision of employment with the organization or company doctor. Organizations vary in their tolerance for workers with a diagnosis of mental illness but it should be borne in mind that the bulk of mental illnesses afflicting workers will be considered minor. These are usually highly amenable to treatment and, on resolution, there is no reason why a worker should not be able to return to full performance and make a valuable contribution to the organization.

Case Study 7: An Issue of Risks and Dangers — Peter

Peter is a train driver in his forties. He takes great pride in his work and one could say he was even "married to it". So much so that it caused a severe rift in his marriage and family life. Feeling more and more neglected, his wife turned to another man for solace and comfort. Not long after that, his wife began to talk about her intention to separate from him. Peter sank into a severe depression and at its worst it was difficult to ascertain if he had lost touch with reality — he began to entertain notions that his colleagues were sabotaging his train. In desperation, he took an overdose to escape from his mental pain. He was found by his wife and brought to hospital. He was commenced on medications and made a fairly good recovery. He recovered well enough to return to work but was requested to change to a non-driving job, much to his annoyance. He protested that he had recovered and that driving trains was his only source of affirmation now that his marriage had broken down. He pleaded that he be allowed to resume driving. He was upset about his psychiatrist's recommendation and tended to downplay his illness.

Comment: A significant suicide attempt often raises sufficient concern for a change of job status to be recommended. Such behavior suggests that an individual is vulnerable to severe perturbation and may act in a similar manner whilst under distress in future. This, coupled with the issue of public safety, often forces a recommendation to err on the side of caution. Pay should ideally not be affected and goodwill and understanding shown on both sides.

Motivations for starting such a program may range from cost savings (a number of studies show cost savings in the longer term), medico-legal protection, worker demands, good public relations, improved worker benefits, to a strong corporate culture pertaining to worker health and well-being Box 6. Regardless of the motivation, three key factors to a successful program are availability, accessibility and attractiveness. Workers have different needs and priorities and a range of products should be available to meet these differing needs. Ease of access is likely to influence the utilization. The recent explosion in the use of interactive health-focused websites on a corporate intranet allows for easy and confidential access to information. On-line and interactive counseling programs are currently under study but it is highly unlikely that these will be able to replace a face-to-face meeting with a counselor or health professional. Programs have to be attractive enough to capture and retain the attention of the user. For example, holding a program during the work week is likely to be better supported than one after working hours; as are programs suggested and requested by a significant proportion of the workers themselves. One of the biggest challenges is the engagement of those workers most likely to benefit from such programs (usually they are also the ones least likely to attend). Not uncommonly, the majority of workers attending certain programs are those who are the most motivated and the healthiest — the ones who are least in need of them!

Two of the commonest deficiencies of such programs is poor assessment of the mental health needs and priorities of the organization and poor evaluation of the actual efficacy of such programs. Traditionally, evaluation has consisted of feedback from the participants. Various studies have shown that these may be poor indicators of actual effectiveness (for example, participants may rate certain courses appealing and helpful but no actual benefit can be demonstrated, or worse a negative effect may result from them).

Self-help resources are less threatening and may result in a higher utilization rate if easily accessible. Changing the theme and focus regularly may help sustain interest and participation. Examples of possible themes are given in Box 7. One of the most popular interventions is the use of stress management talks and workshops. An example of a typical one-day course is shown in Box 7. It has to be acknowledged that these interventions have not been rigorously studied, though anecdotal evidence suggests some benefit.

Box 6.   Getting Started

Find out problems, needs and wants
    Doing a survey and get a baseline
    Personal interviews
Find resources and support
    Speaking with the bosses
Get people
    Designate and train facilitators
    Set up a dedicated committee
Get ideas
    Brainstorm ideas
    Speak to others, see other programs

(Continued)

(*Continued*)

Provide self-help resources
  Resource center
  Resource person
  Intranet website (interactive)
Simple programs to start
  Health talks
  Workshops
  Health check/fair
Promoting interest and motivation
  Theme focus of the month
  Focus on wellness as well as illness
  Reward participation
Review and adjust
  Feedback
  Results and effects
  Rethink carrots and sticks

Box 7.   Stress Management Program and Themes for Talks and Workshops

One-day stress management program
  Stress and its development; recognizing and measuring stress
  Group discussion and break
  Stress and personality; effects of stress; anger and hostility
  Summing up
  Lunch
  Managing individual stress; work stress
  Group discussion and break
  Marriage/Relationships and stress; time management
  Relaxation therapy and guided imagery
  Summing up

(*Continued*)

(Continued)

Themes for talks and workshops

- Stress
- Weight control
- Eating healthily
- Anger
- Worry and depression
- Fear and anxiety
- Enhancing relationships
- Focus on the family
- Stop smoking
- Addictions
- Emotional intelligence
- Back care and ergonomics
- Changing bad habits
- Dealing with family stresses
- Communication
- Moral intelligence
- Music and the mind
- Bringing up children
- Handling changes and transitions
- Surviving trauma
- Beating travel stress
- Knowing yourself
- Successful self-esteem
- Sleeping soundly
- Sexual problems
- Thinking yourself to health

Case Study 8: How One Company Does It — Hewlett-Packard (Singapore)

Hewlett-Packard (Singapore) is part of a multinational organization dealing with computer and office products. It places a strong emphasis on worker wellness and has a clubhouse with a pool and gym. It also has a resource center where videos and books are available for loan. These are accessible on the company's intranet. It allows for part-time work, job sharing, flexi-time and telecommuting as work options subject to management approval (with nature of the job, personality of applicant and whether the option makes business sense as the three key considerations). It offers standard medical and dental benefits and provides a small holiday accommodation subsidy. It has full-time wellness officers and arranges talks, workshops and sporting/family activities. Worker well-being and improvement are emphasized and staff are encouraged to attend workshops and seminars. Although it does not have a specific corporate mental health program, many of the provisions do reduce work stress.

Websites

www.mentalhealth.com *Comprehensive website offering on-line diagnosis for all the mental disorders discussed in this chapter and excellent links*

www.rcpsych.ac.uk/public *Download and print the excellent Royal College of Psychiatrists' (UK) "Help is at Hand" series of leaflets covering all the major mental disorders*

www.nimh.nih.gov *Download brochures, fact sheets and educational information from the American National Institute of Mental Health*

www.cdc.gov/niosh *Download the excellent "Stress at Work" booklet and files on ergonomics. A vast range of occupational health material*

www.intelihealth.com *Excellent source of health information. You may opt for a regular e-mail update on various topics including mental health*

www.apa.org *Website of the American Psychological Association*

References

Asian Business. (1995) Executive stress: A company killer. *Asian Business*, August, 22–26.

Boey KW, Chan KB, Ko YC, *et al.* (1997) Work stress and psychological well-being among the nursing profession in Singapore. *Singapore Med J* **38**: 256–260.

Chan OY, Gan SL, Chia SE. (1997) Sickness absence in private sector establishments in Singapore. *Singapore Med J* **38**: 379–383.

Cooper C. (1981) *Executive Families under Stress.* Englewood Cliffs: Prentice-Hall.

Cooper C, Smith M. (1985) *Job Stress and Blue Collar Work.* London: John Wiley.

de Vries KM, Miller D. (1990) *The Neurotic Organization: Diagnosing and Revitalising Unhealthy Companies.* New York: Harper Business.

Finkelstein SN, Berndt ER, Greenberg PE. (1996) Economics of depression. Prepared for the consensus conference on the undertreatment of depression. January 17–18.

Fones CSL, Kua EH, Ng TP, Ko SM. (1998) Studying the mental health of a nation. *Singapore Med J* 38: 251–255.

Fryer D, Payne R. (1986) Being unemployed. In: Cooper C, Robertson T (eds). *International Review of Industrial and Organizational Psychology.* Chichester: John Wiley.

Goleman D. (1995) *Emotional Intelligence.* New York: Bantam Books.

Goleman D. (1998) *Working with Emotional Intelligence.* London: Bloomsbury.

Greenberg PE, Kessler RC, Nells TL, *et al.* (1996) Depression in the workplace: An economic perspective. In: Feighner JP, Boyer WF (eds). *Selective Serotonin Re uptake Inhibitors: Advances in Basic Research and Clinical Practice,* 2nd edn. New York, NY: John Wiley & Sons Ltd.

Gregory S, von Korff M, Barlow W. (1995) Health care costs in primary care patients with recognized depression. *Arch Gen Psychiatry* 52: 850–856.

Hunter JB, Schmidt FL. (1984) Validity and utility of alternative predictors of job performance. *Psychol Bulletin* 96: 72–98.

Kates N, Greiff B, Hagan D. (1990) *The Psychosocial Impact of Job Loss.* Washington, DC: American Psychiatric Press.

Kessler RC, Frank RG. (1997) Impact of psychiatric disorders on work loss days. *Psychol Med* 27: 861–873.

Kua EH, Tian CS, Lai L, Ko SM. (1989) Work stress and mental distress. *Singapore Med J* 30: 343–345.

Kua EH, Ko SM, Chan P, Nair N. (1996) Women and mental illness. *ASEAN Journal of Psychiatry* 4: 43–51.

Kua EH, Ko SM, Tian CS, *et al.* (1990) A follow-up study of Asian problem drinkers. *Addiction* 85: 571–573.

Kua EH. (2004) Psychiatry in Singapore. *Br J Psychiatry* 185: 79–82.

Land D. (1988) *The Phantom Spouse.* New York: Dodd Mead.

Levinson H. (1978) The abrasive personality. *Harvard Business Review,* May–June, 86–87.

Moore-Ede M. (1993) *The 24-Hour Society*. London: Piatkus.

Murray C, Lopez A. (1997) Global mortality, disability and the contribution of risk factors: Global burden of disease study. *Lancet* **349**: 1436–1442.

Rizzo A, Mendez C. (1990) *The Integration of Women in Management: A Guide for Human Resources and Management Development Specialists.* New York: Quorum Books.

Sherwood M, DeSimone J. (1983) Relocation counseling: Current status and potential. In: Manuso J (ed). *Occupational Clinical Psychology*, pp. 202–214. New York: Praeger.

Siegel D. (1988) Relocation counselling and services. In: Gould S, Smith M (eds). *Social Work in the Workplace: Practice and Principles*, pp. 109–122. New York: Springer.

Spencer LM, Spencer SM. (1993) *Competence at Work*. New York: John Wiley and Sons.

Sternberg R. (1996) *Successful Intelligence*. New York: Simon & Schuster.

Woo M, Yap AK, Oh TG, Long FY. (1999) The relationship between stress and absenteeism. *Singapore Med J* **40**: 9.

Yeo BK, Perera IS, Kok LP, Tsoi WF. (1996) Insomnia in the community. *Singapore Med J* **37**: 282–284.

Zaccaro SJ, Riley AW. (1987) Stress, coping and organizational effectiveness. In: *Occupational Stress and Organizational Effectiveness.* New York: Praeger.

Chapter 9

Musculoskeletal Disorders

Alphonsus Chong,* Naresh S Kumar,*
Eng-Hin Lee*,† and Hee-Kit Wong*

Neck, Shoulder and Upper Limb Problems

Case Study 1

A 32-year-old woman presented with a one-month history of stiffness and aching in the neck and right shoulder. She also had a feeling of tiredness in her right arm and hand with occasional cramps and numbness in the fingers. An examination showed tenderness in her trapezius muscles bilaterally (more on the right), and tenderness in her forearm extensor muscles. There was pain in her neck on extreme lateral rotation and lateral flexion. The neurological examination was normal.

Further questioning revealed that she had been working in her present job as an accounting-machine operator for about three months. In addition to her neck and arm symptoms, she also complained of feeling tired and irritable and was also experiencing some eye strain.

An analysis of her workplace showed that she had to sit with neck bent forwards and tilted to the left at her desk. Her

*University of Orthopaedics, Hand and Reconstructive Microsurgery Cluster,
National University Health System (NUHS), Singapore.
†Corresponding author. E-mail: dosleeeh@nus.edu.sg.

right arm was lifted off the desk while her hand was touching the keyboard of the accounting machine. The height of her desk was found to be too high for her chair, which made it necessary for her to overcompensate for the height by lifting her right arm higher and tilting her torso.

This woman was diagnosed as suffering from repetitive strain injury and a recommendation was made for ergonomic changes to her workplace.

Case Study 2

A 42-year-old carpenter of 20 years presented with severe neck, right shoulder and arm pain that had lasted for two weeks. The pain was aggravated when he turned his neck to the left or looked upwards. He also complained of numbness in his right thumb and index finger.

Clinically, he was found to have tenderness in his right trapezius and interscapular region. There was also tenderness in the right lateral epicondyle with pain on resisted dorsiflexion of his wrist. There was a diminished right biceps jerk with decreased sensation over the C6 dermatome and weakness of his biceps muscle.

Radiographs of the cervical spine showed narrowing of the C5–6 disc space with osteophytic encroachment into the C5–6 neural foramina in the oblique views. A diagnosis of cervical spondylosis and a right tennis elbow (lateral epicondylitis) was made.

He was given medical leave and sent for physiotherapy which saw an improvement in his symptoms. An analysis of his workplace showed that he had to work on a very low workbench. As a result he had to bend forward excessively and extend his neck while he was working. Suggestions were made to improve the ergonomics of his workplace.

Commentary on clinical cases

These two cases illustrate several features of repetitive strain injury (RSI) affecting the neck, shoulder and upper limb. Firstly, in RSI, symptoms arising from multiple body parts are common presenting feature. Second, the time interval between the start of the work and the development of symptoms may vary significantly. This is because other factors such as aging may play a part in the development of the condition and onset of symptoms. Finally, in the overall management of these conditions, changes in the workplace environment and work activities often need to be made for successful management of the problem.

Introduction

Work-related musculoskeletal disorders are common. Workers who spend long hours at a desk, workstation or in a factory have a significant incidence of neck, shoulder and arm pain, aching and tiredness. Work-related factors, including ergonomic conditions, may be factors contributing to the development or aggravation of these symptoms.

Work-related disorders are not recent discoveries. In 1713, Bernardino Ramazzini described the "diseases of clerks and scribes", involving "continuous sitting, repeated use of the hand and strain of the mind". In 1833, Sir Charles Bell described "writer's cramp" which Sir William Gowers later elaborated on in 1888. The current literature attributes many of these conditions to repetitive stress or strain.

The term "repetitive strain injury" is now widely used for these disorders. However, a variety of names have been used in the past and continue to be used, including "work-related musculoskeletal disorders" (WRMSDs), "repetitive stress injuries", "cumulative trauma disorders", "occupational cervico-brachial disorders", "occupational overuse syndrome", "upper extremity musculoskeletal disorders", "upper limb disorders" and "upper limb pain syndromes". This arose because of differences in views on the definition, scope and factors leading to this problem.

RSI is an umbrella term rather than a specific clinical diagnosis. Conditions such as trapezius myalgia, carpal tunnel syndrome and De Quervain's tenosynovitis are included under RSI.

Factors contributing to the development of repetitive strain injury include the following:

 (i) highly repetitive work;
 (ii) work demanding a certain amount of force, exerting force on the arm;
(iii) awkward postures during the execution of certain tasks;
(iv) insufficient rest or recovery time, leading to fatigue;
 (v) an aging workforce with less resilience to wear and tear; and
(vi) job dissatisfaction.

RSI commonly affects young to middle-aged and predominantly female employees engaged in low-paying, monotonous, low-prestige occupations.

Armstrong *et al.* (1987) studied a total of 652 workers from different work sites which included those in electronics, sewing, appliance, bearing fabrication, bearing assembly and investment molding plants. They looked at high-repetition vs. low-repetition jobs as well as high-force and low-force jobs, and found a strong association between wrist and hand tendinitis and the repetitiveness and forcefulness of the work. They also found that women were at a slightly greater risk.

Epidemiology of Repetitive Strain Injury

Musculoskeletal disorders are the second most common work-related disorder (Chen *et al.*, 2005). In one of the earliest accounts of RSI, Hymovich and Lindholm (1966) reported 62 cases out of 160 workers in an electronics assembly plant. This translates into six cases per 200,000 man-hours of work, and 41 lost work days per 200,000 work hours. In another report by Luopajarvi *et al.* (1979), symptoms of pain in the wrist and forearm were found in as many as 56% of assembly line food packers.

A study of localized fatigue in accounting-machine operators by Maeda, Hunting and Grandjean (1980) found that almost 50% of the workers felt tiredness in the arms and hands and over 40% felt pain. In addition, about 30% had neck stiffness with pain and 20% had shoulder stiffness with pain. A significant number also complained of low back and loin pain. It has been suggested that a plant-wide rate of 6 per 200,000 work hours is an acceptable baseline rate for RSI (Putz-Anderson, 1988).

The socioeconomic cost of this disorder is large, as it is associated with loss of productivity and absence from work. In the United States, the average worker's compensation payout ranges from $5000 to $8000, reaching a total of $6.5 billion a year (Baldwin and Butler, 2006).

Common occupations associated with RSI

RSI is common in working-age adults; however, rates are much higher in specific working populations. In addition to machine operators and assembly line workers, many other workers are also subject to RSI. Typists, keyboard operators, musicians, packers, car-penters, brick-layers, construction workers, butchers and even operating room personnel are subject to these symptoms. Chen *et al.* (2006) reported that jobs at the highest risk for upper limb RSI were those classified as clerical, craft-related and machine work. In addition, upper limb disorders with neck and back problems were more common in keyboard related, work involving heavy lifting, and in craft-related occupations which involve gripping or holding tools.

Treatment of Neck and Upper Extremity RSI

Medical treatment of RSI can only be instituted after a careful assess-ment of the patient. A short period of rest away from the workplace may be beneficial, especially in early cases. Rest can also be provided in the form of splinting. The physiotherapist and occupational thera-pist play a major role in the assessment and treatment of patients with RSI. Supplementing with oral medication is sometimes useful.

Analgesics, non-steroidal anti-inflammatory drugs (NSAIDs) or muscle relaxants can be prescribed when necessary. Topical medication such as NSAID ointments/gels may have a beneficial effect. Steroid injections can be given in certain specific conditions such as rotator cuff tendinitis or tenosynovitis. However, care must be taken not to inject the tendon itself as this may lead to tendon rupture. Surgery is seldom indicated in the treatment of RSI. However, in selective cases of severe or intractable problems such as carpal tunnel syndrome or trigger finger, surgical release may be necessary. The appropriate treatment options for each condition will be discussed below, following its description.

Clinical Presentation

In this section, conditions producing neck, shoulder and arm pain will be presented. Some of the conditions which may not be work-related will also be discussed as workers may present with these conditions as well.

Neck pain

The most common complaint is pain in the neck with tightness and pain in the shoulders and interscapular region. This has been labeled "postural neck pain", "fibrositis", "tension neck", among many other names. Occasionally, the pain can be radicular in nature; usually radiating down one arm to the fingers following a dermatomal distribution. This is usually associated with numbness. In these cases, there is nerve root compression which can be due either to nerve impingement by osteophytes in the neural foramina as in cervical spondylosis, or to a cervical disc prolapse. Sluiter, Rest and Frings-Dresen (2001) suggested the following diagnostic criteria for work-related neck pain: for radiating neck complaints, at least intermittent pain or stiffness in the neck and pain or paresthesia in one or more of the upper extremity regions, associated with head movements, for more than four of the past seven days and pain in upper extremity on active or passive cervical rotation. Van Tulder, Malmivaara and Koes (2007) reviewed studies for the treatment of RSI-related neck pain and found exercise therapy to be most beneficial. Other treatment options include a collar, medication (NSAIDs, psychotropic medication), intramuscular lignocaine, epidural methylprednisolone and transcutaneous electrical nerve stimulation.

Patients who have postural neck pain usually have some restriction of neck movement and tenderness in their neck, shoulder or interscapular muscles. Laboratory tests are not helpful. In those patients with radicular symptoms and signs, careful neurological examination can help to localize the level of involvement. Cervical spine radiographs can demonstrate narrowing of the disc space with osteophytic encroachment of the foramina best seen in the oblique views (Figs. 1–3). If symptoms persist despite treatment, a magnetic resonance scan is the most helpful imaging technique for looking at the degree of nerve root and/or spinal cord compression by osteophytes and/or intervertebral discs (Fig. 4).

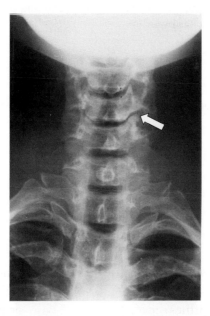

Fig. 1. Anteroposterior radiograph of the cervical spine of a 36-year-old factory worker who complained of neck pain radiating down her left arm, associated with numbness and tingling of her left thumb. It shows narrowing of the C5–6 intervertebral disc space and osteophyte formation at the uncovertebral joints (arrow).

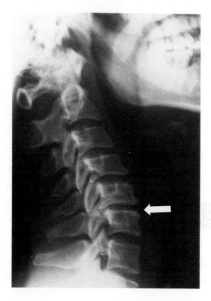

Fig. 2.   Lateral radiograph of the same patient, showing narrowing of the C5–6 intervertebral disc space (arrow).

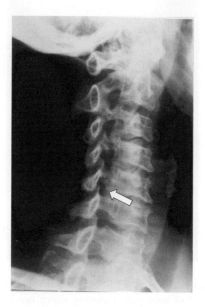

Fig. 3.   Oblique radiograph of the same patient showing narrowing of intervertebral foramen at C5–6 by osteophytes (arrow).

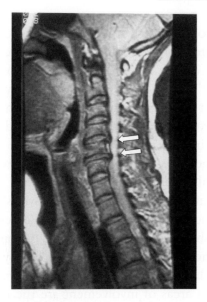

Fig. 4. MRI of cervical spine of the same patient, showing intervertebral disc prolapses at C4–5 and C5–6 (arrows).

Shoulder pain

Pain in the shoulder can be referred from the neck. If it arises in the shoulder, the most common causes are rotator cuff tendinitis (typically presenting as painful arc syndrome), bicipital tendinitis or acromioclavicular joint arthritis. In some cases there can be impingement syndrome. With shoulder pain, a good physical examination can usually identify the cause of the pain. Plain shoulder radiographs are usually not helpful. In chronic cases, a shoulder arthrogram or MRI is sometimes helpful in identifying a rotator cuff tear. Shoulder arthroscopy is now widely used for diagnosis and treatment. Physiotherapy, intra-articular or subacromial steroid injections and arthroscopic decompression have been shown to be beneficial for shoulder RSI (van Tulder, Malmivaara and Koes, 2007).

Arm pain

Pain in the arm can be referred from the neck or shoulder. Pain resulting from problems in the arm itself can arise from the tendons, nerves and vessels.

Tendinitis is commonly seen in the shoulder, elbow and wrist. In the shoulder, rotator cuff tendinitis and bicipital tendinitis have been alluded to. In the elbow, tendinitis at the extensor ("tennis elbow") and flexor ("golfer's elbow") origins are commonly seen. In wrist tendinitis it can affect the flexors and extensors of the wrist, e.g. flexor carpi ulnaris and extensor carpi radialis. Non-steroid anti-inflammatory drugs (NSAIDs) in either topical or oral forms, steroid injections, ultrasound treatment or surgical release in severe cases have been shown to be useful for elbow tendinitis.

Tenosynovitis affects tendons within a synovial sheath. The classical condition called peritendinitis crepitans, first described by Troell in 1918, has been shown to be work-related (Thompson, Plews and Shaw, 1951). Tenosynovitis was first observed by Velpeau in 1818 and he published his findings in his *Traité D'Anatomie Chirurgicale* in 1825. Common areas of involvement are the radial aspect of the wrist (De Quervain's disease, involving the abductor pollicis longus and extensor pollicis brevis) and flexor tendons of the thumb and fingers in the distal palm (trigger finger).

Nerve compression can occur either in the elbow or wrist, giving rise to cubital tunnel syndrome and carpal tunnel syndrome. Symptoms of pain, numbness and tingling are commonly reported in this condition either in the ulnar nerve distribution for cubital tunnel syndrome or in the median nerve distribution for carpal tunnel syndrome. Nerve entrapment syndromes are also fairly classical in presentation. Confirmation can be done by electromyography (EMG) and nerve conduction studies, although these may be normal in mild cases. Splinting is helpful in mild cases. Corticosteroid injection has some effect in the short term, and can help predict symptom resolution following surgery (Edgell *et al.*, 2003). Surgery is an effective treatment option in cases that do not respond to conservative treatment. Minimally invasive surgical techniques to release the nerve entrapment are becoming more widely used.

Apart from tendon and nerve-related problems, workers occasionally present with symptoms related to neuromuscular problems. Although rare, thoracic outlet syndrome should be considered when individuals who do a lot of overhead work complain of numbness and tingling in their hands. Thoracic outlet syndrome is much more difficult to diagnose. Often EMG and nerve conduction studies are not helpful. Angiography is also not helpful in many cases. Radiographs of the cervical spine may occasionally show a cervical rib.

Another rare RSI condition has been described in workers who use vibrating tools such as pneumatic hammers. These workers experience pain, numbness and blanching of their fingers similar to Raynaud's phenomenon. This has been termed "white finger disease" (Lee and Evans, 1984).

How to Distinguish Occupational Neck, Shoulder and Arm Pain from a Non-Occupational Problem

In general, older workers are more prone to experiencing neck, shoulder and arm pain. Due to the aging process and chronic wear and tear, cervical spondylosis and rotator cuff problems are common. In many cases, there is an underlying pathology which is aggravated by repetitive strain. There is no single good method of distinguishing occupational from non-occupational musculoskeletal problems. The following guidelines can be used:

(i)   Symptoms usually develop after working on the same job for some time (usually weeks to months);
(ii) Symptoms disappear after ceasing to do the particular job;
(iii) The type of job is known to produce the set of symptoms that the worker has;
(iv) The worker may have predisposing factors for the symptoms, e.g. age, underlying cervical spondylosis.

Assessment of Clinical Status

Assessment of the clinical status of the worker is based on all the information gathered from the history, physical examination and relevant laboratory investigations. In addition, knowledge of his/her occupation and the mechanics of the actual job will be invaluable.

Whenever possible a precise diagnosis should be made so that correct treatment can be instituted. The severity or chronicity of the problem should also be documented. This can be objectively analyzed in cases where there is wasting or weakness of muscles or neurological impairment. It is also important to determine whether the problem is due to repetitive strain. The guidelines given previously will be helpful.

In addition to the assessment of the worker, it would be useful to assess the workplace as well. This can be done with the help of an occupational therapist. A worker who is sent back to work in the same job which produced the initial symptoms will have a recurrence unless he/she returns to a different job or unless modifications have been made to his/her present job to reduce the risk of RSI.

An assessment of fitness to return to work can be made together with the physiotherapist and occupational therapist. In some cases a work hardening program may be useful to prepare the worker for his/her return to work. In strains and sprains of the musculoskeletal system, healing usually requires three to six weeks. However, in many instances, there is a lack of objective criteria for determining fitness to return to work. In such cases, clinical judgment has to be exercised. In the case of RSI, it is important to make sure that the worker is returning to a job situation that will not provoke a recurrence of symptoms.

Low Back Problems

Case Study 3

A 36-year-old furniture artisan presented with acute low back pain radiating to the back of both thighs. He gave a past history of chronic low back pain of about two years with intermittent episodes of severe symptoms. It was aggravated by bending forward, and he had difficulty straightening his back afterwards. A physical examination showed tenderness over the lower back and paraspinal muscle spasm, with limitation of spinal movements. The straight-leg-raising test was negative and neurological examination of the lower limbs was normal. Radiographs of the lumbosacral spine showed loss of the normal lumbar lordosis, but were otherwise normal. Magnetic resonance imaging of the lumbosacral spine was performed during a previous attack of pain, and this showed degeneration of the intervertebral disc at the L4/5 level. He was given medical leave and treated with analgesics and physiotherapy with rapid resolution of his acute symptoms. An analysis of his workplace showed he was doing detailing work on antique furniture that required him to bend over or squat for long periods at a time.

Case Study 4

A 42-year-old secretary started complaining of low back pain for the past one year after moving to a new office. The pain was worse towards the end of the day and was localized to the lower portion of the back with no radiation to the lower limbs. The pain improved every day after she left the workplace — she had to walk about 0.5 km to get to the bus station and required another half an hour of bus travel to get home. A physical examination revealed a non-tender spinal column with a good range of movement and no paraspinal spasm. Plain radiographs of the lumbosacral spine revealed normal lumbar lordosis but slightly reduced intervertebral disc space at L5/S1. An MRI scan of the lumbar spine revealed mild degeneration of the L5/S1 disc with a high intensity zone in the posterior annulus; the other intervertebral disc levels were normal. An ergonomic assessment revealed that she used a workstation which was too high and that her office chair had a fixed height with a soft cushion and no lumbar support. A change of her office chair to one with an adjustable height and a firmer cushion with lumbar support addressed the problem of her back pain.

Commentary on cases

These two cases illustrate occupation-related back pain. The time interval between the presentation of symptoms and the exposure to painful stimuli varies from person to person; the exposure may also involve heavy physical work in some but not in others. In both cases, suggestions were made to improve the ergonomics of the workplace and the patient showed improvement in symptoms (Schonstein *et al.*, 2003).

Introduction

Low back pain is one of the most common medical conditions. The lifetime incidence is 85% for the whole population at some time during their lives (Hult, 1954; Spengler *et al.*, 1986). The prevalence of back pain in the general population is 30% in a study conducted in Sweden (Bergenudd and Nilsson, 1988). The exact prevalence of low back pain in industry is unknown but it is thought to be higher than in the general population. In a study on large groups of employees in Sweden, Hult found a prevalence of back pain in 60% of the employees (Hult, 1954). Similarly a cross-sectional study conducted on 1562 workers in Ontario, Canada, revealed that the lifetime prevalence of low back pain (LBP) and point prevalence were 60% and 11%, respectively; and all of them at some time in their career required medical care (Lee *et al.*, 2001). It has been estimated that 6.5% to 11% of the workforce in the United States incur back injuries related to industry each year (Spengler *et al.*, 1986; Lee *et al.*, 2001). In the United States, low back pain was second to upper respiratory illness in terms of time lost because of illness (Zuhosky *et al.*, 2007). Back injuries account for approximately 19% to 30% of all workers' compensation claims (Yu *et al.*, 1984; Spengler *et al.*, 1986; Yu and Wong, 1996) with approximately US$14 billion spent in the US in 1976 on the treatment and compensation of low back pain sufferers. It was estimated that the financial effect of compensation for low back pain would surpass US$35 billion in annual expenditures by the end of the 1990s (Spengler *et al.*, 1986).

Risk Factors for Low Back Pain

Individual factors

Age

There is an increase in the incidence and prevalence of back pain with increasing age (Zuhosky *et al.*, 2007). However, back problems in an industrial setting may not be directly related to aging of the lumbar spine. In a study of a large industrial manufacturer in the United States,

Bigos *et al.* (1986a) found the risk of back injury to be significantly higher in employees less than 25 years old. This may reflect the time and experience needed to learn methods for efficient and safe care of the back. Although the rate of injury was high in this younger age group, the claims tend to be low-cost ones, possibly reflecting the greater potential for younger employees to recover from their symptoms more rapidly (Bigos *et al.*, 1986a). Their data also showed that the group most susceptible to high-cost back injuries tended to be in the 31–40 age group, a finding that is common in other back pain studies (Lee *et al.*, 1985; Guo, 2002).

Gender

The incidence of back problems is the same in both genders (Andersson, 1992; Bergenudd and Nilsson, 1988). According to workers' compensation data, males were reported to produce between 76% and 80% of all back compensation claims (Snook, Campanelli and Hart, 1978; Klein, Jensen and Sanderson, 1984). Lately the trend has slightly changed as more women are involved in industrial jobs (Guo, 2002; Waehrer, Lee and Miller, 2005). Overall, women had fewer injuries than men, but women tended to have an increased chance of becoming high-cost injury claimants (Bigos *et al.*, 1986b; Waehrer, Lee and Miller, 2005).

Physical fitness

Workers with poor physical fitness may be at risk of developing back injury. Cady *et al.* (1979), in a prospective study of 1652 firefighters, reported the frequency of subsequent injuries to be 10 times higher for the least fit group than for the fittest group. They concluded that physical fitness and conditioning are important factors in the prevention of back injuries. Walton *et al.* (2003) in their retrospective review of work-related claims in the case of firefighters concluded that "Overexertion due to lack of fitness is a costly source of injury to fire fighters that can likely be reduced through policy intervention". Height and body weight are probably unimportant (Andersson, 1992;

Bigos *et al.*, 1986) although there are reports, and it is logical to assume, that increased height or excessive weight makes an individual more susceptible to back symptoms.

Psychosocial factors

Various studies have shown the importance of education level as a prognostic factor for back pain and other musculoskeletal diseases (Feuerstein, Berkowitz and Huang, 1999; Huang and Feuerstein, 2004). One explanation given was that men with limited education and low-paying jobs were more likely to be performing strenuous labor or work that involved vibration or other stresses on the spine. In a study of the prevalence of back pain in a sample of 575 middle-aged residents of Malmö, individuals with back pain had been less successful in a childhood intelligence test, had a shorter period of formal education and worked at physically more strenuous jobs (Bergenudd and Nilsson, 1988). Other psychosocial factors commonly found in patients with back pain include depression, alcoholism, divorce, job dissatisfaction, inability to establish emotional contacts, family problems, previous back surgery and abnormal Minnesota Multiphasic Personality Inventory (MMPI) scores. However, the question remains as to whether these psychosocial factors are predictive of industrial injury or whether they are only results of the injury (Bigos *et al.*, 1986b).

Radiographic changes

Low back pain is related to structural abnormalities of the lumbosacral spine in only 3% of patients (van Tulder *et al.*, 1997). In a young worker, radiological manifestations of disc degeneration are rarely present. Radiological abnormalities like four or six lumbar vertebrae, transitional vertebrae, increased lumbosacral angle, leg-length difference, spina bifida occulta, tropism, spondylolysis and spondylolisthesis have been shown to occur with equal frequency in back pain patients and in a control group (van Tulder *et al.*, 1997). In an older patient, radiological evidence of disc degeneration may be present and may be clinically important. Traction spurs or disc space narrowing, or both, between the fourth and fifth lumbar vertebrae were associated with an increased incidence of severe low back and leg pain, while transitional vertebrae, Schmorl's nodes, and the disc vacuum sign were not (Frymoyer *et al.*, 1984). Rowe reported that degenerative disc changes were found in 80% of the patients who had lost time from work because of back pain, and in only 20% of the controls without back problems (Rowe, 1982). Other authors have reported disc degeneration to be present equally in both patient and control groups (van Tulder *et al.*, 1997).

Workplace factors

Job type

An increased sickness absence because of low back symptoms has been found in jobs with a high physical demand, jobs with prolonged static work postures, jobs with primarily bent-over postures and jobs with sudden, unexpected, high physical workloads (Andersson, 1992). Certain occupations (Elders and Burdorf, 2001), particularly truck driving, nursing (Waehrer, Lee and Miller, 2005), firefighting (Walton *et al.*, 2003) and materials-handling jobs have been shown to have a high rate of disability. The increased computerization of the industrial sector in recent years has resulted in increased risk factors for musculoskeletal problems specifically related to the nature or design of visual display unit (VDU) work (Yu and Wong, 1996). Workers in government and finance are least likely to be affected. However, a recent meta-analysis showed that there is an increasing trend in complaints of back and neck pain in office workers using computers. This association was however much stronger for the use of the computer mouse and neck pain (IJmker *et al.*, 2007).

Lifting and twisting are specific motions most commonly associated with back pain. Bigos *et al.* (1986b) found materials handling the most common *job* causing injury, and improper lifting the most frequent *cause* of injury in the Boeing Company. Falls accounted for only 10% of back injuries in this study, the distribution reflecting the manufacturing base of the company. Klein, Jensen and Sanderson (1984), using workers' compensation data, found that "overexertions", encompassing lifting, pulling and throwing, led to 72% of compensation claims. Frequent lifting of objects weighing more than 10 kg, sudden maximal effort that is unexpected, lifting heavy objects held away from the body, and failing to bend at the knees when lifting are other specific motions associated with increased risks of low back pain (Lee *et al.*, 2001).

Job factors other than mechanical loading of the spine may be also important. Less physically stressful, but boring and repetitive jobs (assembly line work), and those involving vibration (driving vehicles and operating power tools) have been linked to increased reports of back pain. A study of 672 full-time female operators in three large organizations in Singapore showed that 54% of them had low back pain and 60% had stiffness and discomfort in the neck (Jeyaratnam *et al.*, 1989). Cumulative exposure to repetitive lifting, and use of jackhammers, chainsaws or rotary cultivators have also been reported to be associated with a higher incidence of low back pain (Lee *et al.*, 1985).

Job satisfaction

Workers who are not satisfied with their present occupation, place of employment, or social situation have a higher incidence of low back pain (Bergenudd and Nilsson, 1988). In a longitudinal, prospective study on 3020 aircraft employees, the factors most predictive of subsequent reports of back problems were work perceptions and certain psychosocial responses identified on the MMPI. Subjects who stated that they "hardly ever" enjoyed their job tasks were 2.5 times more likely to report a back injury than subjects who "almost always" enjoyed their job tasks. Bigos *et al.* (1986a,b) reported an interesting correlation between back injuries and a six-monthly employee appraisal rating. Employees with a poor evaluation by one's immediate supervisor appeared to have a greater risk of high-cost back injury (Johnston *et al.*, 2003).

Clinical Presentation

Low back pain can present as:

1. An acute episode
2. Chronic back pain with episodes of acute exacerbation.

Acute onset may follow lifting or pulling activities, and pain may be experienced immediately, often increasing in severity over a few hours. The workman complains of inability to straighten his back, and may notice that his trunk is listed to one side. Pain in the back may be associated with radiation down one or both legs. Such pain can be 'referred' from the intervertebral disc or facet joints of the spine, or 'radicular' due to spinal nerve root impingement from a prolapsed intervertebral disc. 'Referred pain' typically radiates down the back of the thigh to the back of the knee while 'radicular pain' is felt in the dermatome of the affected nerve root, radiates beyond the knee into the foot, and may be associated with paresthesia in the distribution of the affected nerve root. It is important to ask about bladder control to rule out cauda equina compression as a result of a massive central disc prolapse.

A careful physical examination should be performed. Paraspinal muscle spasm, trunk listing and restriction of the degree and direction of spinal movements are frequently observed in a painful spine, and are not specific to any diagnosis. The presence of any spinal deformity is noted. Nerve root tension is assessed by the straight-leg-raising test. A complete neurological examination of the lower limbs, including perianal sensory testing, is done. The hips and sacroiliac joints are routinely assessed during the spinal examination. Sacroilitis, osteoarthritis of the hip and other pathological conditions in these joints have been frequently mistaken for spinal pain. Examination of spinal movements and the straight-leg-raising test can cause severe discomfort in a patient with acute back pain. If the patient is unable to cooperate with a full spinal examination at this stage, he or she should be allowed to rest and the examination should be performed again when the acute pain is better.

More commonly, the onset of back pain is gradual, without any history of a specific injury. Back pain typically comes on when the person sits or stands for some time, when he does lifting or pulling activities, or when assuming certain work positions unique to his profession, e.g. crouching and squatting during welding. The symptoms are reduced or relieved by rest. There is often a previous history of intermittent low back problems. There could be periods of remissions and exacerbations. The pain is truly axial but there may be non-radicular referral of pain to the lower limbs. A clinical examination in this situation will often reveal a reduced range of spine movement, especially forward flexion (which at times could be a voluntary act by the worker). The neurological examination of the lower limb is essentially normal.

Etiology

It is estimated that the back symptoms in about 70% of industrial workers are due to degenerative disease of the lumbosacral spine (Zuhosky *et al.*, 2007). Acute traumatic injury causing fractures or disc disruptions are uncommon and account for less than 5% of patients with back symptoms. More commonly, acute back symptoms occur against a background of chronic intermittent back problems from degenerative disease (Zuhosky *et al.*, 2007). Cumulative stresses or sudden unaccustomed heavy lifting may cause ligamentous sprain, rupture of the annulus fibrosus, or disc prolapse in these patients. Less common causes of back pain are spondylolisthesis, ankylosing spondylitis and developmental conditions like spondylolysis. Spinal infections and neoplasms are uncommon causes of back pain, but must be suspected in the presence of progressive unrelenting back pain that is not relieved by rest and particularly if associated with fever or general malaise.

Diagnostic and Laboratory Tests

Radiographs of the lumbosacral spine are commonly done for low back pain, although the results are normal in most instances. It has been reported that structural abnormalities are present in only 3% of patients, and the maximum detection rate for radiological abnormalities related to back pain is 10% or less (Rowe, 1982; van Tulder *et al.*, 1997). Immediate radiographs for a patient with acute back pain are generally not helpful and are certainly not cost-effective (van Tulder *et al.*, 1997). Most back pain settles within a short period and radiographs are done if symptoms persist or when directed by abnormal physical findings. Evidence of degenerative disease is present more frequently in older individuals (Frymoyer *et al.*, 1984; van Tulder *et al.*, 1997). Degeneration, defined by the presence of disc space narrowing, osteophytes and sclerosis, is associated with nonspecific low back pain with odds ratios ranging from 1.2 to 3.3. Spondylolysis and spondylolisthesis, spina bifida, transitional vertebrae, spondylosis, and Scheuermann's disease did not appear to be associated with low back pain (van Tulder *et al.*, 1997). It must be emphasized that disc degeneration can occur without producing significant symptoms. Lateral radiographs of the spine in flexion and extension may demonstrate unusual mobility of a spinal segment consistent with 'segmental instability'.

Magnetic resonance imaging (MRI) adds a new dimension to the diagnosis of spinal lesions, particularly degenerative disc disease (Figs. 5–7). Although the cost of this investigation is still high there is a definite role for MRI in the evaluation of acute low back pain after the failure of a fair trial of conservative management. For chronic low back pain, MRI has a definite role in studying the discs and their anatomy (van Tulder *et al.*, 1997). For spinal injuries and infections, MRI is an essential investigational modality.

Investigations like full blood counts, including the erythrocyte sedimentation rate, and bone scans are done as directed by clinical evaluation, or when there is a need to exclude inflammatory, infective or neoplastic causes of back pain.

Treatment

Non-operative

An episode of acute low back pain should be treated with analgesics, a short period of rest, followed by early return to work. Shortwave

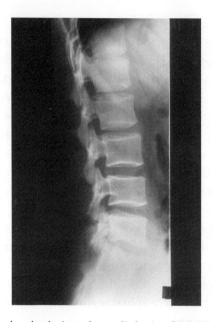

Fig. 5. Loss of lumbar lordosis and retrolisthesis of L5/S1 are present on this lateral lumbosacral spine radiograph of a 24-year-old worker involved in moving heavy drums of chemicals. No other bony abnormalities are noted on the radiograph. He complained of intermittent episodes of acute low back pain that had been troubling him for two years. The pain radiated down the back of both thighs, but there were no signs of nerve root tension or neurological deficits on physical examination.

diathermy, intermittent lumbar traction and trunk exercises are generally helpful, and are started as early as can be tolerated. Prolonged bed rest is not recommended as it may lead to further "de-conditioning" of the spinal musculature (Johnston *et al.*, 2003; Schonstein *et al.*, 2003; Irwin *et al.*, 2007). Resolution of the acute symptoms can be expected in nine out of ten patients within one month.

Educating the worker in back pain prevention and care of the back should be an integral part of the treatment of back pain, with emphasis on patient responsibility, workplace ergonomics and home self-care treatment of acute low back pain. Duties or activities should be modified to allow early return to work and minimize the risk of

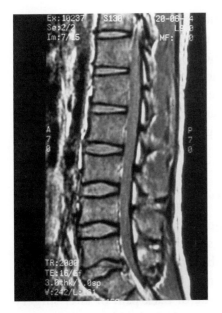 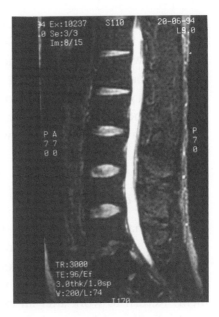

Figs. 6 and 7.　MRI of the lumbosacral spine showing degenerative changes in the intervertebral disc at L5/S1 associated with protrusion of the disc posteriorly. There was no compression of the dural sac and the spinal nerve roots. This patient was treated conservatively, and was advised on posture and ergonomics. In spite of a job modification, his symptoms progressed. He was advised to have a discectomy and lumbar interbody fusion at L5/S1.

prolonged disability (Johnston *et al.*, 2003; Schonstein *et al.*, 2003; Irwin *et al.*, 2007).

Operative

Surgery may be necessary for specific pathologies like intervertebral disc prolapse, spondylolisthesis or spinal stenosis; and is indicated only after an adequate period of conservative therapy has failed to relieve the symptoms (Hodges *et al.*, 2001; Irwin *et al.*, 2007). Common surgical procedures are microdiscectomy for lumbar disc prolapse; laminotomy or laminectomy for lumbar spinal stenosis; and spinal decompression, fusion, and instrumentation for spondylolisthesis. The operative treatment and post-operative follow-up will be the same as that for the general population (Hodges *et al.*, 2001; Irwin *et al.*, 2007). However, differences have been reported in the post-operative rehabilitation period between occupational and non-occupational back pain. The rehabilitation period is prolonged when an industrial related accident is linked as an etiological factor (Hodges *et al.*, 2001).

A healthcare guideline on the management of acute low back pain in adults is available at http://www.guideline.gov under "Adult Low Back Pain".

Assessment of Clinical Status

The vast majority of low back injuries are not serious, and most employees can return to work in a short time. In general, a worker with acute back strain could probably return to work within a few weeks. If he is a heavy laborer, he may require 3–4 weeks of treatment. Return to work after an episode of back pain or after surgery can be facilitated by a period of lighter duties, with restrictions on repeated bending, stooping and twisting. Most patients go on to complete recovery. Absenteeism and disability from low back pain are more likely to occur when there is less availability of a lighter job during recovery from back pain. It is now known that a positive employer approach to the rehabilitation process and management's ability to provide lighter working conditions during convalescence is associated with a higher probability of return to work (Johnston *et al.*, 2003; Schonstein *et al.*, 2003; Irwin *et al.*, 2007).

The importance of early return to work cannot be overemphasized. The longer the worker stays away from work, the less likely he is to return to the workforce. Workers with back complaints who are away from work for over six months have only a 50% chance of ever returning to work. If they are off work for over one year, this possibility drops to 25%, and if they are away for more than two years it is almost zero (Schonstein *et al.*, 2003).

Many patients who remain symptomatic will have continuing complaints but without any objective physical signs. A 5–10% impairment rating is usually given to this group of patients. Patients with true radiculopathy and those who have had back surgery should never be expected to return to heavy work. Typical impairment ratings given following discectomy are 10% for a perfect result or 20% for those with continued symptoms.

Prevention of Low Back Pain

It would be ideal if risk factors could be used to identify individuals at risk for low back pain. Unfortunately the epidemiology of this problem is complex, making early identification and screening difficult. Attempts at preventing low back pain have not met with great success. Preventive strategies commonly used in occupational back injury include the appropriate selection of new employees, training in manual handling techniques, and ergonomic modification of workplaces and tasks (Snook, Campanelli and Hart, 1978; Bigos *et al.*, 1992; IJmker *et al.*, 2007).

Job applicants may be screened in the hope of identifying and bypassing those potential workers at increased risk for developing low back pain. The most commonly used procedure is the pre-employment history and physical examination. It is estimated that 10% of workers who will get low back problems can be identified from a pre-employment medical history and examination. The best predictor is a history of back problems, but potential employees often will not volunteer such information (Rowe, 1982; Bigos *et al.*, 1991; Bigos *et al.*, 1992). Routine pre-employment low back radiographs have no medical predictive value (Rowe, 1982; Frymoyer *et al.*, 1984; van Tulder *et al.*, 1997).

Pre-employment strength testing has been used with the hope of reducing the risk of back injury by matching the worker's strength to the requirements of the job. Using an isometric simulation of the job, Bigos *et al.* found that a worker's likelihood of sustaining a back injury increased when job-lifting requirements approached or exceeded the individual's strength capacity (Bigos *et al.*, 1992). However, questions on types of effective strength tests, the number of tests, risk to the job applicant during the tests and determination of the amount of 'protective' strength remain unresolved. In contrast, Bigos *et al.* (1991) found no significant difference in comparing the strength of injured versus non-injured individuals of similar age and sex, doing similar tasks.

Education and training on lifting methods have been employed to reduce the incidence of back pain and injury. Knowledge of ergonomics is essential in reducing the level of stress on the spine so that a job can be done safely without exacerbating or causing back symptoms (Stobbe, 1996). This would also allow continued work or a rapid return to work for those having back symptoms. Constant vigilance adopting safe techniques of materials handling is important. Instruction can be given to workers in the form of workgroup instructions, as part of regular health talks or with the participation of 'back schools'.

Where possible, the workplace should be altered to better fit the abilities of the worker. Changing the height of workbenches, reducing the weight or size of objects being manipulated and altering the position or mechanics of machinery or tools are some measures which may help make the workplace more "back-friendly" (Stobbe, 1996; Schonstein *et al.*, 2003). Other possible approaches include elimination of manual handling tasks, use of mechanical aids and reorganization of work schedules to ensure a more even distribution of hazardous activities between employees (Stobbe, 1996; Zuhosky *et al.*, 2007; Irwin, 2007).

References

Armstrong TJ, Fine LT, Goldstein SA, *et al.* (1987) Ergonomic considerations in hand and wrist tendinitis. *J Hand Surg* **12A**: 830–837.

Andersson G. (1992) Factors important in the genesis and prevention of occupational back pain and disability. *J Manipulative Physiol Ther* **15**(1): 43–46.

Baldwin ML, Butler RJ. (2006) Upper extremity disorders in the workplace: Costs and outcomes beyond the first return to work. *J Occup Rehabil* **16**: 303–323.

Barton NC. (1989) Repetitive strain disorder. *Br Med J* **299**: 405–406.

Bell C. (1833) *Partial Paralysis of Muscles of the Extremities: The Nervous System of the Human Body*. Washington: Duff Green, p. 211.

Bergenudd H, Nilsson B. (1988) Back pain in middle age; occupational workload and psychologic factors: An epidemiologic survey. *Spine (Phila Pa 1976)* **13**(1): 58–60.

Bigos S, Spengler D, Martin N, *et al.* (1986a) Back injuries in industry: A retrospective study. II. Injury factors. *Spine (Phila Pa 1976)* 11(3): 246–251.

Bigos S, Spengler D, Martin N, *et al.* (1986b) Back injuries in industry: A retrospective study. III. Employee-related factors. *Spine (Phila Pa 1976)* 11(3): 252–256.

Bigos S, Battié M, Spengler D, *et al.* (1991) A prospective study of work perceptions and psychosocial factors affecting the report of back injury. *Spine (Phila Pa 1976)* 16(1): 1–6.

Bigos S, Battié M, Fisher L, *et al.* (1992) A prospective evaluation of pre-employment screening methods for acute industrial back pain. *Spine (Phila Pa 1976)* 17(8): 922–926.

Cady L, Bischoff D, O'Connell E, *et al.* (1979) Strength and fitness and subsequent back injuries in firefighters. *J Occup Med* 21(4): 269–272.

Chen Y, Turner S, McNamee R, *et al.* (2005) The reported incidence of work-related ill-health in Scotland (2002–2003). *Occup Med (Lond)* 55(4): 252–261.

Chen Y, McDonald JC, Cherry NM. (2006) Incidence and suspected cause of work-related musculoskeletal disorders, United Kingdom, 1996–2001. *Occup Med (Lond)* 56(6): 406–412.

Edgell SE, McCabe SJ, Breidenbach WC, *et al.* (2003) Predicting the outcome of carpal tunnel release. *J Hand Surg Am* 28(2): 255–261.

Elders L, Burdorf A. (2001) Interrelations of risk factors and low back pain in scaffolders. *Occup Environ Med* 58(9): 597–603.

Feuerstein M, Berkowitz S, Huang G. (1999) Predictors of occupational low back disability: Implications for secondary prevention. *J Occup Environ Med* 41(12): 1024–1031.

Frymoyer J, Newberg A, Pope M, *et al.* (1984) Spine radiographs in patients with low-back pain. An epidemiological study in men. *J Bone Joint Surg Am* 66(7): 1048–1055.

Gowers WR. (1888) *A Manual of Diseases of the Nervous System*, Vol. 2. London: Churchill, pp. 656–676.

Guo H. (2002) Working hours spent on repeated activities and prevalence of back pain. *Occup Environ Med* 59(10): 680–688.

Hodges SD, Humphreys SC, Eck JC, *et al.* (2001) Predicting factors of successful recovery from lumbar spine surgery among workers' compensation patients. *J Am Osteopath Assoc* 102(2): 78–83.

Huang G, Feuerstein M. (2004) Identifying work organization targets for a work-related musculoskeletal symptom prevention program. *J Occup Rehabil* 14(1): 13–30.

Hult L. (1954) Cervical, dorsal and lumbar spinal syndromes; a field investigation of a non-selected material of 1200 workers in different occupations with special reference to disc degeneration and so-called muscular rheumatism. *Acta Orthop Scand* **17**(Suppl): 1–102.

Hymovich L, Lindholm M. (1966) Hand, wrist and forearm injuries. *J Occup Med* **8**: 575–577.

IJmker S, Huysmans M, Blatter B, *et al.* (2007) Should office workers spend fewer hours at their computer? A systematic review of the literature. *Occup Environ Med* **64**(4): 211–222.

Ireland DCR. (1988) Psychological and physical aspects of occupational arm pain. *J Hand Surg* **13B:** 5–10.

Irwin R, Zuhosky J, Sullivan W, *et al.* (2007) Industrial medicine and acute musculoskeletal rehabilitation. 5. Interventional procedures for work-related lumbar spine conditions. *Arch Phys Med Rehabil* **88**(3 Suppl 1): S22–28.

Jeyaratnam J, Ong CN, Kee WC, *et al.* (1989) Musculoskeletal symptoms in VDU operators. In: Smith MJ, Salvendy G (eds). *Work with Computers: Organisational, Management, Stress and Health Aspects,* Vol. 1, pp. 330 –337. Amsterdam: Elsevier Science Publishers.

Johnston J, Landsittel D, Nelson N, *et al.* (2003) Stressful psychosocial work environment increases risk for back pain among retail material handlers. *Am J Ind Med* **43**(2): 179–187.

Klein B, Jensen R, Sanderson L. (1984) Assessment of workers' compensation claims for back strains/sprains. *J Occup Med* **26**(6): 443–448.

Lee EH, Evans JG. (1984) Vibration-induced white finger disease: A case report. *Can J Surg* **27**(5): 513–514.

Lee P, Helewa A, Goldsmith C, *et al.* (2001) Low back pain: Prevalence and risk factors in an industrial setting. *J Rheumatol* **28**(2): 346–351.

Lee P, Helewa A, Smythe H, *et al.* (1985) Epidemiology of musculoskeletal disorders (complaints) and related disability in Canada. *J Rheumatol* **12**(6): 1169–1173.

Luopajarvi T, Kuorinka I, Virolainen M, Holmberg M. (1979) Prevalence of tenosynovitis and other injuries of the upper extremities in repetitive work. *Scand J Work Environ Health* **5**(Suppl 3): 48–55.

Maeda K, Hunting W, Grandjean E. (1980) Localised fatigue in accounting-machine operators. *J Occup Med* **22**: 810–816.

Putz-Anderson V. (1988) *Cumulative Trauma Disorders: A Manual for Musculoskeletal Diseases of the Upper Limbs.* London: Taylor and Francis.

Rowe M. (1982) Are routine spine films on workers in industry cost- or risk-benefit effective? *J Occup Med* **24**(1): 41–43.

Schonstein E, Kenny D, Keating J, Koes B. (2003) Work conditioning, work hardening and functional restoration for workers with back and neck pain. *Cochrane Database Syst Rev* **1**: CD001822.

Sluiter J, Rest KM, Frings-Dresen MHW. (2001) Criteria document for evaluating the work-relatedness of upper extremity musculoskeletal disorders. *Scand J Work Environ Health* **27**(Suppl 1): 1–102.

Snook S, Campanelli R, Hart J. (1978) A study of three preventive approaches to low back injury. *J Occup Med* **20**(7): 478–481.

Spengler D, Bigos S, Martin N, *et al.* (1986) Back injuries in industry: A retrospective study. I. Overview and cost analysis. *Spine (Phila Pa 1976)* **11**(3): 241–245.

Stobbe T. (1996) Occupational ergonomics and injury prevention. *Occup Med* **11**(3): 531–543.

Stone WE. (1983). Repetitive strain injuries. *Med J Aust* **2**(12): 616–618.

Thompson AR, Plews LW, Shaw EG. (1951) Peritendinitis crepitus and simple tenosynovitis. A clinical study of 544 cases in industry. *Br J Indust Med* **8**: 150–160.

van Tulder M, Assendelft W, Koes B, Bouter L. (1997) Spinal radiographic findings and nonspecific low back pain: A systematic review of observational studies. *Spine (Phila Pa 1976)* **22**(4): 427–434.

van Tulder M, Malmivaara A, Koes B. (2007) Repetitive strain injury. *Lancet* **369**: 1815–1822.

Walton S, Conrad K, Furner S, Samo D. (2003) Cause, type, and workers' compensation costs of injury to fire fighters. *Am J Ind Med* **43**(4): 454–458.

Waehrer G, Leigh J, Miller T. (2005) Costs of occupational injury and illness within the health services sector. *Int J Health Serv* **35**(2): 343–359.

Yu T, Roht L, Wise R, *et al.* (1984) Low-back pain in industry: An old problem revisited. *J Occup Med* **26**(7): 517–524.

Yu I, Wong T. (1996) Musculoskeletal problems among VDU workers in a Hong Kong bank. *Occup Med (Lond)* **46**(4): 275–280.

Zuhosky J, Irwin R, Sable A, *et al.* (2007) Industrial medicine and acute musculoskeletal rehabilitation. 7. Acute industrial musculoskeletal injuries in the aging workforce. *Arch Phys Med Rehabil* **88**(3 Suppl 1): S34–39; quiz S40–48.

Chapter 10

Hepatobiliary and Gastrointestinal Disorders

Tar-Ching Aw,*,§ Lily LF Aw†
and J Malcolm Harrington‡

Introduction

Occupational exposures can affect the hepatobiliary system and the gastrointestinal tract. Ingestion of corrosive chemicals will have a direct effect on the upper gastrointestinal tract. The gastrointestinal tract also functions as a means of absorbing ingested toxic substances. However, there are in-built defense mechanisms of the gastrointestinal tract that can reduce the likelihood of systemic absorption. Some compounds are poorly absorbed through the gastrointestinal tract, and others may be removed by diarrhea and/or vomiting. Systemic absorption of chemicals leads to its distribution to other sites, and can result in effects on other target organs. The liver is an important organ for the detoxification of systemically absorbed chemicals, and is therefore a prime site for toxic damage.

*Department of Community Medicine, Faculty of Medicine and Health Sciences, UAE University, Al-Ain, United Arab Emirates.
†Lily Aw Pasir Ris Family Clinic and Surgery, Singapore.
‡Emeritus Professor of Occupational Medicine, The University of Birmingham, Edgbaston, Birmingham, United Kingdom.
§Corresponding author. E-mail: tcaw@uaeu.ac.ae

The efficacy of detoxification by the liver varies, depending on the substances involved. It is possible that attempts at detoxification will result in metabolites that may have other toxic or carcinogenic properties, e.g. conversion of a procarcinogen into a direct carcinogen. Interaction between occupational and non-occupational chemical agents can also result in additive or synergistic effects on the liver, e.g. exposure to chlorinated organic solvents and alcohol ingestion. In the evaluation of liver and gastrointestinal damage from exposure to chemicals, information on non-occupational risk factors such as alcohol consumption and medications is essential.

Pathophysiology of Liver Disease

Hepatic Response to Toxic Exposures

Two basic precepts should be remembered when considering the response of a target organ to external assault. First, humans evolved in an environment of clean air but contaminated food and water. Thus, the gastrointestinal system has a better protective mechanism than the respiratory system. Second, the more specialized the target organ, the more limited is its range of responses to external damage.

In the case of the liver, its metabolic role means that it can double as a detoxification factory to some extent. Furthermore, the relatively unspecialized nature of its cellular function means that its power of regeneration following damage is formidable. However, this ability to regenerate at a cellular level is not matched by a similar ability to repair lost architecture, and so continued damage can lead to cirrhosis. To continue the analogy: the liver can replace the bricks but may not necessarily use them to recreate a building of the same shape.

The liver is the largest visceral organ and has a major role in body metabolism. It produces bile, which assists in the digestion of fats, and the liver itself processes amino acids, glucose, fatty acids and glycerol. The liver also has a further function of detoxification, though it does not have the toxicological lexicon to distinguish poison from food. It performs its digestive functions on the majority of toxic chemicals through its widely varied enzymic activity in two main ways: degradation and conjugation.

In general, the main objective is to produce water-soluble by-products which are then capable of being used as nutrient material, or, in the case of foreign (non-nutrient) agents, render them capable of urinary excretion. Whilst some foreign materials, particularly the metallic poisons such as lead, cadmium and mercury are directly toxic, others only achieve their toxic potential after metabolic transformation. For example, carbon tetrachloride (CCl_4) becomes toxic only when it has been acted upon by a hydroxylation enzyme system to produce the highly reactive $-CCl_3$ radical.

The degradation enzyme systems are chemical reactions involving oxidation, reduction or hydration, and, as in the case of carbon tetrachloride, can result in unstable intermediates capable of damaging the hepatocytes. Conjugation is a more complex reaction usually involving glucuronic acid but again the objective is to produce the polar and less fat-soluble compounds. The metabolism of trichloroethylene is a good example. Following absorption, trichloroethylene is converted into chloral hydrate, which is further metabolized by one of two routes. One involves rapid reduction to trichloroethanol and the other is a slower oxidation to trichloroacetic acid (TCA). Trichloroethanol is not water-soluble and further metabolic transformation by conjugation with glucuronic acid is required to produce a water-soluble conjugate capable of being excreted through the urinary tract.

The liver also possesses two other characteristics of relevance to its role of detoxification. The first is the phenomenon of enzyme induction. Inducing agents are factors that increase the levels of the relevant metabolic enzymes and thus improve or speed up the detoxification process (or enhance the production of secondary toxins). In small doses, many toxic chemicals can cause enzyme induction. Ethanol, phenobarbitone and the pesticide DDT are prime examples. Ethanol induces hepatic enzymes which increase the metabolism of trichloroethylene, particularly at high levels of exposure; it also enhances the breakdown of 1,1,1,-trichloroethane at high and low levels of exposure (Kaneko, Wang and Sato, 1994). Heavy drinkers may be more susceptible than others to the toxic effects of chlorinated hydrocarbon exposure because of damage to liver cells from ethanol, resulting in a reduced liver capacity to metabolize other hepatotoxic chemicals.

The other characteristic of note concerns the liver architecture itself. Not only is it less well-regenerated than the individual hepatocytes; the structure of the hepatic lobule means that the liver cells closest to the hepatic venules receive blood with a lower oxygen content than those closest to the portal tracts. The centrilobular hepatocytes are therefore more vulnerable to toxic (and anoxic) conditions than the periportal cells. Centrilobular necrosis is thus an early sign of hepatic damage.

Finally, pre-existing liver disease will render the liver less capable of dealing with some new xenobiotic assault and this is of particular importance when undertaking health assessments of workers who, during their job, may be potentially exposed to hepatotoxins. Whilst ethanol (and viral hepatitis) are the most important causes of liver disease, chronic exposure to certain drugs such as the anti-convulsants phenobarbitone and phenytoin results in liver enzyme induction, potentially increasing the hepatotoxic metabolism of other xenobiotic exposures. But enzyme induction does not always result in a deleterious effect. It can stimulate other pathways for the production of non-toxic metabolites. In the event of pre-existing liver disease, reduced hepatic function may also lead to reduced conversion of a substance into a toxic metabolite. The outcome of these competing effects is heavily dependent upon the nature of the absorbed toxic substance, and the pre-existing condition of the liver.

Mechanisms for Liver Disease

Liver disease in occupational health practice does not differ to any great extent in its presenting features from those confronting a gastroenterologist in any hospital clinic. In broad terms, the hepatocytes can be damaged (hepatocellular effect) and/or the transport mechanism to or from the hepatocytes may be blocked (obstructive effect), or there can be an increase in bilirubin to the liver following severe destruction of erythrocytes (hemolytic effect). All these mechanisms can lead to jaundice.

Hepatocellular effect

The steps in the process of hepatocellular damage are illustrated in Fig. 1.

Obstructive effect

Obstruction to the outflow of bile from the liver to the gallbladder or from the gallbladder to the duodenum can result in cholestasis manifesting clinically as jaundice. Cholestasis (Greek for "stagnation of bile") can be pre-hepatic, intra-hepatic or post-hepatic. The mechanism of bile transport can be swamped at the pre-hepatic stage by an excessive production of unconjugated bilirubin from hemolysis. Hepatic causes include hepatocellular damage itself, e.g. from

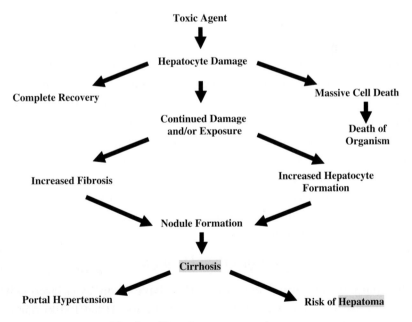

Fig. 1.   Hepatic response to damage.

exposure to carbon tetrachloride; and conjugation process defects or intra-hepatic obstruction as in viral hepatitis. Post-hepatic cholestasis is usually mechanical and non-occupational (e.g. tumors, gallstones, stricture of the bile ducts).

Cholestasis can occur following inadvertent ingestion of methylene dianiline in humans (see the Epping jaundice in Case Study 1). Dinitrophenol, methylenedianiline and the organic arsenicals cause acute cholestatic jaundice that begins with fever, chills and pruritus. Most patients recover uneventfully. Cholestasis with steatosis and hepatic perisinusoidal fibrosis have been reported in workers exposed to a variety of chemicals including benzene, xylene and vinyl chloride monomer (Cotrim *et al.*, 2004).

Long-term parenteral administration of supplements containing manganese has led to raised blood levels of manganese and accompanying cholestasis (Fell *et al.*, 1996). However, similar effects have not been noted in occupational exposure to manganese or its compounds. The halogenated hydrocarbon 1,1-dichloroethylene has caused cholestasis in rats (Moslen, Poisson and Reynolds, 1985) but this has never been reported in humans.

Hemolytic effect

While not having a direct effect on the liver, agents that cause hemolysis can lead to jaundice from an increase in circulating unconjugated bilirubin. Hemolysis can be due to congenital or acquired factors, and the extrinsic causes of rapid red blood cell destruction include occupational exposure to chemical agents, e.g. phosphine or arsine gas. Individuals with glucose-6-phosphate dehydrogenase (G6PD) deficiency are also susceptible to hemolyis on exposure to naphthalene, sulphur drugs and following consumption of fava beans.

Etiologic Agents Causing Liver Damage

The main occupational exposures that have been associated with liver disease are chemicals and infectious agents. Table 1 summarizes some of the chemical agents and the types of toxic effect on the

Table 1.   Chemical Agents Causing Hepatotoxicity

Toxic Effects	Chemical Agents	
	Occupational	Non-Occupational
I. Zonal degeneration	Arsenic	Aspirin (salicylates + viral infection leading to Reye's syndrome) Chloroform (also from occupational exposure) Ethanol (can also be diffuse or focal)
	Carbon tetrachloride Nitrobenzene Paraquat Yellow phosphorus Trichloroethylene Trinitrotoluene	
II. Focal degeneration	Infections: Viral hepatitis, typhoid, tularemia, brucellosis (may be occupational or non-occupational)	
		Drug effect: Tetracyclines, and methotrexate
III. Massive necrosis		Drug effect: Halothane, phenytoin and isoniazid
IV. Cholestatic jaundice	Dinitrophenol Methylenedianiline	

liver. The data in the table are based mainly on case reports or epidemiological studies in humans supported by findings from animal studies.

Chemical Agents

Some hepatic toxins act by causing acute disease at the time of exposure. This is usually due to a particularly heavy exposure, but for a few chemicals such as yellow phosphorus (although cases of poisoning are now very rare), even a relatively small exposure can have a cata-strophic effect with massive hepatic cell death. Today, most occupational exposures are relatively low and any effect is therefore likely to result from chronic low-level exposure leading to chronic hepatotoxicity.

Halogenated hydrocarbons

This is the most important group of hepatotoxic chemicals and many are, or have been, in widespread use in industry mostly as chlorinated derivatives of aliphatic or aromatic bases. As a rule of thumb, for the chlorinated benzene derivatives, increasing the extent of chlorination tends to lower the overall toxicity whereas for saturated aliphatic and some aromatic hydrocarbons, the reverse is true.

Chloroform is an example of an aliphatic agent belonging to this group of hepatotoxic agents. It has a long history of use as an anesthetic agent and is known to cause chemical hepatitis and encephalopathy. There is an interesting case report where relatives of a comatosed female laboratory worker were able to identify chloroform as the cause of her hepatic encephalopathy by examining the workplace and the available material safety data sheets (Lin *et al.*, 2005).

Among the aromatic derivatives, chlorinated naphthalene and the chlorodiphenyls are particularly potent causes of liver damage. The toxicity of polychlorinated biphenyls (PCBs) and polychlorinated dibenzofurans (PCDFs) is dependent on the number and also on the location of chlorine atoms in the molecule.

Aliphatic halogenated hydrocarbons are capable of producing severe acute centrilobular necrosis. Carbon tetrachloride (CCl_4) is the classic example. The damage is first noted in the endoplasmic reticulum with vacuolation and ribosome detachment. Whilst the mitochrondria remain intact, lipid droplets appear intracellularly and gross fatty changes occur in the lobular mid-zone. The toxicity of CCl_4 is enhanced by earlier treatment with enzyme-inducing drugs but diminished by a previous low-protein diet. Death from exposure to CCl_4 is usually caused by renal failure rather than hepatic failure. The hepatotoxic effects of other chemicals in this group are usually less marked, but their fat solubility ensures their widespread dissemination in the bone marrow and central nervous system where the clinical effects of toxicity may be more obvious or the long-term sequelae more serious.

Trichloroethylene and tetrachloroethane exposure have also been known to cause acute liver failure. On an equivalent amount basis, 1,1,1-trichloroethane is probably one of the least toxic of the halogenated hydrocarbon solvents in common industrial use.

Alcohols

Alcohols have a predilection for the liver. The effect of ethanol on the liver is the best known and understood. Exposure is primarily dependent on lifestyle, with limits being suggested for sensible alcohol consumption. The current advice (2009) from the UK Department of Health is that, for men, alcohol intake should be no more than 3–4 units a day; and for women, no more than 2–3 units per day. The difference in levels recommended for men and women is due to factors including differing proportions of body fat (thereby affecting storage and clearance of alcohol from the body) and differing rates of metabolism for alcohol. One unit is equivalent to half a pint of beer (250 ml); a measure of spirits (25 ml); a measure of fortified wine (50 ml) or a glass of ordinary wine (80 ml). The advice for pregnant women and those trying to conceive is that alcohol intake should be avoided. Advice is also provided on not mixing alcohol with medications or recreational drugs, not drinking and driving or when operating machinery, and discouraging alcohol consumption for those with mental health problems such as depression.

Fatty liver is common in those who have a prolonged history of excessive alcohol intake and this can progress to a diffuse hepatitis and eventually liver cirrhosis. Genetic susceptibility has been suggested as an explanation for the different amounts of alcohol required to cause liver effects in individuals (Alcolado, 1994). Ethyl alcohol is metabolized to acetaldehyde and then to acetate. Highly reactive free radicals are also produced, and the liver damage from alcohol consumption is thought to be due to acetaldehyde and the free radicals. A high proportion of individuals of Chinese ethnic origin have a genetically determined lack of alcohol dehydrogenase and aldehyde dehydrogenase (Thomasson *et al.*, 1993). An increase in blood levels of unmetabolized acetaldehyde causes "facial flushing", tachycardia and headaches (Kim *et al.*, 2005). These symptoms may discourage further alcohol intake, and thus act as a protective factor against acute alcohol effects. An analysis of data in a study on sewage workers in Paris showed an increased mortality from malignant and non-malignant liver disease. This is probably a result of alcohol consumption but exposure to chemicals and infectious agents may also be a contributory factor (Wild *et al.*, 2006).

Nitro compounds

Nitrated compounds, particularly the aromatic ones, can cause hepatocellular damage. Trinitrotoluene, which is used in the munitions industry (and therefore a cause of acute injury following explosion) has been linked to an increased risk of aplastic anaemia and also causes fatalities from centrilobular liver necrosis. Nitrobenzene also causes jaundice, from hepatocellular damage and from excessive hemolysis. 1,1-Dimethylhydrazine is used as a rocket fuel and can cause centrilobular necrosis while 1,2-dimethylhydrazine has no commercial applications and is classified as a Group 2A carcinogen (probably carcinogenic to humans) by the International Agency for Research on Cancer (IARC). Another nitro compound, 5-nitro-o-toluidine, has been shown to cause dose-related reversible liver damage in exposed workers (Shimizu *et al.*, 2002).

Metals and metalloids

Metals and metalloids reported to cause hepatic damage in humans include arsenic, selenium, thallium and phosphorus. Yellow phosphorus, used in the manufacture of "strike-anywhere" matches, is largely of historical interest. It was used because of its ability to ignite readily; hence it was also included in napalm (used in the Vietnam War). It gained notoriety in occupational health when workers in the East End of London (Bow) developed "phossy jaw" from work exposure to the element. It also causes acute yellow atrophy of the liver. Phosphorus compounds are used today for the production of pesticides (organophos-phates), fireworks and detergents. Control of occupational exposure to the ingredients of these products in modern factories today have diminished the likelihood of "phossy jaw" and acute yellow atrophy.

Pharmacological Agents

Idiosyncratic reactions of the liver occasionally occur following drug absorption. Some examples of the drugs involved are isoniazid, halothane, phenytoin, methyldopa, and propylthiouracil (Lee, 1993). The basis for these reactions is not well understood. Some of the drugs in combination apparently act synergistically to cause liver damage, e.g. alcohol and acetaminophen, rifampicin and isoniazid. Genetic factors, immunological responses and variable reactions to toxic metabolites have all been invoked to explain the effects. A good example of a drug hypersensitivity reaction affecting the liver is that of halothane administered in patients as an anesthetic, resulting in acute liver atrophy in a small proportion of patients. One explanation proposed for this effect is that toxic metabolites cause an immune response in predisposed individuals. The release of hepatic proteins cause further liver damage (Crawford, 1986). Occupational exposure to anesthetic agents in nurses and other operating theatre and intensive care staff have been investigated with regard to spontaneous abortions but there has been no indication of a link to hepatotoxic effects.

Specific chemicals

4,4-Methylenedianiline (MDA)

Case Study 1: Epping Jaundice and MDA

In February 1965, a medical student reported sick at his hospital with a history of severe upper abdominal pain of two days' duration. He was mildly jaundiced. In the succeeding few weeks, 83 other cases of jaundice were noted in the relatively small area of Epping in South East England. The medical student did not live in Epping but had been visiting relatives there within the relevant "incubation" period.

A detailed review confirmed the outbreak and the medical student's case helped to identify a dietary factor rather than an environmental one (Kopelman et al., 1966a). All the affected cases had consumed a particular type of wholemeal bread. Enquiries at the bakery traced the flour — some of which was unused. The sacks were contaminated with 4,4'-methylenedianiline (MDA). This chemical, used as a hardening agent for epoxy resins, had leaked from its containers onto sacks of flour while being transported together in the same truck. The original investigators fed some of the remaining contaminated flour to laboratory animals. Hepatocellular damage was noted, including portal inflammation, eosinophilic infiltration, cholangitis and cholestasis (Kopelman et al., 1966b).

At that time there had been no previous report of human poisoning by MDA but subsequent animal studies confirmed the hepatotoxic properties of MDA and showed that this aromatic amine causes hepatocellular carcinoma. Epidemiological studies of workers occupationally exposed to MDA have not demonstrated a similar degree of hepatotoxicity but case reports indicated that the target organs of interest are the liver and the bladder. One report suggested a link with retinopathy.

A follow-up of the 84 cases, 24 years later, was not able to show any clear-cut, long-term sequelae although one individual died of a biliary tract carcinoma and two others have had some visual disturbances (Hall, Harrington and Waterhouse, 1992). One individual remains intolerant of dietary fat.

The relevance of these findings to those who have occupational exposure to MDA is uncertain. Workplace exposures are generally of a lower dose and longer duration, with a different route of entry into the body. Nevertheless, in the absence of good occupationally related epidemiology, all accidental exposures to workplace toxins merit follow-up, particularly where animal evidence suggests that the agent may have serious long-term effects such as carcinogenicity.

N,N-Dimethylformamide (DMF) $[(CH_3)_2NC(O)H]$

This is an amide derivative of formic acid used as a solvent in industry. It causes fatty degeneration of the liver and hepatocellular necrosis, with the severity of liver damage related to the extent of exposure (Hamada *et al.*, 2009). The pathological effects present clinically as gastrointestinal symptoms, alcohol intolerance and jaundice in severe cases. Liver function abnormalities include elevated serum aminotransferases, alkaline phosphatase and bilirubin. The toxicity of DMF is a result of an intermediate produced from a minor metabolic pathway involving the cytochrome P450 enzyme system. The intermediate metabolite is thought to be methyl isocyanate — the same agent that was responsible for the effects on the community in the Bhopal disaster.

Dimethylformamide was among several hepatotoxic agents implicated in an outbreak of fulminant toxic hepatitis in workers involved in industrial waste disposal in Korea (Cheong *et al.*, 2007). One fatality from liver failure occurred amongst the five workers affected. The other chemicals were pyridine, dimethylacetamide and methylenedianiline.

Infectious Agents

Table 2 lists the main infectious agents which can cause liver damage and the occupational groups at risk. Laboratory workers who have to process organisms for research or diagnostic purposes, or work on potentially infected biological samples, may be exposed to a variety of infectious agents in the course of work activity. Research staff in genetic engineering laboratories and laboratory and post-mortem technicians in the healthcare industry are also at risk.

The hepatitis viruses (hepatitis A, B, C, D and E) cause acute hepatitis and in some cases this may progress to chronic liver disease (Teo, 1992).

Hepatitis A is an enterovirus transmitted by the oro-faecal route. It appears to be an occupational health hazard for sewage workers. Outbreaks have also occurred in institutions for the mentally handicapped. A formalin-inactivated vaccine is available to protect against this infection. Primary immunization involves a single dose given intramuscularly with a booster administered any time between six to 12 months later.

Table 2.   Infectious Agents Affecting the Liver

Infectious Agents/Diseases	Occupations at Risk
Dengue hemorrhagic fever	Forestry workers
Hepatitis A	Sewer workers
Hepatitis B	Pathologists, laboratory staff, other healthcare personnel
Hepatitis C	Healthcare and laboratory staff
Leptospirosis (*L. icterohaemorrhagiae, L. hardjo*)	Sewer workers
Malaria (*Plasmodium falciparum, vivax, malariae*)	Workers who have to travel and work in endemic areas
Melioidosis (*Burkholderia pseudomallei*)	Farmers
Yellow fever	Workers who have to travel and work in endemic areas
Q fever (*Coxiella burnetii*)	Farm workers
Schistosomiasis (*S. mansoni, S. japonicum*)	Agricultural workers, civil construction workers (e.g. dams, irrigation projects)

Hepatitis B causes infection that can result in full recovery or lead to chronic carrier status. The carrier state carries with it a risk of liver malignancy and there is a residual risk of transmission of the infection to others through contact with blood or body fluids or from sexual activity.

Hepatitis C is now thought to be responsible for more than 75% of what was previously termed post-transfusion non-A, non-B hepatitis. Hepatitis D and E seem less likely to be occupationally acquired. (For further information, see the chapter on occupational infections.)

Hepatic Carcinogens

Occupational groups such as workers in the restaurant and beverage trade, journalists and seafarers have an increased risk of liver cancer. This is likely to be due to consumption of alcoholic drinks — ethyl alcohol being a recognized liver carcinogen in humans. It has been designated a human carcinogen (Group 1) by the International Agency for Research on Cancer (IARC). Agents causing primary hepatocellular tumors can be arbitrarily separated from hepatotoxic agents. The latter group can, in some cases, cause sufficient damage over a long enough time to lead to cirrhosis. About one-fifth of cirrhosis patients subsequently develop hepatomas and in the United Kingdom approximately 70% of all hepatomas develop in cirrhotic livers. The incidence of cirrhosis varies greatly from country to country, so these figures should only serve to illustrate that previous liver damage appears to be an important precursor of many primary liver cancers.

In Central Africa, for example, where hepatomas are common, aflatoxin may be a more important etiological factor than ethanol. Experimental animal hepatomas can be produced by a variety of compounds obtained from molds. Aflatoxin B1 from the mold *Aspergillus flavus* and *Aspergillus parasiticus* produced liver tumors when fed to rats and newborn mice, but not adult mice. This aflatoxin is present in moldy peanuts and other grain. In China, by contrast, the high incidence of liver cancers seems more related to previous infection with the hepatitis B virus. Other chemicals causing liver tumors in experimental animals include dialkylnitrosamines, urethanes and polychlorinated biphenyls (PCBs).

Angiosarcoma of the liver is a rare malignancy consisting of malignant endothelial cells supported by a reticular framework. The classic occupational example of angiosarcoma of the liver due to vinyl chloride monomer is described in the following case study. Cases have also arisen in patients 15–25 years after receiving thorium dioxide (Thorotrast) for contrast angiography. Thorium therapy has also resulted in cholangiocarcinomata (a bile duct tumor that has been linked with parasitic infestations such as *Clonorchis sinensis* and *Opisthorchis viverrini*). Chronic exposure to inorganic arsenical compounds is also thought to cause angiosarcoma of the liver (Neugut, Wylie and Brandt-Hauf, 1986).

Case Study 2: Vinyl Chloride Monomer (VCM) and Angiosarcoma of the Liver

VCM was first synthesized in 1835 and has been in commercial production for the past 60 years. Nearly all the monomer is used in the production of vinyl chloride homopolymer and copolymer resins. In the early days of production, control of the gaseous VCM was not particularly stringent. This may have been in part due to the mistaken belief that VCM was relatively safe, as it had been trialed at one time for possible use as an anesthetic agent. Concentrations in the vicinity of the polymerization reactor vessels frequently reached 3000 ppm and, during the process of cleaning the chambers, the workforce might have been exposed to levels of 4000 ppm. By the mid-1960s, certain curious effects of exposure had been noted in the workers who cleaned the reactor vessels. A number of them had developed acro-osteolysis, some had Raynaud's phenomenon and a few had periportal fibrosis. Animal experiments in the early 1970s revealed more disturbing findings. Liver angiosarcoma and mammary adenocarcinoma were noted in mice and rats. These results appeared in the literature between 1974 and 1977 (Maltoni et al., 1974).

In 1974, more than 40 years after the introduction of vinyl chloride, two occupational physicians working at the BF Goodrich plant in Louisville, Kentucky, reported three cases of liver angiosarcoma in the workforce of the polyvinyl chloride resin plant. One case had cleaned reactor vessels (Creech and Johnson, 1974). Further reports of this exceedingly rare tumor rapidly followed both in North America and Western Europe. The latent period for the tumor appeared to be about 15 to 20 years.

Introduction of measures to control the workplace concentration of VCM was swift. Within three years of the first human report of angiosarcoma, occupational hygiene standards throughout the developed world were reduced to between 1 and 5 ppm and compliance was good. By the late 1980s, the number of new cases of angiosarcoma reported had peaked and was beginning to decline. In total, perhaps less than 100 cases have occurred worldwide but the effect of the VCM story on the chemical industry invoked a salutary lesson. No chemical agent can be considered "safe" until proven to be so, and no new chemical since this episode has been assumed to be without serious hazard.

The VCM story is not over. Other possible cancer sites have been suggested — such as the brain, lung, hemopoietic and lymphatic systems — but the evidence is not conclusive. An updated analysis of VCM-exposed European workers showed a marked exposure response for all liver cancers including angiosarcoma and hepatocellular

Vinyl chloride $CH_2=CHCl$

Acrylamide $CH_2=CH \cdot CONH_2$

Fig. 2. Chemical structures of vinyl chloride and acrylamide.

carcinoma, but no obvious link with other cancers (Ward *et al.*, 2001). The similarity in chemical structure between VCM and acrylamide (Fig. 2) had raised the suspicion that acrylamide might also be a human carcinogen.

Clinical Presentation

The clinical presentation in patients of occupational liver damage is no different from that of other non-occupational liver disease. The features depend on the underlying pathology, e.g. whether there is acute or chronic liver damage, and whether there is infection, liver atrophy or malignancy. In the early stage of liver disease, symptoms may be vague, e.g. poor appetite, intolerance of fatty foods and tiredness. Jaundice is often not apparent until the late stage of liver disease where sufficient liver function has been compromised. When this happens, other clinical effects may also manifest. Clinical features include edema and ascites from lack of serum proteins, bleeding tendencies because of insufficient clotting factors, gynecomastia from the inability of the liver to metabolize estrogens, and hematemesis from esophageal varices.

Acute Hepatitis

Acute toxic hepatitis is now rare. The main reason for this is the replacement of many of the more hepatotoxic substances used in industry by less toxic substitutes. The few cases that still occur are mainly due to accidental overexposure to fumes, splashes of large quantities of liquid chemicals onto the skin or intentional overexposure by ingestion rather than exposures in normal working environments. Symptoms akin to acute viral hepatitis (but without a fever) begin within 12 to 48 hours of exposure. The prognosis depends on the dose absorbed and can therefore vary from massive hepatic necrosis and death to complete recovery within four to six weeks.

Chronic Hepatitis

Prolonged, often asymptomatic, exposure to hepatotoxic agents can lead to chronic liver disease that usually presents as an end-stage liver disease such as cirrhosis. Teasing out a possible occupational component can be extremely difficult, if not impossible. Indeed, cirrhotic liver disease is more likely than not to be non-occupational. Hepatocellular carcinoma resulting from chronic hepatitis B or hepatitis C infection is an example of the neoplastic sequelae of occupational exposure or the cirrhotic process.

Confirming Occupational Exposure

A key element in the investigation for possible occupational liver disease is the confirmation of exposure to a hepatotoxic agent. This may be suspected from the history provided by the patient. An occupational history of poor systems of work leading to frequent skin contact with organic solvents or working in poorly ventilated areas with solvent vapor is important as a clue to the etiology of the disease. Work involving high exposure to gases is also relevant. This was the case for the workers who had to clean out the polymerization chambers where vinyl chloride monomer (VCM) was being polymerized to polyvinyl chloride (PVC). High levels of residual VCM gas were present. Lack of provision and/or use of personal protective equipment is also a relevant factor in the occupational history.

Environmental hygiene records may be available which could confirm high levels of exposure to the suspected hepatotoxic chemicals. Evaluation of hygiene records will require comparison of the readings against some occupational exposure standard. In the United Kingdom, the Health and Safety Executive produces an annual update on such standards (document EH40/00). In the United States, such standards are available from the American Conference of

Governmental Industrial Hygienists (ACGIH) in the form of a booklet on threshold limit values and biological exposure indices (ACGIH, 2010). The US Occupational Safety and Health Administration (OSHA) also produces permissible exposure levels (PELs) for exposure to chemicals in the workplace. In Germany, equivalent standards are produced by the Deutsche Forschungsgemeinschaft. These documents will help in the interpretation of hygiene measurements regarding the extent of exposure. However, the basis of the standards set is not necessarily data pertaining to the likelihood of liver damage. Some of the standards are based on toxic effects on other target organs, and others are produced by extrapolation from animal studies with the introduction of different safety factors, or from case reports which unfortunately often lack good exposure data.

Occasionally, biological monitoring results may be available to indicate absorption of hepatotoxins from several different sources of exposure. Chlorinated hydrocarbons such as trichloroethylene, perchloroethylene, and 1,1,1-trichloroethane can be detected from analysis of blood and breath samples. Trichloroethylene is metabolized to trichloroacetic acid (TCA) and trichloroethanol, both of which are detectable in urine as an indicator of exposure. In contrast, only a small fraction of perchloroethylene is metabolized to TCA. Hence, detection of TCA in urine is of limited value for perchloroethylene exposure, except possibly for end-of-shift samples taken at the end of a working week when urinary levels may be expected to be at the highest level. Other examples of biological monitoring data for hepatotoxic chemicals are venous blood levels of aromatic compounds such as toluene and styrene, or urinary levels of metabolites such as hippuric acid in those exposed to toluene, methyl hippuric acid for xylene exposure, and mandelic acid in workers exposed to styrene. Documentation of excessive exposure with an appropriate time interval between exposure and effect are essential in deciding on an occupational cause for liver damage.

Differential Diagnoses

Although there appears to be a bewildering array of workplace hepatotoxins, a clinician faced with a patient with liver disease is, in most cases, dealing with a non-occupational etiology. Cases of acute hepatitis or fulminant hepatic failure are usually due to viruses, drugs or mycotoxins. The acute nature of the disease means that the only occupational etiology that usually could be countenanced is a history of accidental acute overexposure to a known hepatotoxin. The absence of such a history would, in the vast majority of cases, preclude an occupational etiology.

A jaundiced patient likewise is more likely to have a familial disease, a hemolytic disorder, or have been taking drugs capable of causing cholestasis, than to have liver disease of an occupational etiology. Nevertheless, there is no substitute for a good occupational history and if a suspicion exists, laboratory investigations may provide evidence of toxic exposure.

A patient presenting with cirrhosis is a similar example. The etiology depends quite heavily on geographic location. In the Western world, alcohol and hepatitis from other causes account for most of the cases, although a sizable minority is cryptogenic. In the Far East, hepatitis B and C would be a much more likely cause. It would be the exclusion of alcohol and viral infections that spurs the clinician to delve further into possible occupational exposures but the chances of finding a relevant workplace exposure are, thankfully, small these days.

Laboratory Investigations

Detection of abnormal liver structure

Investigation of structural abnormalities of the liver by biopsy, special radiological techniques, radioisotope studies including scans, and ultrasound methods have been used mainly in the clinical evaluation of patients with liver damage. These investigations are not warranted for regular health surveillance of occupational groups.

Liver function tests

Standard liver function tests include the determination of serum levels of a range of liver enzymes that may be released from damaged hepatocytes into the bloodstream. This includes gamma-glutamyl transpeptidase (GGT), alanine aminotransaminase (ALT) and aspartate aminotransaminase (AST), alkaline phosphatase (ALP) and lactate dehydrogenase (LDH). In addition, serum bilirubin, albumin, globulin and cholesterol are often included. Of all these parameters, the one most used for exposure to chemical agents is GGT, and this is usually in the context of detecting excessive alcohol consumption. This may be in an occupational or non-occupational setting. GGT has been attempted as a biological effect measure for exposure to organic solvents and other hepatotoxic chemicals. The main limitation in its use is its high sensitivity and low specificity as an indicator of liver injury. Of the other enzymes mentioned, raised LDH levels are not specific to liver cell injury. Raised serum levels may also occur from sources such as the heart, lungs and muscle tissue.

In a study of VCM-exposed workers, 13 of 271 workers had persistent liver function abnormalities (Ho *et al.*, 1991). These abnormalities include raised GGT alone, or with either raised AST or ALT, or had in addition raised ALP. Some workers showed an improvement in liver function within six months of removal from further VCM exposure. A follow-up of the patients showed no consistent pattern of liver function abnormalities. Another investigation into workers exposed to relatively low levels of VCM and ethylene dichloride showed raised ALT and AST levels, but not GGT (Cheng *et al.*, 1999). Hsieh *et al.* (2003) in Taiwan reported a possible synergistic effect between those with hepatitis B and C infection and occupational exposure to VCM and 1,2-ethylene dichloride. A possible synergistic effect for liver function abnormalities between hepatitis B infection and exposure to dimethylformamide was also reported by Luo *et al.* (2001). The laboratory findings from the different studies point to the difficulty of using liver function tests for biological effect monitoring of individuals exposed to VCM.

In the Epping jaundice saga, individuals who had ingested methylenedianiline inadvertently had elevated serum alkaline phosphatase as the main liver function abnormality.

Bile acid clearance

Clearance of bile acids has shown some promise of being a useful indicator of chemical hepatic injury (Tamburro and Liss, 1986). Bile acids are synthesized and cleared only by the liver, and serum levels can be analyzed by radioimmunoassay. Bile acid clearance can detect both acute and chronic liver damage and levels are related to the severity of effect.

D-glucaric acid excretion

The excretion of urinary D-glucaric acid has been proposed as an indicator for biological effect monitoring in operating theater workers exposed to anesthetic agents (Franco and Fonte, 1994). Absorption of anesthetic gases can lead to the induction of liver microsomal enzymes such as the mixed-function oxidases. Halothane, nitrous oxide and isoflurane are anesthetic agents that can increase urinary D-glucaric acid.

Compensation for Liver Disease

Most countries have lists of agents that can cause occupational disease and for which state compensation is payable. In the United Kingdom, hepatitis B is by far the most important infectious agent resulting in tens of cases per year. For the chemical hepatotoxins, there are only a handful of claims in any year.

Viral hepatitis is a prescribed occupational disease in the United Kingdom and benefits may be paid under the Industrial Injuries Scheme, where viral hepatitis occurs following occupational contact with human blood or blood products or a source of viral hepatitis. The latter could include patients suffering from hepatitis B or carriers of the disease.

Angiosarcoma of the liver, as well as acro-osteolysis of the terminal phalanges of the fingers and non-cirrhotic portal fibrosis are conditions which are included in the UK prescribed diseases list (Department for Work and Pensions, 2009; Industrial Injuries Advisory Council, 1993). The relevant occupational activity for consideration of benefits under this scheme is work involving or work near the polymerization of vinyl chloride monomer.

Liver damage from exposure to carbon tetrachloride or chloroform fumes or vapor is also listed as a prescribed disease.

Fitness for Work

Employees with liver disease should be protected where possible from workplace exposure to hepatotoxins to a greater extent than other employees unless there is good clinical and laboratory evidence that their previous liver disease has resolved. Astbury and Southgate in 2007 provided specific guidance on a range of gastrointestinal and liver disorders in relation to particular problems with specific occupations or work activity.

For specific hepatic infections such as hepatitis B, e-antigen positive chronic carrier status would represent a risk of person-to-person transmission. This is relevant for healthcare workers involved in exposure-prone procedures. The risk of transmission for hepatitis B carriers depends on the viral load, which is measured in terms of genome equivalents per milliliter (see Case Study 3).

Patients with ileostomies and colostomies may be seen by occupational physicians for advice on fitness for work. The advice given is often inconsistent and concerns may revolve around suitability for jobs requiring food handling, problems with manual handling, working in hot environments and perceived increased sickness absence. Ileostomy patients tend to have a lower sickness absence rate (Wyke, Edwards and Allan, 1988). With good personal hygiene and proper systems of work, there is no increased risk of spread of infection from or to a stoma patient from work activity. Lifting heavy objects or excessive bending may damage the stoma, and as for working in hot environments, stoma patients may experience some difficulty. In hot climates, as in the tropics and in the desert climate of the Middle East, adequate occupational advice should include instructions on rehydration (Wyke *et al.*, 1989).

Case Study 3: A Healthcare Worker with Markers of Hepatitis B Infection

Routine screening of a pediatrician in a hospital's intensive care unit reveals the presence of markers of hepatitis B infection. The occupational health department is asked for advice on the fitness of the healthcare *worker to continue in his work. An opinion on fitness for work would depend on several considerations. First, the specific results on the markers of infection. Was surface antigen (s-Ag) or e-antigen (e-Ag) detected? According to the UK Department of Health guidelines, an individual with s-Ag but not e-Ag would need to have the hepatitis B viral load determined. Those with a hep B viral load >10^3 genome equivalents/ml would be excluded from performing exposure-prone procedures (EPPs). The second consideration is in regard to the nature of the work. This requires an assessment of the work activities. A pediatrician in an intensive care unit may not be involved in exposure-prone procedures. The UK Department of Health guidance indicates that neither general nor neonatal/special care pediatrics are likely to involve EPPs (pediatric surgeons are a different case). Phlebotomy, arterial cutdown, cardiac catheterization and procedures where the operator's hands are always clearly visible are not considered EPPs. In this case the pediatrician is unlikely to pose a significant risk from regular intensive care work and can be allowed to continue in his vocation. However, in some countries, there are national laws that require that for issuance of work visas, a foreign worker (in healthcare or other jobs) is required to demonstrate the absence of carrier state not only for hepatitis B but also for other infections such as HIV.*

Exposures Affecting Other Parts of the Gastrointestinal Tract

Oesophagitis, Peptic Ulcer and Gastritis

Ingestion of corrosive chemicals causes severe esophageal and gastric damage. The extent of the damage depends in part on the specific chemical involved, the pH of the solutions ingested, the amount ingested, and the presence of food in the upper gastrointestinal tract. Severe gastric damage from chemicals is more likely to result from intentional ingestion as in suicide attempts, rather than from inadvertent occupational exposures. Ingestion of small quantities of workplace chemicals can follow poor hygiene practices at work, such as eating or drinking at worksites where chemicals are handled, or consuming food and drink without adequate cleaning of the hands after contact with chemicals. Some hexavalent chromates when ingested have been reported to cause gastroenteritis with possible hepatic and renal effects (Langard and Norseth, 1986). Carbon disulphide used in the viscose rayon industry has been described as causing gastrointestinal and metabolic disturbances in addition to the neurotoxic and cardiotoxic effects. In studies on cattle, arsenical herbicides have caused hemorrhagic gastritis with midzonal hepatic necrosis (Dickinson, 1992). Non-occupational causes of gastritis include chronic use of aspirin, excessive alcohol intake and smoking.

Psychological stress including stress in the workplace can aggravate duodenal ulcers and ulcerative colitis (Jenkins, 1989). Machine-paced work has been shown to lead to high levels of job stress with accompanying symptoms of gastrointestinal and other symptoms (Wilkes, Stammerjohn and Lalich, 1981). Groups viewed as belonging to high-stress occupations include teachers, air traffic controllers, tax officers and dentists. Self-reported sickness absence in teachers indicate that bowel symptoms are a common complaint (Travers and Cooper, 1993). In addition to gastrointestinal symptoms, stress can also cause fatigue and sleeplessness, and the long-term effects may include ulcers, heart disease, hypertension and asthma (Baker, 1988).

Shift workers have an increased incidence of digestive disorders and peptic ulcers. However, the specific contribution of diet, smoking, alcohol intake, stress and irregular mealtimes to the condition in these workers has not been determined (Waterhouse, Folkard and Minors, 1992). Harrington (1978) concluded that there is a balance of good epidemiological evidence linking gastrointestinal disorders, particularly gastric and duodenal ulcers, with shift work.

Case Study 4: Ingestion of Metallic Mercury

A child bit on a mercury thermometer while his temperature was being taken. The thermometer broke, causing the mercury to be released and the child to swallow some of it. The clinic staff were concerned about gastrointestinal absorption and the risk of mercury poisoning from the mercury ingested. An occupational health department was contacted. What advice should the occupational health staff give?

Metallic mercury, as opposed to compounds of mercury, is not readily absorbed through the gastrointestinal tract (WHO, 1991). Less than 0.01% of the ingested dose is absorbed (Lauwerys, 1983). Ingested *metallic mercury* will therefore be excreted after passing through the gastrointestinal tract. Or at most it will cause some local mucosal irritation leading to vomiting and/or diarrhea. The risk of acute or chronic mercury poisoning from this incident is low. The best advice therefore is reassurance, and perhaps recommending the use of a non-mercury-based thermometer for children in the future. There is probably a greater risk of harm to health from the broken glass of the thermometer than the mercury swallowed.

Pancreatitis and Pancreatic Cancer

Pancreatitis is known to be associated with gallstones, heavy alcohol consumption and some medications (Anon, 1994). Effects on the pancreas from occupational exposures are rare. A transient increase in serum amylase indicating some effect on the pancreas has been linked to exposure to the pesticide malathion (Dagli and Shaikh, 1983). Other organophosphate pesticides have also produced acute pancreatitis after ingestion (Lee, 1989; Marsh, Vukov and Conradi, 1988).

Pancreatic cancer has a high case-fatality rate. In a population-based case-control study of occupational factors related to pancreatic cancer in Shanghai, there was a suggestion of an association between the malignancy and exposure to mineral oils, solvents, metals and textile dusts (Ji *et al.*, 1999). There was also an elevated risk in electricians, and the researchers speculated on the possible role of electromagnetic fields.

In a meta-analysis covering 23 different occupational agents, it was noted that excess pancreatic cancer was associated with exposure to nickel and nickel compounds, and possibly to some chlorinated hydrocarbons (Ojarjärvi *et al.*, 2000).

However, an earlier review of the factors linked to pancreatic cancer concluded that the evidence on coffee consumption was negative; that fat intake is a risk factor and this is associated with obesity and diabetes; and that there is no convincing evidence for the etiological role of specific occupational or environmental agents (Weiderpass *et al.*, 1998).

Peritoneal Mesothelioma and Cancer of the Colon

Asbestos exposure can lead to mesothelioma of the pleura and peritoneum. Asbestos cement workers have also been shown to have a slightly increased risk of colorectal cancer (Jakobssen, Albin and Hagmar, 1994). The site affected is primarily the proximal part of the colon. Elevated mortality odds ratios were observed for cancer of the colon in a study on chemists and laboratory professionals employed in the US Department of Agriculture (Dosemeci *et al.*, 1992). Reviews of a cluster of colorectal cancers in polypropylene production workers and carpet manufacturing workers using polypropylene concluded that the weight of existing evidence pointed to a chance finding rather than a causal association (Lagast, Tomenson and Stringer, 1995, 1994). An association with colon polyps and colorectal cancer was also noted in an analysis of health claims data from workers at a perfluorooctanesulfonyl fluoride facility (Olsen *et al.*, 2004). A non-significant excess of certain gastrointestinal tract malignancies including cancer of the colon, esophagus and liver was noted in a study on over 14,000 aircraft maintenance workers exposed to trichloroethylene and a variety of other organic solvents and chemicals. The conclusion from the study was that there was no causal link between trichloroethylene exposure and the malignancies because the associations were not significant; there was no clear dose-response relationship; and there were inconsistent findings between males and females (Blair and Hartge, 1998). In a cohort study of 15 million inhabitants from five Nordic countries, there was an increased risk of colon cancer related to sedentary work. However, there did not appear to be any protective effect from physical activity (Pukkala *et al.*, 2009).

Other Gastrointestinal Effects

Gastroenteritis is common in laboratory technicians working in research and hospital laboratories, particularly those handling and processing microorganisms regularly. Sewer workers have a higher prevalence of gastrointestinal disorders. Other rare conditions include gas-filled cysts in the gastrointestinal tract caused by exposure to trichloroethylene (Fleming, 1992). There are case reports suggesting a possible link between phenoxyacetic acid pesticides and gastric non-Hodgkin's lymphoma (Hardell, 1992). A study on uranium-processing workers indicated that exposure to cutting fluids was associated with an increase in laryngeal cancer, and that kerosene exposure increased mortality from several gastrointestinal cancers. A causal link was suggested by the finding that cancers increased with duration and level of exposure (Ritz, 1999).

Conclusion

There is a wide variety of etiological agents encountered in the course of work activities that can cause damage to the liver and gastrointestinal tract. A careful occupational history with a documentation of exposure, an understanding of the nature and properties of chemical and physical agents, and consideration of the differential diagnoses will aid the clinician in reaching the correct diagnosis. The appropriate treatment can then be provided and relevant preventive measures taken.

Acknowledgments

Thanks are due to Ms. Lynnette Ee-Sing Tan from the Yong Loo Lin School of Medicine, National University of Singapore; and Ms. Juliet Sher-Kit Tan from the Duke-NUS Graduate Medical School Singapore for their help with the literature search.

References

Alcolado J. (1994) Genetic markers in alcoholic liver disease. *Br Med J* **308**: 341–353.

American Conference of Governmental Industrial Hygienists. (2009) *Threshold Limit Values for Chemical Substances and Physical Agents and Biological Exposure Indices. 2010.* Cincinnati: ACGIH.

Anonymous. (1994) Drug-induced pancreatitis: An underconsidered problem. Current problems in pharmacovigilance. *Committee on Safety of Medicines/Medicines Control Agency.* **20**: 2–3.

Astbury C, Southgate JL. (2007) Gastrointestinal and liver disorders. In: Palmer KT, Cox RAF, Brown I (eds). *Fitness for Work: The Medical Aspects,* 4th edn. Oxford: Oxford University Press.

Baker DB. (1988) Occupational stress. In: Levy BS, Wegman DH (eds). *Occupational Health: Recognizing and Preventing Work-related Disease.* Boston: Little, Brown Co.

Blair A, Hartge P. (1998) Mortality and cancer incidence of aircraft maintenance workers exposed to trichloroethylene and other organic solvents and chemicals: Extended follow-up. *Occ Env Med* **55**: 161–171.

Cheng TJ, Huang ML, You NC *et al.* (1999) Abnormal liver function in workers exposed to low levels of ethylene dichloride and vinyl chloride monomer. *J Occ Env Med* **41**(12): 1128–1133.

Cheong HK, Kin EA, Choi JK *et al.* (2007) Grand rounds: An outbreak of toxic hepatitis among industrial waste disposal workers. *Environ Health Perspect* **115**: 107–112.

Cotrim HP, De Freitas LA, Freitas C *et al.* (2004) Clinical and histopathological features of NASH in workers exposed to chemicals with or without associated metabolic conditions. *Liver Int* **24**: 131–135.

Crawford JS. (1986) Halothane and the liver. *Br Med J* **293**: 334–335.

Creech JL, Johnson MN. (1974) Angiosarcoma of the liver in the manufacture of polyvinyl chloride. *J Occup Med* **16**: 150–151.

Dagli AJ, Shaikh WA. (1983) Pancreatic involvement in malathion–anticholinesterase insecticide intoxication: A study of 75 cases. *Br J Clin Pract* **37**: 270–272.

Department for Work and Pensions. (2009) *DB1 — A Guide to Industrial Injuries Disablement Benefits.* http://www.dwp.gov.uk/publications/specialist_guides (retrieved 20 April 2010).

Department of Health, UK. (2006) *Immunisation Against Infectious Disease,* 3rd edn. London: The Stationery Office.

Department of Health, UK. (2007) Health clearance for tuberculosis, hepatitis B, hepatitis C and HIV: New healthcare workers. http://www.dh.gov.uk/publications (retrieved 20 April 2010).

Department of Health, UK. (2009) Alcohol advice. http://www.dh.gov.uk/publications (retrieved 20 April 2010).

Dickinson JO. (1992) Toxicity of the arsenical herbicide monosodium acid methane arsenate in cattle. *Am J Vet Res* **33**: 1889–1892.

Dosemeci M, Alavanja M, Vetter R *et al.* (1992) Mortality among laboratory workers employed at the US Department of Agriculture. *Epidemiology* **3**: 258–262.

Edwards G. (1996) Sensible drinking. *Br Med J* **7022**: 312–331.

Fell JME, Reynolds AP, Meadows N, *et al.* (1996) Manganese toxicity in children receiving long-term parenteral nutrition. *Lancet* **347**: 1218–1221

Fleming LE. (1992) Unusual occupational gastrointestinal and hepatic disorders. In: Shusterman DJ, Blanc PD (eds). *Occupational Medicine: State of the Art Reviews.* Philadelphia: Hanley Belfus, Inc.

Franco G, Fonte R. (1994) Advances in evaluating liver response to operating theatre work: Urinary D-glucaric acid as an index of effect. *Occup Med* **44**: 12–16.

Hall AJ, Harrington JM, Waterhouse JAH. (1992) The Epping jaundice outbreak: A 24 year follow up. *J Epi Comm Health* **46**: 327–328.

Hamada M, Abe M, Tokumoto Y *et al.* (2009) Occupational liver injury due to N,N-dimethylformamide in the synthetics industry. *Intern Med* **48**: 1647–1650.

Hardell L. (1992) Primary gastric lymphoma and occupational exposures. *Lancet* **340**: 186–187.

Harrington JM. (1978) *Shift Work and Health: A Critical Review of the Literature.* London: HMSO.

Health Safety Executive. (2000) *EH40/00 Occupational Exposure Limits 2000.* London: HMSO.

Health Safety Executive. (1996) *A Guide for Employers on Alcohol at Work.* Sudbury: HSE Books.

Ho SF, Phoon WH, Gan SL, Chan YK. (1991) Persistent liver dysfunction among workers at a vinyl chloride monomer polymerisation plant. *J Soc Occup Med* **41**: 10–16.

Hsieh HI, Wang JD, Chen PC, Cheng TJ. (2003) Synergistic effect of hepatitis virus infection and occupational exposures to vinyl chloride monomer and ethylene dichloride on serum aminotransaminase activity. *Occup Environ Med* **60**: 774–778.

Industrial Injuries Advisory Council. (1993) *Periodic Report 1993. A Review of Recent Activity of the Industrial Injuries Advisory Council Concerning Work-related Ill Health*. London: HMSO.

IARC. (2009) IARC strengthens its findings on several carcinogenic personal habits and household exposures. http://www.iarc.fr/en/media-centre/pr/2009/pdfs/pr196_E.pdf (retrieved 20 April 2010).

Jakobsson K, Albin M, Hagmar L. (1994) Asbestos, cement, and cancer in the right part of the colon. *Occup Environ Med* **51**: 95–101.

Jenkins R. (1989) Mental health of people at work. In: Waldron HA (ed). *Occupational Health Practice*, 3rd edn. London: Butterworths.

Ji BT, Silverman DT, Dosemeci M, *et al*. (1999) Occupation and pancreatic cancer risk in Shanghai, China. *Am J Ind Med* **35**: 76–81.

Kaneko T, Wang PY, Sato A. (1994) Enzymes induced by ethanol differently affect the pharmacokinetics of trichloroethylene and 1,1,1-trichloroethane. *Occup and Environ Med* **51**: 113–116.

Kim JS, Kim YJ, Kim TY, *et al*. (2005) Association of ALDH2 polymorphism with sensitivity to acetaldehyde-induced micronuclei and facial flushing after alcohol intake. *Toxicology* **210**: 169–174.

Kopelman H, Robertson MH, Sanders PG, Ash I. (1966a) The Epping jaundice. *Br Med J* **1**: 514–516.

Kopelman H, Scheuer PJ, Williams R. (1966b) The liver lesion of the Epping jaundice. *Queensland J Med* **35**: 553–564.

Lagast H, Tomenson J, Stringer DA. (1995) Polypropylene production and colorectal cancer. *Occup Med* **45**: 69–74.

Langard S, Norseth T. (1986) Chromium. In: Friberg L, Nordberg GF, Vouk V (eds). *Handbook on the Toxicology of Metals*, 2nd edn. Amsterdam: Elsevier Science Publishers.

Lauwerys R. (1983) Mercury. In: Parmegianni L (ed). *Encyclopaedia of Occupational Health and Safety*, 3rd edn. Geneva: International Labor Office.

Lee HS. (1989) Acute pancreatitis and organophosphate poisoning: A case report and a review. *Singapore Med J* **30**: 599–601.

Lee WM. (1993) Review article: Drug-induced hepatotoxicity. *Aliment Pharmacol Therap* **7**: 477–485.

Lin CH, Du CL, Chan CC, Wang JD. (2005) Saved by a material safety data sheet. *Occup Med* **55**: 635–637.

Luo JC, Kuo HW, Cheng TJ, Chang MJ. (2001) Abnormal liver function associated with occupational exposure to dimethylformamide and hepatitis B virus. *J Occup Environ Med* **43**: 474–482.

Maltoni C, Lefeming G, Chieco P, Carrett ID. (1974) Vinyl chloride carcinogenesis: Current results and perspectives. *Med Lav* **65**: 421–444.

Marsh WH, Vukov GA, Conradi EC. (1988) Acute pancreatitis after cutaneous exposure to an organophosphate pesticide. *Am J Gastroenterol* **83**: 1158–1160.

Moslen MT, Poisson LR, Reynolds ES. (1985) Cholestasis and increased biliary excretion of insulin in rats given 1,1 -dichloroethylene. *Toxicology* **34**: 201–209.

Neugut AI, Wylie P, Brandt-Rauf PW. (1986) Occupational cancers of the gastrointestinal tract, part II: Pancreas, liver, and biliary tract. In: *Occupational Cancer and Carcinogenesis — State of the Art Reviews* ed. Brandt-Rauf PW. **2**: 137–154.

Ojajärvi IA, Partanen TJ, Ahlbom A, *et al.* (2000) Occupational exposures and pancreatic cancer: A meta-analysis. *Occup Environ Med* **57**: 316–324.

Olsen GW, Burlew MM, Marshall JC, *et al.* (2004) Analysis of episodes of care in a perfluorooctanesulfonyl fluoride production facility. *J Occup Environ Med* **46**: 837–846.

Pukkala E, Martinsen JI, Lynge E, *et al.* (2009) Occupation and cancer — follow-up of 15 million people in five Nordic countries. *Acta Oncol* **48**: 646–790.

Ritz B. (1999) Cancer mortality among workers exposed to chemicals during uranium processing. *J Occup Environ Med* **41**: 556–566.

Shimizu H, Kumada T, Nakano S, *et al.* (2002) Liver dysfunction among workers handling 5-nitro-o-toluidine. *Gut* **50**: 266–270.

Tamburro CH, Liss GM. (1986) Tests for hepatotoxicity: Usefulness in screening workers. *J Occ Med* **28**: 1034–1044.

Teo GG. (1992) The virology and serology of hepatitis: An overview. *CDR Review* **2**: 109–114.

Thomasson HR, Crabb DW, Edenberg HJ, Li TK. (1993) Alcohol and aldehyde dehydrogenase polymorphisms and alcoholism. *Behav Genet* **23**: 131–136.

Travers CJ, Cooper CL. (1993) Mental health, job satisfaction and occupational stress among UK teachers. *Work and Stress* **7**: 203–219.

Ward E, Boffetta P, Andersen A, *et al.* (2001) Update of the follow-up of mortality and cancer incidence among European workers employed in the vinyl chloride industry. *Epidemiology* **12**: 710–718.

Waterhouse JM, Folkard S, Minors DS. (1992) *Shift Work, Health, and Safety: An Overview of the Scientific Literature 1987–90. HSE Research Report 31/1992.* London: HMSO.

Weiderpass E, Partanen T, Kaaks R, *et al.* (1998) Occurrence, trends and environmental etiology of pancreatic cancer. *Scand J Work Environ Health* **24**: 165–174.

WHO International Programme on Chemical Safety. (1991) *Inorganic Mercury. Environmental Health Criteria 118.* Geneva: WHO.

Wild P, Ambroise D, Benbrik E *et al.* (2006) Mortality among Paris sewage workers. *Occup Environ Med* **63**: 168–172.

Wilkes B, Stammerjohn L, Lalich N. (1981) Job demands and worker health in machine-paced poultry inspection. *Scand J Work Environ Health* **7**: 12–19.

Wyke RJ, Edwards FC, Allan RN. (1988) Employment problems and prospects for patients with chronic inflammatory bowel disease. *Gut* **29**: 1229–1235.

Wyke RJ, Aw TC, Allan RN, Harrington JM. (1989) Employment prospects for patients with intestinal stomas: The attitude of occupational physicians. *J Soc Occ Med* **39**: 19–24.

Chapter 11

Auditory Disorders

KG Rampal,* Ailin Razali[†,§] and Noor Hassim Ismail[‡]

Introduction

Noise is a major health hazard in the workplace and with industrialization there has been a marked increase in noise in workplaces. Auditory disorders as a result of exposure to noise in these workplaces, in particular noise-induced hearing loss (NIHL), are a common health problem among workers exposed to high levels of noise. However, this hearing loss goes undetected until it has an impact on how the worker functions in his day-to-day life. While more and more evidence is emerging that NIHL might be reversible or at least arrested in its early stages via pharmacological interventions, prevention of NIHL should best remain as the *modus operandi*. Knowledge regarding NIHL, therefore, should be edified at every level; including the workers, employers, engineers, policy makers and especially the health professionals.

*Department of Community Medicine, Perdana University Graduate School of Medicine, Kuala Lumpur, Malaysia.
†Department of ORL-HNS, Kulliyyah of Medicine, International Islamic University Malaysia, Kuantan, Malaysia.
‡Department of Community Health, Faculty of Medicine, Universiti Kebangsaan Malaysia, Kuala Lumpur, Malaysia.
§Corresponding author. E-mail: ailin.razali@gmail.com

Epidemiology

Blacksmith's deafness occurring as a consequence of employment (Fosbroke, 1831) and boilermakers having difficulty in hearing at church or at public meetings (Barr, 1886) were reported as early as the 1800s. The World Health Organization in their study of the burden of disease in 2000 estimated that 16% of the disabling hearing loss in adults (over 4 million disability-adjusted life years or DALYs) can be attributed to occupational noise and ranges from 7% to 21% in various subregions. The effects of exposure to occupational noise are larger for males than females in all subregions and are greater in the developing regions (Nelson *et al.*, 2005). Dobie (2007), in describing the burden of hearing loss in the United States, while considering age to be the most significant factor in hearing loss, attributes about 10% of adult hearing loss to occupational noise. He emphasizes that noise exposure is the most significant preventable cause of hearing loss and stresses the need for stricter enforcement of noise control measures (Dobie, 2007). In the United Kingdom, 2% of working-age adults reported severe hearing difficulty and its risk increased with the number of years exposed to noise. It was estimated that 153,000 men and 26,000 women had severe hearing difficulty attributable to noise at work (Palmer *et al.*, 2002). Of the 3392 cases of work-related diseases reported to the Norwegian Labour Inspectorate in 2006, 59% (1987) of the cases were of NIHL (Samant *et al.*, 2008).

Auditory disorders in individuals working in various industrial sectors and occupations have been studied over the years. Fishermen in small-scale fisheries with current or previous exposures to noise had poorer hearing thresholds on pure tone audiometry as compared to controls. There was a significant difference in the absolute amplitudes of the distortion product otoacoustic emissions (DPOAE) in fishermen with current and previous exposures to engine noise when compared with controls (Paini *et al.*, 2009). The prevalence of hearing loss of more than 20 dB at 1–4 kHz was found to be 4%, 17% and 27% among administrative personnel, flight deck personnel and flight deck engineers in a Nimitz-class aircraft carrier (Rovig, Bohnker and Page, 2004). A study on Finnish Air Force pilots found that the hearing of pilots corresponded to approximately the 80th percentile and was 9–13 dB better than the 50th percentile of industrial workers due to a larger number of risk factors among industrial workers (Kuronen *et al.*, 2004).

The effect of aircraft noise on hearing and auditory pathways studied in 112 airport employees by audiometry and brainstem-evoked potentials showed a typical NIHL pattern of a dip at 3–4 kHz and a moderate hearing loss at frequencies of 6–8 kHz. Among these employees, the overall prevalence rate of high-frequency hearing loss was 41.9% with the highest incidence of 65.2% in maintenance workers continuously exposed to noise (Chen and Chen, 1992). Among 6000 employees in a large healthcare facility, abnormal hearing patterns were observed in 59 (19%) of 308 workers exposed to potentially hazardous noise levels. There were 36 cases of NIHL documented from occupational exposure at this hospital (Yassi *et al.*, 1991). NIHL and annoyance due to noise was more frequent among those in shipbuilding (average noise level of 98 dBA) as compared to those in the machine shop (85.5 dBA) of a shipyard (van Dijk, Verbeek and de Fries, 1987).

Ultrasound from high-intensity ultrasonic devices may interact with biological tissues to produce thermal effects, mechanical disruption or cavitation (Wiernick and Karoly, 1985). Sound and ultrasound emitted by these ultrasonic devices exceeding known hygienic limits for frequencies 10–20 kHz have a negative influence on auditory function in the high frequency range. While there was no abnormality in the hearing range of 0.5–8 kHz, there was an elevation of threshold in the 10–20 kHz range in a study of 55 operators exposed to industrial ultrasonic devices of frequencies 0.5–20 kHz. Reference hearing levels of 189 non-exposed persons were used (Grzesik and Pluta, 1983).

Workers exposed to occupational vibration are also often exposed to excessive noise levels. Sympathetic vasoconstriction has been considered to be responsible for vibration white finger (VWF). It has been suggested that vasoconstriction in the cochlear and peripheral blood vessels may be due to a common mechanism in NIHL and VWF. A study of lumberjacks who had used a chainsaw for three consecutive years for a minimum of 500 hours a year showed NIHL increased with duration of exposure to chainsaw noise. However, with equal noise exposure, NIHL was about 10 dB greater in lumberjacks with VWF than those without VWF. The higher NIHL in VWF subjects suggests this may occur through vasoconstriction of the cochlear vessels (Pyykkö *et al.*, 1981). In another study of 122 noise-exposed forest workers, along with exposure to noise and aging, the presence of VWF and an elevated diastolic pressure were found to be major factors responsible for generating sensorineural hearing loss (Pyykkö, Pekkarinen and Starck, 1987). Vibration and noise may have the effects of combined exposures on the auditory system.

NIHL and vestibular disturbances can coexist. NIHL and balance disturbance with Meniere-type symptoms appeared to be significantly higher among 18 senior army officers exposed to impulse noise for a long duration. Endolymphatic hydrops may be the underlying pathophysiologic mechanism in these cases (Ylikoski, 1988). A study of 60 subjects with exposure to high levels of intermittent noise from firearms compared with 115 healthy subjects showed that those with more severe hearing loss at higher frequencies (4 kHz and 6 kHz) had more body sway, estimated as movement from the center of gravity in the horizontal plane, than those with less severe hearing loss (Juntunen *et al.*, 1987). Simultaneous mechanical damage to both the cochlear and vestibular partitions by intense impulse noise may be responsible for the subclinical disturbance of the vestibular system among subjects with impulse-noise-induced hearing loss (Ylikoski *et al.*, 1988).

Equal noise exposure is generally considered to cause symmetrical hearing loss. However, lateral difference in noise exposure may not lead to a difference in hearing loss in the ears. Shingle sawyers characteristically exposed to noise from the left side had symmetrical hearing loss (Chung *et al.*, 1983). The asymmetrical NIHL in this group was small, suggesting that if significant asymmetry occurred, other contributing factors need to be explored. In 1461 audiometric records of claims for NIHL, 69 (4.7%) had a well-defined pattern of hearing loss where the asymmetry at 2 kHz was more than 20 dBA. There were worse hearing thresholds in the left ear in 82.6% of them. This asymmetry could not be accounted for by medical, occupational and non-occupational histories. Inter-aural asymmetry at 4 kHz, where the left ear was twice as often the worse ear in males and 1.5 times in females, was demonstrated in four noise-exposed populations (Pirila *et al.*, 1991). Right- or left-handedness was not found to be a significant factor for the poorer hearing in the left ear when 211 left-handed subjects were compared with a matched control group of right-handed subjects (Prilla *et al.*, 1991). While the actual cause is not known there has been a suggestion that there may be a difference in susceptibility to noise, with the left ear more susceptible than the right.

Etiology

Auditory disorders that arise in the workplace have predominantly been those caused by noise and vibration. A prerequisite to understanding noise and its effects on the auditory system is an understanding of the physics of sound and the mechanism of hearing.

Physics of Sound

Noise is sound unwanted, undesirable and most times damaging, and bearing no information and varying in intensity randomly in time. However, wanted sound can also be harmful if it is exposed for too long and too loudly. The very variability of sound can render objective descriptions of noise difficult. Hence, many descriptors of sounds have been proposed in order to quantify them, including decibel values, weighing scales and equivalent levels, to name a few examples.

Sound is produced by vibration of an object causing alternate waves of compression and rarefaction. It needs to be transmitted through a medium, and travels best in solids, followed by liquids and air (or gases). Sound waves become weaker as they move away from the source. These sound waves will evoke the impulse of hearing when they reach the ear. Sound waves possess various physical characteristics including frequency, amplitude and complexity, while their psychological counterparts are pitch, intensity and timbre, accordingly.

Frequency

Frequency is the number of times a waveform repeats itself per unit time. It is expressed in cycles per second (hertz, Hz) where 1 Hz = 1 cycle per second. Wavelength is the distance between peaks or troughs of the sound wave. Wavelength is inversely related to frequency.

Amplitude

The amplitude of sound is the magnitude of displacement of the waveform from the equilibrium to the peak or trough. Amplitude gives rise to the loudness, or intensity, of a sound. A sound unit, measured in dB, is perceived as intensity or loudness.

Timbre

The complexity of a sound gives it some identifiable characteristics that are known as timbre. This characteristic of sound is a combination of at least five acoustic parameters including the spectrum of the stimulus, its waveform, the sound pressure, the frequency location of the spectrum, and the temporal characteristics of the sound; resulting in what is termed as spectral energy.

Sound Measurement

The amplitude of a sound wave is typically expressed in pascal (Pa). While 0.00002 Pa (or 20 μPa) is generally considered to be the minimum detectable level of sound, the greatest sound pressure level that can be tolerated is 10 million times over! Since it is difficult to cope with this wide range of numbers, the logarithmic scale is used to express the ratio of these intensities. Logarithms compress a wide range of numbers into a smaller scale. All ratio scales must have an arbitrary zero, i.e. a reference point, and on the decibel scale the standardized reference point is 20 μPa. The following formula is used to calculate the sound level in decibels (dB):

$$20 \log_{10} (p_1/p_2), \quad \text{with } p_2 \text{ being the reference point.}$$

Thus a scale of 200,000,000:20 has been effectively compressed into one with a more manageable range of 140 to 0 dB. Decibels are relative units of measure and thus cannot be added or subtracted arithmetically. Another important concept to grasp here is the relative change in sound pressure. The inverse square law states that as the distance is doubled from the source of sound (or exposure time is halved, for example), the sound pressure will decrease to half its original value. And because of its logarithmic property, a doubling of sound power will lead to a 3 dB rise (and, vice versa, halving it will lead to a 3 dB decrease). This will explain why decreasing half the exposure time will actually lead to a 3 dB decrease (3 dB exchange rate). Hence the 3 dB exchange rate is more suitable.

Equivalent sound pressure level

Sound from various noisy sources varies during a working day. In an attempt to objectively quantify a worker's exposure to noise, especially for the sake of legislation and enforcement purposes, a time-weighted energy average that represents the total sound energy experienced over a given period of time has been used. The equivalent level or $L_{eq(t)}$ is the average sound energy received during time t. The popularity of L_{eq} is twofold: (1) it makes it possible to compare widely different sound exposures as a total amount of energy exposed, and (2) because it uses a 3 dB trading relationship, it allows a more accurate analysis of the hazards posed by noise.

Weighting network

Weighting networks or scales attempt to overcome the frequency variability of sound measurement and analysis equipment. With three standardized weighting scales A, B and C and the more recently developed D and Z, it may be therefore useful to look at alternatives to the A-weighting scales. The major drawbacks of A-weighting is that readings resemble the response of the ear, measuring only pure tones and only at relatively low levels (i.e. about 40 dB) and moderate frequencies. A-weighting is thus used mainly because it has been incorporated into most commercially available sound level meters, and because it has been around for as long as it has (based on the findings by Fletcher and Munson, 1933). Until other scales have been validated, it may be advisable to continue using the A-weighting scale.

Frequency analysis

Frequency analysis is conducted to determine the intensity of sound by individual frequency. This helps in determining noise source for effective engineering controls to be instituted. An octave band analyzer is used to determine the intensity at each of the frequencies.

Types of noise

Sound can be classified as infrasonic (less than 20 Hz), audible (20–20,000 Hz) and ultrasonic (greater than 20,000 Hz). Noise in the frequency range of 125 Hz to 8000 Hz is particularly important because this is the range that most speech frequencies fall into. A diagrammatic representation of this is shown in Fig. 1, marked by the blue-shaded area, termed as the "long-term average speech spectrum" (LTASS), or often known as the speech banana.

The LTASS demarcates where sounds of speech fell within the audiogram, in order to better understand how each and every frequency within the speech spectrum, or the speech banana (most usually from 250 Hz to 8000 Hz for many languages), is important for speech detection and discrimination. For many languages such as English or Malay, the consonants give meaning, whereas vowels give strength to the words. Hence, by the very strictest principles of speech and audiology, each and every frequency within the speech spectrum is important.

This would be where the methods of averaging a hearing threshold come into conflict with the above-mentioned concept. A person thus needs to be able to hear all frequencies well, and not just, for example, up to 3 kHz as with the American Academy of Otolaryngology — American Medical Association (AAO-AMA) classification. Without the ability to hear, say, the fricatives (such as /sh/, /f/) and plosives (alveolar plosives such as /t/, /d/), a person will have significant

DIAGRAMMATIC REPRESENTATION
OF COMMON SOUNDS

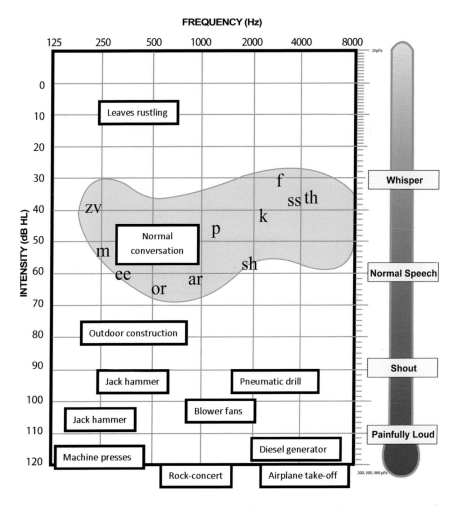

Fig. 1. A diagrammatic representation of everyday sounds in an intensity/ frequency graph. The speech spectrum falls into the shaded area.

difficulty understanding most if not all of speech. The usual tenet that speech frequency lies mostly in the 2000 Hz region is an anecdotal fact that should not be propagated just to justify the need to come up with an easy and manageable method of classifying hearing impairments.

Generally there are four types of noise: continuous or steady state, fluctuating, intermittent and impulse noise (Fig. 2). Continuous or steady state noise is sound whose quality and intensity are practically constant over a period of time. It generally varies less than 3 dB. Examples of sources of steady state noise include electrical generators, printing machines and weaving machines.

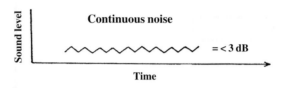

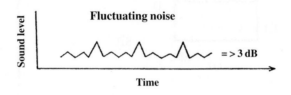

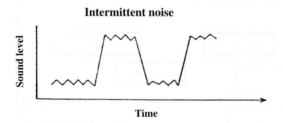

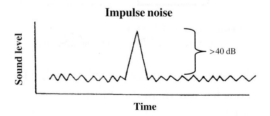

Fig. 2.   Types of noise.

Fluctuating noise is continuous noise where the intensity of noise varies more than 3 dB. Intermittent noise is sound whose intensity drops to the ambient level several times. These drops in intensity are for periods of one second or more. An example is the sound of a chainsaw cutting logs. Impulse noise or impact noise is sound with a sudden change of intensity of at least 40 dB. It is of short duration, generally less than half a second. Any type of noise can damage the ear, although there are some studies that have proven that high-frequency noise is generally more destructive to the hair cells.

Hearing Mechanism

The ear can be divided into the outer, middle and inner ear (Fig. 3). The outer ear is made up of the pinna and the external auditory meatus. It helps conduct sound to the middle ear, amplifies certain frequencies (1–3 kHz) to about a 20 dB sound pressure level (SPL) and, bilaterally, is the main player in our ability to localize distant sources of sound. The middle ear is a cavity connected to the outer ear by the tympanic membrane and the inner ear by the oval and round windows. It has three bones (ossicular chain) comprising the

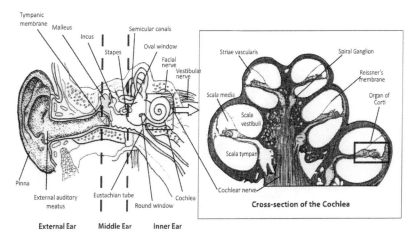

Fig. 3. Diagram of the external, middle and inner ear, with a cross-section view of the cochlea.

malleus, incus and stapes. These ossicles conduct sound waves from the external ear to the cochlea. The middle ear's main function is to overcome the impedance mismatch in relaying relatively small amounts of sound energy from the air to the fluid medium of the labyrinth while maintaining the same amount of sound energy. The middle ear, via the stapedius muscle, also protects the inner ear from impulsive, loud noise.

The cochlea and the semi-circular canals in the inner ear are responsible for hearing and balance, respectively. The cochlea, essentially a tube coiled around a central pillar of bone, resembles a snail shell. It is further divided into three chambers (scalae vestibuli, media and tympani) by the basilar membrane and the vestibular membrane. All three chambers are filled with fluid that will vibrate when the ossicles in the middle ear passes its energy through the oval window. The organ of Corti (Fig. 4) with about 24,000 hair cells lies resting on the basilar membrane. The displacement of these hair cells are responsible for triggering the action potential that will then be relayed to the final processing center at the temporal lobe where it will be interpreted as meaningful sounds.

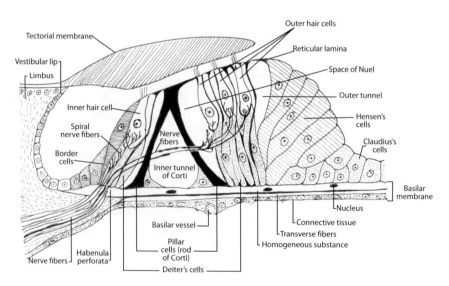

Fig. 4. Organ of Corti.

For physiological purposes the ear can be divided into the conducting apparatus and the sensorineural apparatus. The conducting apparatus comprises the outer ear, the tympanic membrane, the ossicular chain and labyrinthine fluids. The sensorineural apparatus comprises the organ of Corti in the cochlea, the auditory division of the acoustic nerve and its central connections.

Sound can be transmitted to the inner ear in three modes. The most common route is when sound energy is transmitted to the oval window from the vibrating tympanic membrane by the ossicular chain. Sound can be transmitted directly across the middle ear when waves fall on the round window if there is a large perforation in the ear drum. It is also transmitted by bone conduction when sound energy is transmitted to the inner ear through the bones of the skull.

In the most common route the middle ear serves as a transformer device matching the acoustic resistance of the air in the outer ear to that of the labyrinthine fluids. Within the cochlea, vibrations in the cochlear fluid are processed such that the frequency, intensity and relationships in time of the sound are transmitted to the auditory nerve. The cochlear nerve carries sensory information from the hair cells of the organ of Corti to the brain. The direction from which the sound originates is assessed by correlating differences in the two sides of the head (differences in loudness and time of reception).

Effects of Noise

The effects of noise can be auditory and non-auditory. Noise can be a nuisance and cause speech interference at 30–80 dBA. It can cause conductive hearing loss if the tympanic membrane is ruptured or the ossicles are dislocated as a result of loud impulse noise from an explosion. Noise-induced sensorineural hearing loss or NIHL occurs as a result of prolonged exposure at 85–120 dBA. Whole-body effects have been seen at intensities of noise greater than 130 dB. NIHL is the most significant problem facing employees in noisy workplaces. The damaging effects of noise depend on overall intensity of the noise, total duration of exposure, frequency characteristics of the noise and susceptibility of the individual.

Noise-induced hearing loss

The effect of noise on hearing may be temporary or permanent. The effect is a change in threshold hearing levels, and if temporary and reversible on cessation of noise exposure, it is called temporary threshold shift (TTS). If the loss is irreversible it is permanent threshold shift (PTS). As the cochlea is a mechanical analyzer that codes frequency into tonotopic stimuli, its mechanical structure and impedance are critical for maintaining a faithful representation of sound vibrations along the cochlear partitions. Hence, any damage within the cochlea will have implications on one's hearing ability.

Temporary threshold shift (TTS) is transitory hearing loss with normal hearing being restored after cessation of noise exposure. Time to recovery from TTS varies. TTS occurs as early as after two minutes of exposure. The higher the intensity and duration of exposure, the higher the TTS. TTS is maximum at about half an octave higher than the frequency of noise. TTS occurs at 75 dB and 70 dB at the lower and higher frequencies, respectively.

Recovery from TTS begins immediately after cessation of exposure with most of the recovery occurring within 16 hours. If loss of hearing due to TTS is less than 30 dB, recovery is usually within 16 hours. However, if the loss is greater than 50 dB, recovery is only rapid after the first day. In some cases auditory evoked responses had full recovery as late as after 30 days. While it has been suggested that TTS is an antecedent and must occur before permanent hearing loss occurs, there is insufficient evidence for this.

NIHL is irreversible permanent hearing loss with no recovery on cessation of exposure. The hearing loss typically commences at the 4 kHz frequency and extends to other frequencies with continued exposure. The dip is typically bilateral and symmetrical. Permanent hearing loss may occur without prior onset of TTS.

Case Study 1

A 44-year-old male has been working as a shovel operator in an auto-motive factory for 14 years. He was examined in conjunction with the audiometric testing program that had recently been introduced in his workplace. There was no history of ear discharge, head injury or any exposure to loud noise outside of his work. Otoscopic examination revealed normal ear canals and intact tympanic membrane bilaterally. Rinne's test was positive and Weber's test showed no lateralization. Pure tone audiometry revealed dips in the 4 kHz region with no air-bone gap in both ears (Fig. 5). He was diagnosed with noise-induced hearing loss

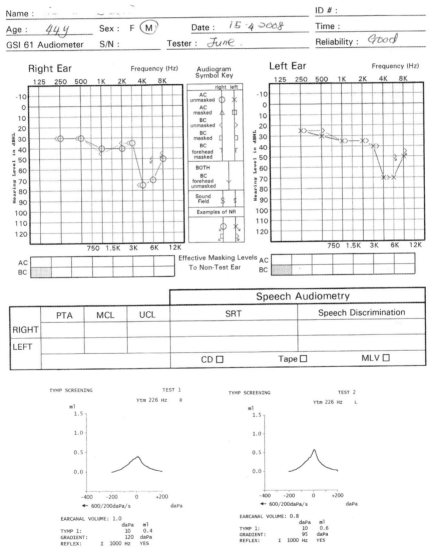

Fig. 5. Audiogram of a 44-year-old with bilateral noise-induced hearing loss.

based on his history of exposure to noise, the dips at the 4 kHz frequency and the absence of an air-bone gap.

Pathophysiology of noise-induced hearing loss

The basic mechanisms involved in noise-induced hearing loss can be broadly classified into mechanical damage and metabolic stress. Among the various mechanical processes, loud noises affect the delicate sensory structures in the cochlea where there will be obvious physical and structural changes to the major cellular systems within the organ of Corti.

Metabolic stress results from excessive mitochondrial activities, excitotoxic neural swelling, and reduction in cochlear blood flow, all of which will increase free radical production. Normally the cochlea's inner-ear defenses counter the damage by reactive oxygen species (ROS) and free radicals but with excessive sound stimulation these defenses are overwhelmed, injuring the hair cells and nerve endings (Henderson *et al.*, 2006). Both processes are detailed below (Fig. 6).

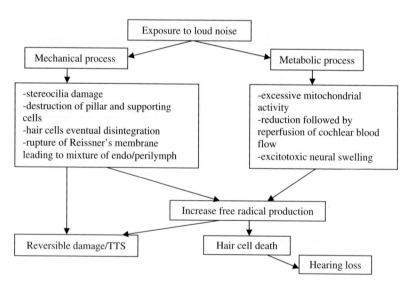

Fig. 6.   A flow-chart illustrating the pathophysiology of NIHL.

Mechanical processes

The various mechanical processes that could cause damage to the hair cells as a result of noise exposure include:

1. Violent fluid motion in the cochlear partition from exposure to loud noise, causing the tips of the stereocilia on the outer hair cells to be removed from their points of insertion with the tectorial membrane. In addition, the stereocilia may be broken, fused or have broken tip links that lead to loss of structural integrity and further reduce their ability to act as mechanoelectrical transducers due to the loss of permeability of protein transduction channels in the surrounding cell membrane.
2. Damage to pillar cells and supporting cells (Deiters's and Hensen's). The loss of these cells will interfere with the local impedance of vibration along the organ of Corti.
3. Damage to the hair cells either directly by detaching the organ of Corti or tearing of the basilar membrane, or indirectly from the damage of the supporting cells.
4. Rupture of the Reissner's membrane with mixing of the endolymph and perilymph, resulting in damage to the hair cells.

The above processes are usually seen when the exposure is to high-intensity noise levels and NIHL is of rapid onset. There is, however, a window of opportunity where a respite from the assaulting noise can lead to recovery, making the hearing loss reversible. However, the more common sustained, prolonged exposure to noise will more often cause damage resulting from metabolic exhaustion, where the increased metabolic activity as well as glycogen depletion and ischemia possibly induced by changes in the cochlear microcirculation will eventually result in cell death via necrosis or apoptosis.

Metabolic processes

The metabolic processes that could damage hair cells as a result of noise exposure include:

1. Overstimulation of the outer hair cells, making them require more energy. The hair cells may then be more susceptible to injury by

ischemia. Vesiculation and vacuolation in the endoplasmic reticulum of the hair cells and swelling of the mitochondria will lead to eventual rupturing of the cell membrane and hair cell loss.

2. Hair cell loss may be due to metabolic exhaustion as a result of disruption of enzyme systems essential for energy production, biosynthesis of protein and ion transport.

3. A significant rise in the intra-cellular calcium levels in the outer hair cells has been documented. This will lead to cytoskeletal breakdown, membrane defects and DNA damage. The consequence of these damages will be loss of body cell stiffness.

4. Injury to the stria vascularis causes disturbances in Na^+, K^+ and ATP level concentrations. This causes inhibition of the active transport process and energy utilization by the sensory cells. The damaged sensory cells create small lesions in the reticular membrane with intermixing of the endolymph and cortilymph and spread of damage to other sensory cells.

5. Reduction in the cochlear blood flow can occur and this will lead to an increased level of ROS in the cochlea.

6. Glutamate excitotoxicity will cause swelling and rupturing of the dendritic terminals of the auditory nerve's afferent fibres.

The region of the organ of Corti about 8 to 10 mm from the basal end (tonotopically corresponding to the 4 kHz region of the audiogram) is viewed to be uniquely vulnerable to noise, which causes the typical notch around the 4000 Hz region in NIHL. Several theories have been offered on why NIHL initially involves frequencies surrounding the 4000 Hz region, and they include:

1. The harmonic amplification theory: The physical structure of the ear canal creates a resonance and amplifies frequencies at 2–3 kHz. Hence, although occupational noise is mostly broadband, the energy that is mostly transmitted to the cochlea is in the 2–3 kHz region. Maximum hearing loss usually occurs about one or half an octave above the exposure frequency.

2. The absolute sensitivity theory: The ear is most sensitive in the 4000 Hz region, as evidenced by many established psychoacoustic studies.

3. The biomechanical theory: From a biomechanical point of view, the energy that is being transferred from the middle ear into the endolymph is greatest as it goes through the first bend of the cochlea. The hair cells located at the first bend are those representing approximately 4 kHz.

4. Middle ear muscle contraction: Chronically intense loud sounds will make the middle ear muscles contract and reduce only the transmission of low-frequency energy into the cochlea, as opposed to the acute contraction of the muscles which will block the transmission of sound across all frequencies.

Other auditory effects of noise

Acoustic trauma is usually caused by exposure to sudden loud sounds. Below is an illustrative example.

Case Study 2

A 31-year-old male factory worker was a victim of an explosion in the workplace. He came to the clinic five days following the explosion with complaints of hearing loss in both ears and a ringing noise in the left ear. These complaints began immediately after the explosion. On examination of the ear, there was a small traumatic perforation of the tympanic membrane in the right ear and an intact tympanic membrane in the left ear. Pure tone audiometry revealed bilateral severe hearing loss. Tympanometry was flat (type B) in the right ear and normal (type A) in the left ear. His hearing level was monitored regularly and a marked improvement in hearing level was noted three days later.

An examination two and a half months later revealed a healed tympanic membrane and that his hearing had returned to normal. He was diagnosed and managed as a case of acoustic trauma with temporary threshold shift.

Tinnitus (ringing noise in the ears) usually presents immediately after noise exposure and may become permanent on continued exposure. Tinnitus due to noise exposure is usually perceived as a high-pitched sound.

Vertigo only occurs after exposure to very extreme noises. Temporary vertigo has been described after exposures to noise of unsilenced jet engines. Temporary or even permanent vertigo can follow firearm explosions. Vertigo does not occur with ordinary industrial noise exposure. Presbycusis due to aging, occurring at high frequencies, is additive to NIHL. "Socioacusis" is a term that has been coined for hearing loss due to causes other than age and noise.

Non-auditory effects of noise

Increased noise levels also produce stress reactions with variations in heart rate, blood pressure, respiration, blood glucose and lipid levels. Increased gastrointestinal motility and peptic ulcers have also been reported. Studies have suggested that excessive noise above 55 dBA produce annoyance and a reduction in efficiency.

Diagnosis

The diagnosis of occupational NIHL is based on a history of exposure to noise in the workplace and not elsewhere, a clinical examination excluding other causes of hearing loss and an NIHL audiologic profile.

History Taking and Clinical Examination

An occupational history should include detailed, chronological information on current and all previous employment (particularly with respect to noise exposure, including part-time jobs held). Information on hobbies and other environmental exposures should also be elicited. The medical history must determine whether the employee has or had ear disease and whether he has taken ototoxic drugs, e.g. streptomycin. The clinical examination of the ear must exclude the presence of wax, infection and perforation of the tympanic membrane.

Pure tone audiometry

Pure tone audiometers have been used for more than 100 years as devices for measuring hearing threshold (Martin, 1975) and are the reigning "gold–standard" in assessing hearing threshold. Pure tone audiometry (PTA) is indispensable both for the screening (air conduction) and diagnosis (both air and bone conduction) of NIHL.

During PTA, pure tones are delivered to the ear through a suitable earphone, the most common being the supra-aural headphones. Insert earphones could improve the result as they would reduce the incidence of ear canal collapse and improve inter-aural attenuation. Circumaural headphones are occasionally used when the background ambience noise cannot be attenuated, e.g. when a soundproof room is unavailable. The frequencies tested range from 125 Hz to 8 kHz (testing at least 0.5, 1, 2, 3, 4 and 6 kHz) at intensities from 0 dB to 120 dB in 5 dB steps. Here we establish a threshold intensity of pure tone, above which the pure tone will be detected and below which it will not. Note that the unit used is dB HL (decibel hearing level) and not dBA or dB SPL. The response may however vary from one testing session to another, depending on the skill of the tester, motivation of the worker and the presence of ambient noise. The usual intra-personal variability is 10 dB HL across all frequencies.

PTA testing in the workplace is used to establish the hearing status of employees, to identify individuals especially susceptible to noise, to monitor hearing loss during the period of employment and to regulate a hearing conservation program.

Baseline audiometry is conducted at the time of first entry into the workforce (we recommend this to be included as part of the pre-employment examination) to evaluate the hearing level of the individual and to use it as a reference for comparison with future audiometric tests. Periodic audiometry is performed at regular intervals (annually or biennially) to monitor for hearing loss among workers in noisy areas. It is suggested that end-of-employment audiometry be performed to assess the amount of hearing loss (if any) that could have occurred during employment. The employee should not have been exposed to high noise levels in the past 16 hours for baseline audiometry and 12–14 hours for periodic audiometry.

Audiometers used for PTA must conform to national or international standards. Instructions for calibration should be followed strictly. Background noise levels should be low and set standards must be met. Audiometric testing should be carried out by trained personnel supervised by medical practitioners. These requirements have sometimes been incorporated into regulations (Factories and Machinery Department, 1989).

Audiologic profile of NIHL

The audiologic profile of NIHL is the presence of sensorineural hearing loss, which reflects cochlear lesions, most pronounced in the high-frequency region between 3 kHz and 6 kHz of the audiogram. The greatest amount of hearing loss is initially around the 4 kHz region (4 kHz dip or notch), although the maximum notch could be anywhere in the 3–6 kHz region. Another important feature is the recovery pattern in the 8 kHz region, which is why the frequency of 8 kHz should be included in any hearing test. It is a cardinal sign of NIHL when seen in individuals with a positive history of noise exposure. The audiometric configuration is bilaterally symmetrical. Continued exposure results in a growth in size of the 4 kHz notch, spreading to adjacent higher and lower frequencies. Higher frequencies (6 kHz and above) are generally affected to a greater extent than lower frequencies (2 kHz and below). In very advanced cases the 1 kHz frequency may be affected but rarely to a great extent.

The damage and profile is usually bilateral and symmetrical although differences may appear due to unequal ear susceptibility, different initial hearing thresholds and specific conditions of work. The audiologic profile of advanced NIHL is similar to other high-frequency sensorineural hearing loss due to cochlear and supracochlear lesions. An audiogram without a cochlear reserve (no air-bone gap) excludes high-frequency conductive hearing loss.

A simple method of categorization can be used to classify employees:

1. Where the hearing thresholds at all frequencies are less than 25 dB HL, the individuals are said to have normal hearing.

2. Where there is a 25 dB loss or more at any one frequency, individuals are said to have hearing loss.

3. Where there is a 25 dB loss or more in the 4 kHz region (including 3 and 6 kHz) plus a recovery pattern at 8 kHz, these individuals are said to have hearing loss that is suggestive of early NIHL. Although there is no legislation on follow-up actions pertaining to this, it would be advisable for these workers to be notified that there are already early signs of NIHL so that due preventive measures can be carried out.

4. Where there is an average loss of 25 dB or more affecting the frequencies 0.5, 1, 2 and 3 kHz, and the individuals have a history of noise exposure, they are said to have hearing impairment from NIHL. The workers need to be notified of their audiological findings, and measures, such as ensuring that the workers are not exposed to noise above 85 dB for more than eight hours, by engineering manipulation or administratively rotating their workstations, must be taken. The importance of wearing personal protective equipment (PPE) should be reiterated. Annual audiograms are a must and the workers should be sent for further referrals when necessary.

5. Where there is an average increase of 10 dB or more in the frequencies 2, 3 and 4 kHz, and the individuals have a history of noise exposure over time, standard threshold shift (STS) is said to have been established and the workers need to be notified, provided with retraining and refitting of hearing protectors and sent for further referrals. The establishment of STS needs to be confirmed within a certain period of time (which varies with different countries) and is a form of compromise to detect NIHL early.

6. Where there is an average loss of 50 dB or more affecting the frequencies 0.5, 1, 2 and 3 kHz, and the individuals have a history of noise exposure, the employees should be eligible for disability benefits.

A decision on whether a hearing impairment is due to noise should be made by the medical practitioner only after reviewing the medical and occupational history, ear examination and audiograms (which should be repeated using diagnostic methods).

Fitness for Work

Normal hearing is difficult to define as there is a wide individual variation in the degree to which hearing impairment causes hearing disability. Moreover, unlike a blind person, an individual with defective hearing has a hidden disability. The deaf and those who are hard of hearing need to be excluded only from a minority of jobs. There are very few jobs where perfect hearing is essential and these are jobs with highly specific auditory requirements, e.g. radio operators and civil airline pilots. The fairest way to judge the employability of a hearing impaired person is to test his hearing ability in the intended working environment. While auditory disorders seldom lead to time off work, they may have an impact on efficiency and safety.

Other auditory disorders that can affect an individual's fitness for work include tinnitus, ear discharge, balance disturbances and problems with barometric pressure differences. While the decision on the auditory requirement for fitness for work is usually left to examining medical practitioners, specific international and national regulations provide general guidance on this matter.

Medical examinations for employees in civil aviation are carried out by those authorized by local civil aviation authorities in accordance with International Civil Aviation Organization (ICAO) guidelines (Harding and Mills, 1983). While pilots rarely lose their license due to hearing loss, audiometry is performed every five years up to 40 years of age and then every three years. The maximum hearing loss allowed in either ear is 35 dB at 0.5, 1 and 2 kHz and 50 dB at 3 kHz.

Forced whisper tests for assessing hearing acuity have been carried out in routine examinations of serving armed forces personnel. In the United Kingdom, if the sum of the hearing threshold is greater than 85 dB at 0.5, 1 and 2 kHz and more than 124 dB at 3, 4 and 6 kHz, the individual is usually unfit for entry.

For policemen and firefighters the screening test for hearing ability is for a forced whisper to be heard separately by each ear at 20 feet. In the rail industry it is considered unsafe to employ a person dependent on hearing aids for footplate duties on main lines. On entry, for those in footplate and safety grades, hearing loss must be less than 20 dB at 0.5, 1 and 2 kHz and 30 dB on follow-up examinations (Coles and Sinclair, 1988a). While defective hearing does not disqualify individuals from having ordinary licenses, for drivers of heavy goods vehicles and public service vehicles, hearing defects are considered contraindications to driving where communication by telephone in an emergency poses a problem. The Medical Commission on Accident Prevention in the United Kingdom recommends that licenses for heavy goods vehicles and public service vehicles drivers should not be granted or renewed if the hearing is so bad that it interferes with the proper discharge of duties (Raffle, 1985).

Similarly, drivers of public service vehicles and taxis are regarded unfit for work if they are unable to communicate with passengers (British Medical Association, 1983). Deafness, perforation of the tympanic membrane and persistent discharge are causes for rejection under the United Kingdom Health and Safety Executive Diving Operations at Work Regulations 1981 (Botheroyd and Jones, 1988).

Assessment for other auditory disorders

While tinnitus does not directly affect fitness for work it may be associated with psychological upset including insomnia that may be severe and incapacitating, affecting work performance.

Otitis media and otitis externa may affect individuals' ability to use earplugs. Hygiene conditions required in the food industry may preclude them from working in the preparation or selling of food (Coles and Sinclair, 1988a).

Middle ear disease can affect flying and diving. Acute disorienting episodes from vestibular disorders coming on without warning may be a potential danger to employees themselves or to others at work (Coles and Sinclair, 1988b). For those who have due warning, episodes are not dangerously disorienting, or for who do not work in hazardous areas, they are not a problem. This group is however liable to recurrent or unpredictable absence from work. This group may be at risk when working with or near potentially hazardous machinery, where attacks are related to or induced by heights, and when working in a potentially dangerous environment, e.g. with molten metal, caustic acids and alkali. Having a sense of orientation is important for divers and those who have a high level of responsibility for the safety of others, e.g. those in control of vehicles on the road, work sites, farms and in the air.

There might be a need for the workers to undergo full medical surveillance to monitor the effects of noise on the cardiovascular system specifically and the workers' stress level in general.

Hearing handicap

The American Academy of Otolaryngology provides guidelines on assessment of hearing handicap. It suggests an average hearing level of 26 dB at 500, 1000, 2000 and 3000 Hz as the onset of handicap (AAO, 1979).

The Factories and Machinery (Noise Exposure) Regulations 1989 in Malaysia use a similar level. The rationale for using these frequencies is that these were felt to contribute most to understanding speech. In assessing handicap according to this guideline, the hearing threshold at 500 to 6000 Hz is assessed. The average hearing threshold at 500, 1000, 2000 and 3000 Hz is calculated for each ear. The percent monaural impairment in each ear is assessed by subtracting 25 dB from the average hearing threshold at 500, 1000, 2000 and 3000 Hz calculated for each ear and multiplying it by 1.5. The hearing handicap of an individual is assessed using the percent monaural impairment measurements of both ears. The hearing handicap is determined by multiplying the percent monaural impairment of the better ear by 5 and adding it to the percent monaural impairment of the poorer ear and dividing this total by 6.

An example using the PTA configuration of the previous example and an additional example with a much worse impairment are calculated (Table 1).

Hearing impairment can be classified into various categories: normal (not worse than 20 dB HL), mild (20 to 40 dB HL), moderate (41 to 70 dB HL), severe (70 to 90 dB HL) and profound (more than 90 dB HL). Deafness is a term that is to be avoided as there is no clear cut-off point to decide when a person becomes "deaf".

Table 1.   Hearing Handicap of Patient in Sample Cases 1 and 2

Frequency	Left Ear	Right Ear
Sample Case 1		
250	10	15
500	35	20
1000	25	15
2000	40	40
3000	50	55
4000	45	45
6000	40	35
8000	35	35
Average (0.5,1,2,3)	37.5	32.5
Percent monoaural	$(37.5 - 25) \times 1.5 =$ 18.75 (poorer ear)	$(32.5 - 25) \times 1.5 =$ 11.25 (better ear)
Hearing handicap	$[(11.25 \times 5) + 18.75]/6 =$ 12.5%	
Sample Case 2		
250	45	55
500	55	55
1000	70	65
2000	75	75
3000	75	75
4000	75	80
6000	80	80
8000	80	80
Average (0.5,1,2,3)	68.75	67.5
Percent monoaural	$(68.75 - 25) \times 1.5 =$ 65.6 (poorer ear)	$(67.5 - 25) \times 1.5 =$ 63.75 (better ear)
Hearing handicap	$[(63.75 \times 5) + 65.6]/6 =$ 64.1%	

While assessment of hearing handicap is based on an individual's hearing, the degree of disability associated with it must take into consideration other work-related factors, including the importance of the auditory function in his job. Guidelines for total disability due to hearing handicap vary from country to country. They generally

require that hearing cannot be restored by hearing aids before benefits are provided. Hearing loss as a result of presbycusis is sometimes
adjusted for in assessing occupational hearing loss.

Table 2 lists the comparative methods in some countries for
assessing disability.

Table 2 illustrates that a method for calculating disability in order
to compensate workers fairly has yet to be perfected. The use of questionnaires has largely been rejected because of its high level of
subjectivity (high variability). Perhaps a method to consider would be
assessing speech perception in quiet as well as in noisy environments
and how much is compromised as a result of the worker's hearing

Table 2.   Methods of Calculating Disability from Hearing Impairment

Formula	Frequencies (kHz)	Low Fence	High Fence	Weight Between Ears
AAO-1979	0.5, 1, 2, 3	25	92	5:1
AAOO-1959	1, 2, 3	25	92	5:1
NIOSH-FECA	1, 2, 3	25	92	5:1
Wisconsin State Formula	0.5, 1, 2, 3, 4, 6	35	92	4:1
British Society of Audiology	1, 2, 4	25	92	5:1
The British "Black Book"	1, 2, 3	—		
DHSS	1, 2, 3	40		4:1
Compensation for Occupational Injuries and Diseases Act 1993	0.5, 1, 2, 3	25		5:1
Workers' Compensation Board, Ontario	0.5, 1, 2, 3	35		5:1
Workers' Compensation Board, Quebec	0.5, 1, 2			
Ireland	0.5, 1, 2, 4	20	100	4:1
SOCSO Malaysia	0.5, 1, 2, 3	25	100	5:1

AAO: American Academy of Otolaryngology
AAOO: American Academy of Ophthalmology and Otolaryngology
NIOSH: The National Institute for Occupational Safety and Health
FECA: Federal Employees' Compensation Act
DHSS: The Department of Health and Social Security (UK)
SOCSO: Social Security Organization (Malaysia)

impairment. The hearing-in-noise test (HINT) is now equipped with many languages validated for commercial use, and has the potential to better diagnose disability resulting from hearing impairment.

Prevention of NIHL

Although the potential of therapeutic intervention, where repair could be initiated after noise injury but before actual permanent cell death sets in, is very real, preventing the onset of NIHL is still the *modus operandi*. It is imperative that a hearing conservation program (HCP) be instituted in noisy workplaces. Where regulations do not exist for the need to have a HCP, a proactive stance must be taken.

Hearing Conservation Program

Elements of an effective HCP include a noise survey, efforts to reduce noise exposure through noise control (engineering controls or administrative controls), personal hearing protectors if these controls are not sufficient to reduce exposure, medical examinations including PTA testing, informing employees of the hazards of noise, and proper record keeping.

Noise survey

A hearing conservation program should always begin with a preliminary noise survey. The objective of the preliminary noise survey is to identify areas in the workplace where workers are exposed to hazardous noise levels. The preliminary noise survey should be able to provide information on whether a noise problem exists, the extent of the problem and identify areas that would need a detailed noise survey. The detailed noise survey obtains information on noise levels at various workstations so as to develop guidelines for engineering and administrative controls. It will also define areas where hearing protection is necessary and identify those employees who would be included in the audiometric testing program (Olishifski and Stanford, 1988). Noise surveys would need to be conducted using approved sound level meters set for the A-scale, slow response. Information obtained during this survey would provide information on whether workers are exposed to levels above the "action levels" and "permissible exposure levels" (PELs) that have usually been fixed by regulations on hazards in the workplace.

Action levels and PELs have generally been based on threshold limit values (TLVs). The TLV for noise refers to sound pressure levels and duration of exposure that represent conditions to which it is believed that nearly all workers may be repeatedly exposed without adverse effects on their ability to hear and understand normal speech. The TLVs are issued by the American Conference of Governmental Industrial Hygienists (ACGIH) as recommendations or guidelines for the control of potential health hazards (ACGIH, 2009). They have been incorporated into regulations or used as standards in various countries, e.g. the action level is an equivalent continuous sound level of 85 dBA or a daily noise dose equal to 0.5 and the PEL an equivalent continuous sound level of 90 dBA or a daily noise dose of 1 under the Factories and Machinery (Noise Exposure) Regulations 1989 in Malaysia. It must be recognized that the application of a TLV will not protect all employees from adverse effects of noise exposures. They have been used to provide guidance on the duration of exposure permissible. The criteria for acceptability of noise are a societal decision. It has been suggested that reducing the permissible exposure level of noise to 85 dBA from 90 dBA would protect 99% instead of 96% of the working population from incurring NIHL over the average lifetime. Social and economic concerns are generally taken into account in specifying PELs used in the standard setting. In some countries such as the Netherlands, Norway and parts of Canada, the PEL has already been reduced to 85 dBA.

Engineering controls

Noise control through engineering controls is the most important control measure in a hearing conservation program. Other measures are implemented only when engineering controls are not possible. It is the only method that controls the noise level while others control exposure to noise. Although the initial cost of putting engineering controls in place is high, it must be realized that this is not a recurrent expenditure. Complete knowledge of the process is necessary to decide whether noise should be controlled at the source or in the path. Measures of controlling noise at the source include replacing or substituting equipment with less noisy equipment, moving the source further from the operator, reducing vibration with vibration-absorbing material, and using silencers for air and gas flows. Measures of noise control in the path include acoustical shields, barrier walls, and partial or total enclosures of the source of noise. In essence, noise control could involve equipment replacement, equipment relocation, vibration isolation, surface damping, barriers, enclosures, mufflers and source redesign (Bruce, 1979).

Administrative controls

When engineering controls are not feasible, administrative controls can be introduced to reduce individual employee exposures. The "equal energy principle" allows a trade-off between noise level and time of exposure. The permitted duration of exposure depends on permissible exposure levels or a daily dose of 1 (Table 3). If exposure

Table 3.   Permitted Duration of Exposure According to Permissible Exposure Level (8 h TWA and Dose)

8-hour TWA dBA			
5 dB Exchange Rate	3 dB Exchange Rate	Dose	Number of Hours of Exposure Per Day
80	80	0.25	16
85	83	0.5	8
90	86	1.0	4
95	89	2.0	2
100	92	4.0	1
105	95	8.0	1/2 (30 min)
110	98	16.0	1/4 (15 min)
115	110	32.0	1/8 (~7 min)
120	113	64.0	1/16 (~3 min)
125	116	128	1/64 (~1 min 30 sec)
130	119	256	1/128 (<1 min)

levels vary during the day, the daily noise dose needs to be calculated to ensure the daily noise dose is less than 1, i.e. in compliance with the regulation.

In Malaysia, for example, following the guidelines set by the American Medical Association — Occupational Safety and Health Administration (AMA-OSHA), the 3 dB exchange rate is actually being taken into consideration by the fact that even though 120 dB would allow about three minutes of exposure, the cut-off point is still set at 120 dB, as calculations using the 3 dB exchange rate reveal that by 119 dB SPL, the allowable exposure time is less than a minute.

Administrative controls may be implemented by switching employees in high noise areas with those in low noise areas after a certain period of time has elapsed. It could also involve scheduling operating times so as to minimize the number of employees exposed to high noise levels.

Hearing protectors

Hearing protection is instituted to supplement these control measures. The primary objective in using hearing protectors is to economically reduce hazardous exposures to safety levels at the ears of employees to prevent hearing loss (Camp, 1979). Hearing protectors, e.g. ear plugs, ear muffs and helmets, must be made available to all those exposed to noise levels at or above 85 dB at no cost to employees. Employees should be able to select the hearing protectors and be provided training in its use and care. Proper fitting of hearing protectors because of the large variation in ear canal diameter and shape is important. Problems are sometimes encountered in finding ear plugs that fit and custom fitted ear plugs may be necessary. The type of hearing protector used will depend on the attenuation factor (noise reduction rate, NRR) and spectral characteristics of the noise environment the employees work in. We need to be aware that the NRR stated by the companies supplying the hearing protectors will often be much reduced when compared to the field performance and the difference can be quite substantial. The wearing of double protection (for example, ear muffs together with ear plugs) is also strongly recommended, especially in work environments exceeding 110 dBA. There are also many interesting developments in the technology of hearing protectors, such as high-tech headphones with noise-canceling technology and wireless connectivity making vital communication among colleagues possible.

Audiometric testing program

Audiometry is not a substitute for noise control. However, an audiometric testing program including baseline, periodic and end-of-employment audiometry is extremely useful in a hearing conservation program. Supervision of personnel, approved and calibrated audiometers and approved booths are essential.

Diagnosis of NIHL is made when noise exposures are definite and other causes are excluded. While NIHL is generally included in the list of compensable occupational diseases, the quantum of compensation varies depending on the amount of handicap. Where guidelines on assessing handicaps have not been developed, the AAO guidelines could be used.

High-frequency audiometry (8–16 kHz) has been suggested as a tool that can be used to detect early NIHL, which has been shown to be present even before the occurrence of hearing loss at the "conventional" frequencies around the 4 kHz region. A study by Hallmo, Borchgrevink and Mair (1995) has shown that extended high-frequency hearing loss (EHF, hearing loss right up to 18,000 Hz) is noted in workers exposed to noise regardless of their age group. However, the use of high-frequency audiometry is still very much limited by the reliability and repeatability of these instruments, and data regarding this is still quite limited.

Another tool that could be used for the early detection of NIHL is otoacoustic emission (OAE). OAEs are sounds that are emitted by the outer hair cells, and there are typically three types of otoacoustic emission that can be clinically utilized: spontaneous emission, transient evoked (TEOAE) and distortion product (DPOAE). Detection of OAE only takes a few seconds, and as it is an objective test the patient's cooperation is not needed. It is also very vulnerable to noxious stimuli such as intense noise, ototoxic medication or solvents or hypoxia and tends to be affected much earlier before any change can be detected in pure tone audiometry. However, the use of OAE in hearing conservation programs still needs more studies (especially longitudinal ones) to determine its clinical utility (Shupak *et al.*, 2007). We feel that at this point in time OAE is best used as an adjunct to the current screening audiogram, especially in workers with still-normal hearing levels, more for the detection of TTS.

Record keeping

Proper record keeping of exposure and hearing status information is crucial for monitoring and medico-legal purposes. Records should be kept for at least 30 years for future medico-legal purposes.

Potential pharmacological treatment of NIHL

The impact of these recent advances in establishing the pathophysiological changes brought upon by noise on the cochlea is substantial. We can now identify the points of intervention that could reduce the damage by noise, and they include:

1. Limiting the formation of ROS, either by providing exogenous antioxidants or by stimulating the production of endogenous antioxidants by sound-conditioning or cross-tolerating with heat (Paz *et al.*, 2004; Niu, Shao and Canlon, 2003).
2. Ameliorating lipid peroxidation and cell damages.
3. Ensuring the cochlear blood flow during and after noise exposure is not compromised.

Interventions such as antioxidant agents, vasodilators, neurotrophic factors (NTFs), steroids, calcineurin inhibitors, caspase inhibitors, c-Jun N-terminal kinase (JNK) inhibitors, and Src protein tyrosine kinase (Src-PTK) inhibitors (Henderson *et al.*, 2006) have all been shown to be at least partially effective in preventing hair cell death and subsequent hearing loss. Given the various points of intervention along the cell death pathways, there is an abundance of potential therapeutic targets. The most effective strategy may include targeting initiating events and early molecular processes, thus maintaining a cell in a relatively "normal" physiological state (Le Prell *et al.*, 2007).

Training and education

Noise is an old problem in most industrialized countries and employees are aware of the auditory hazards associated. This may not be so in developing countries. Informing workers of the auditory disorders that can occur as a result of noise exposure is important for the success of a hearing conservation program. "Right to know" is slowly arriving in developing countries.

Conclusion

The problem of auditory disorders in the workplace, particularly NIHL, is not new. While measures for its prevention appear simple and clear cut, the implementation of these measures is riddled with socioeconomic constraints. Knowledge and awareness of this occupational disease will essentially be the main catalyst for all quarters to comply with the hearing conservation program. While self-regulation is mooted as the way to move forward in promoting occupational health, this may not be so in the majority of developing countries. This is compounded by the problem of NIHL not having an immediate impact on workers' health and as such is not felt to be important enough to be addressed in the midst of competing risks. Stricter enforcement of existing legislation then becomes the cornerstone of conserving the hearing of the working population of the world.

Acknowledgment

The authors acknowledge with thanks Prof. Pakeer Oothman Sayed Ahamed, Professor in Parasitology, Department of Basic Medicial Sciences, Kulliyyah of Medicine, IIUM for drawing the figures in this chapter.

References

American Academy of Otolaryngology Committee on Hearing and Equilibrium and American Council of Otolaryngology Committee on the Medical Aspects of Noise. (1979) Guide for the evaluation of hearing handicap. *JAMA* **241**(19): 2055–2059.

ACGIH. (2009) *2009 TLVS and BEIs: Threshold Limit Values for Chemical Substances and Physical Agents and Biological Exposure Indices.* Ohio: ACGIH.

Barr T. (1886) Enquiry into the effects of loud sounds upon the hearing of boilermakers and others who work amid noisy surroundings. *Proc Glasgow Phil Soc* 17: 223–239.

Botheroyd EM, Jones WEO. (1988) Diving (regulations and medical standards of fitness to dive). In: Edwards FC, *et al.* (eds). *Fitness for Work: The Medical Aspects*, pp. 67–89. Oxford: Oxford University Press.

British Medical Association. (1983) *Notes for Guidance of Doctors Completing Medical Certificates in Respect of Applicants for Heavy Goods and Public Service Vehicle and Taxi Drivers Licences.* London: British Medical Association.

Bruce RD. (1979) Reduction of noise at the source. *Otolarygol Clin North Am* 12(3): 563–568.

Camp RT. (1979) Hearing protectors. *Otolaryngol Clin North Am* 12(3): 569–584.

Chen TJ, Chen SS. (1992) Effects of aircraft noise on hearing and auditory pathway function of aircraft employees. *J Occup Med* 34(6): 613–619.

Chung DY, Mason K, Willson GN, Gannon RP. (1983) Asymmetrical noise exposure and hearing loss among shingle sawyers. *J Occup Med* 25(7): 541–543.

Coles RRA, Sinclair A. (1988a) Hearing. In: Edwards FC *et al.* (eds). *Fitness for Work: The Medical Aspects*, pp. 67–89. Oxford: Oxford University Press.

Coles RRA, Sinclair A. (1988b) Vestibular disorders. In: Edwards FC *et al.* (eds). *Fitness for Work: The Medical Aspects*, pp. 90–100. Oxford: Oxford University Press.

Dobie RA. (2007) The burdens of age-related and occupational noise-induced hearing loss in the United States. *Ear Hear* 29(4): 545–577.

Factories and Machinery Department Malaysia. (1989) *Factories and Machinery (Noise Exposure) Regulations 1989.*

Fosbroke J. (1831) Pathology and treatment of deafness. *Lancet* 19: 645–648.

Grzesik J, Pluta A. (1983) High-frequency hearing risk of operators of industrial ultrasonic devices. *Int Arch Occup Environ Health* 53(1): 77–88.

Hallmo P, Borchgrevink HM, Mair IWS. (1995) Extended high-frequency thresholds in noise-induced hearing loss. *Scand Audiol* 24: 47–52.

Harding RM, Mills FJ. (1983) Is the crew fit to fly? *Br Med J* 287: 114–116; 192–195.

Henderson D, Bielefeld EC, Harris KC, Bo HH. (2006) The role of oxidative stress in noise-induced hearing loss. *Ear Hear* 27: 1–19.

Juntunen J, Matikainen E, Ylikoski M *et al.* (1987) Postural body sway and exposure to high-energy impulse noise. *Lancet* 2(8553): 261–264.

Kuronen P, Toppila E, Starck J, *et al.* (2004) Modelling the risk of noise-induced hearing loss among military pilots. *Int J Audiology* 43: 79–84.

Le Prell CG, Yamashita D, Minami SB, *et al.* (2007) Mechanisms of noise-induced hearing loss indicate multiple methods of prevention. *Hear Res* 226(1–2): 22–43.

Martin FN. (1975) Pure tone audiometry. In: *Introduction to Audiology*, pp. 69–123. Englewood Cliffs NJ: Prentice Hall.

Nelson DI, Nelson RY, Concha-Barrientos M, Fingerhut M. (2005) The global burden of occupational noise-induced hearing loss. *Am J Ind Med* 48: 1–15.

Niu X, Shao R, Canlon B. (2003) Suppression of apoptosis occurs in the cochlea by sound conditioning. *NeuroReport* 14: 1025–1029.

Olishifski JB, Stanford JJ. (1988) Industrial noise. In: Plog BA (ed). *Fundamentals of Industrial Hygiene*, 3rd edn. pp. 163–204. USA: National Safety Council.

Paini MC, Morata TC, Corteletti LJ, *et al.* (2009) Audiological findings among workers from Brazilian small-scale fisheries. *Ear Hear* 30(1): 8–15.

Palmer KT, Griffin MJ, Sydall HE, *et al.* (2002) Occupational exposure to noise and the attributable burden of hearing difficulties in Great Britain. *Occup Environ Med* 59: 634–639.

Paz Z, Freeman S, Horowitz M, Sohmer H. (2004) Prior heat acclimatition confers protection against noise-induced hearing loss. *Audiology and Neurootology* 9: 306–309.

Pirila T, Sorri M, Jounio-Ervasti K, *et al.* (1991) Hearing asymmetry among occupationally exposed men and women under 60 years of age. *Scand Audiol* 20(4): 217–122.

Pirila T, Jounio-Ervasti K, Sorri M. (1991) Hearing asymmetry among left-handed and right-handed persons in a random population. *Scand Audiol* 20(4): 223–226.

Pyykkö I, Starck J, Farkkila M, *et al.* (1981) Hand-arm vibration in the aetiology of hearing loss in lumberjacks. *Brit J Indust Med* 38: 281–289.

Pyykkö I, Pekkarinen J, Starck J. (1987) Sensory-neural hearing loss during combined noise and vibration exposure. *Int Arch Occup Environ Health* 59: 439–454.

Raffle A. (ed). (1985) *Medical Aspects of Fitness to Drive: A Guide for Medical Practitioners*, 4th edn. London: Medical Commission on Accident Prevention.

Rovig GW, Bohnker BK, Page JC. (2004) Hearing health risk in a population of aircraft carrier flight deck personnel. *Mil Med* **169**(6): 429–432.

Samant Y, Parker D, Wergeland E, Wannag A. (2008) The Norwegian Labour Inspectorate's registry for work-related diseases: Data from 2006. *Int J Occup Environ Health* **14**: 272–279.

Shupak A, Dror T, Zohara S, *et al.* (2007) Otoacoustic emissions in early noise-induced hearing loss. *Otol Neurotol* **28**: 745–752.

van Dijk FJ, Verbeek JH, de Fries FF. (1987) Non-auditory effects of noise in industry. V. A field study in a shipyard. *Int Arch Occup Environ Health* **59**(1): 55–62.

Wiernick C, Karoly WJ. (1985) Ultrasound: Biological effects and industrial hygiene concerns. *Am Ind Hyg Assoc J* **46**(9): 488–496.

Yassi A, Gaorieau D, Gillespie I, Elias J. (1992) The noise hazard in a large health care facility. *J Occup Med* **33**(10): 1067–1070.

Ylikoski J. (1988) Delayed endolymphatic hydrops syndrome after heavy exposure to impulse noise. *Am J Otol* **9**(4): 282–285.

Ylikoski J, Juntunen J, Matikainen E, *et al.* (1988) Subclinical vestibular pathology in patients with noise-induced hearing loss from intense impulse noise. *Acta Otolaryngol (Stckh)* **105**(5–6): 558–563.

Chapter 12

Eye Injuries and Other Disorders

Laurence S Lim* and Tien-Yin Wong[†,‡]

Case Study 1

A 21-year-old construction worker was struck in the right eye by a large piece of metal while he was hammering. He experienced a sudden drop in his vision and quickly presented to the accident and emergency department. On examination, his visual acuity was 6/60 in his right eye, and 6/6 in his left. There was gross hyphema in the anterior chamber of his left eye. The intraocular pressure was raised to 25 mmHg. An X-ray of the right orbit showed no orbital fracture or intraocular foreign body. He was admitted for observation and management. When the hyphema had partially cleared, an examination of his retina showed multiple areas of retinal hemorrhage and edema (commotio retinae). His visual acuity improved to 6/18 at discharge. On questioning, he admitted to non-compliance with use of eye protection equipment at the worksite.

Case Study 2

A 33-year-old electrician was connecting wires in the ceiling when the end of a wire poked his left eye. Although he felt no pain or visual loss, he

---

*Singapore National Eye Centre, 11 Third Hospital Avenue, Singapore.
†National University Health System, Singapore Eye Research Institute,
Singapore National Eye Centre.
‡Corresponding author. E-mail: tien-yin-wong@nuhs.edu.sg

consulted a family doctor after work, and was referred to the accident and emergency department. On examination, his visual acuity was 6/6 in both eyes. There was a vertical 2 mm partial-thickness corneal laceration in his left eye (Figs. 1 and 2). The rest of the eye examination was

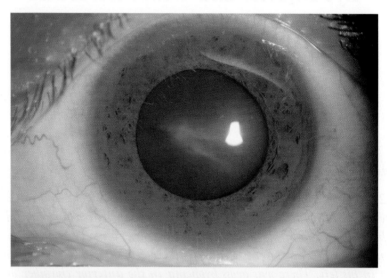

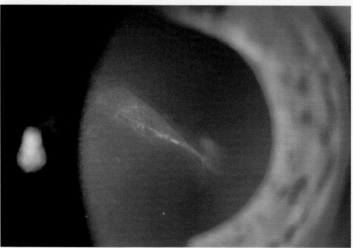

Figs. 1 and 2.   Partial-thickness corneal laceration in a 33-year-old electrician who was poked in the left eye by the end of a wire. Surgical repair is usually not necessary.

unremarkable and an X-ray of the left orbit revealed no intraocular foreign body. He was started on prophylactic topical antibiotic eyedrops and followed up at the outpatient clinic. At the three-month follow-up, his visual acuity remained 6/6 and a corneal scar was seen at the site of the laceration.

Introduction

Occupational eye injuries and other disorders are important for three reasons. First, they cause disproportionately more morbidity than similar injuries elsewhere. A small foreign body lodged in the cornea can inflict significant discomfort and potentially lead to sight-threatening complications (e.g. corneal infection). Second, they occur in the adult working population and therefore carry significant socioeconomic implications, including time off work, loss of income and long-term disability in cases of blindness. Third, work practice legislation and environmental modification offer the potential for primary prevention, which is not possible in other settings (e.g. injuries at home).

In this chapter, we will first discuss occupational eye injuries, the most common and important work-related eye problem seen in clinical practice, and then briefly deal with less common, non-traumatic, work-related ocular disorders.

Occupational Eye Injury

Epidemiology

Work-related eye injuries are significant causes of ocular morbidity. In the United States, these injuries are major components of the 2.5 million ocular injuries that are estimated to occur each year (National Society to Prevent Blindness, 1980). Various case series and eye registry data in the US have indicated that 14–48% of all ocular trauma are work-related (Baker *et al.*, 1996; Dannenberg *et al.*, 1992; Morris *et al.*, 1987; Schein *et al.*, 1988; White *et al.*, 1989). In Australia, a study estimated that 42% of ocular injuries were work-related (Fong, 1995), while in the United Kingdom, another study puts the proportion of occupationally

related eye injury at 70% (MacEwen, 1989). The wide variations in estimates result partly from a lack of well-defined populations at risk in all
these studies and an inability therefore to calculate incidence rates, which
are a better indication of risk of injury.

Data on the incidence rates of eye injury in the workplace are limited (Tielsch, 1995; Wong, 2009). One source of data is from
hospitalization records, which typically capture severe injuries requiring hospital admissions. A retrospective chart review of 812
consecutive patients with open globe injuries treated at the
Massachusetts Eye and Ear infirmary between 1999 and 2008 found
that 18% were attributable to workplace injuries. (Kanoff, 2010). A
study based on hospital discharge data estimated an annual incidence
of 1.7 and 3.0 ocular injuries per 100,000 employed persons when
ocular trauma was the principal reason and secondary reason for hospital admission, respectively (Baker *et al.*, 1996). Less severe injuries
not requiring hospitalization are not captured in that study. However,
from a public health perspective, perhaps less severe injuries are even
more important, as they are more prevalent, can potentially lead to
blinding complications (e.g. trauma-related corneal ulcers) and incur
both the cost of medical care (direct costs) and time lost from work
(indirect costs). Of equal significance is the fact that minor eye injuries
are often preventable by the use of simple protective eyewear or by
modifying worksite environments. The National Institute for
Occupational Safety and Health (NIOSH) estimated that more than
80% of work-related eye injuries could be classified as minor (Centers
for Disease Control, 1984). Studies that include severe injuries exclusively are therefore only partially representative of the size and impact
of the problem.

Incidence rates regarding less severe work-related injuries are less
readily available. One study based on persons treated in the emergency
departments in Dane County, Wisconsin, estimated an incidence of
55 work-related eye injuries per 100,000 persons, 20 to 30 times
higher than the rate of severe injuries requiring hospital admission
reported in Baker's study (Karlson, 1986). Population-based studies
yield an even higher rate; one study in New England observed the
annual incidence of work-related eye injuries to be approximately
600 per 100,000 persons (Glynn, 1988).

The epidemiology of work-related ocular trauma has also been reported in other countries. In Italy, a national insurance database which registers all casualties that cause work disabilities exceeding three days estimated an annual incidence of 370 injuries per 100,000 persons (Cruciani *et al.*, 1997). In Scotland, the incidence of hospitalized ocular trauma was estimated to be 8.14 per 100,000 persons, of which about 70% were work-related injuries (Desai *et al.*, 1996).

Data on work-related ocular trauma from Asian populations, which was previously lacking compared to Western populations (Negrel, 1998), has begun to emerge from a number of large population-based studies. A prospective survey in the emergency department of a large hospital in Singapore indicated that half of all ophthalmic cases presenting to the department were due to trauma, of which 70% were work-related (See, 1998). Grinding, cutting metal and drilling were the specific activities in more than 90% of these injuries. More alarming was the fact that less than 20% used some form of eye protection equipment, with another 30% who were provided with protective equipment, but did not use them at the time of injury (Voon *et al.*, 1998). In India, the Aravind Comprehensive Eye Survey of 5150 adult subjects (Nirmalan *et al.*, 2004) elicited a history of ocular trauma in either eye from 4.5% of the population, with agricultural labor the commonest setting (46.9%). Similarly, the Andhra Pradesh Eye Disease Study reported the age- and gender-adjusted prevalence of a history of ocular trauma as 7.5% in the rural setting, of which 55.9% were work-related, and 3.9% in the urban setting (Dandona *et al.*, 2000; Krishnaiah *et al.*, 2006). Extrapolation of these estimates to the Indian population gives an indication of the magnitude of the problem, with approximately 6 million people with a history of work-related ocular trauma and more than 600,000 blinded as a result.

Data from the Singapore Malay Eye Study are consistent with the estimates in an urban setting, with a history of ocular trauma given in 5%. Interestingly, more than 90% of those with a history of ocular trauma worked indoors (unpublished data). The only estimate to data of the incidence of ocular trauma in Asia is from rural Nepal. In this study, the crude incidence of ocular trauma was 0.51 per 1000 population at risk per year (Khatry *et al.*, 2004). Of these, 68% were classified as "severe" at the initial presentation, and 75% of these were lacerating injuries.

Demographic Information

Like other work-related diseases, ocular injuries occur most often in the young, working adult population (Baker *et al.*, 1992). In particular, they tend to occur in the age group of 20–30 years. This has been observed consistently in both descriptive (Dannenberg *et al.*, 1992; MacEwen, 1989; Morris *et al.*, 1987; Schein *et al.*, 1988) and controlled epidemiological studies (Baker *et al.*, 1996 Brain *et al.*, 2010; Dandona *et al.*, 2000; Glynn, 1988; Jafari, 2010; Karlson, 1986; Khatry *et al.*, 2004; Krishnaiah *et al.*, 2006; Nirmalan *et al.*, 2004; Tielsch, 1989; Wong, 1999). Three-quarters of work-related open globe injury reported in one study were among persons under 40 years of age (Dannenberg *et al.*, 1992). This high incidence may reflect the placement of younger workers in more hazardous jobs, their increased susceptibility from lack of regard for safety practices or, simply, inexperience.

A higher risk in males has been found in every population-based study of ocular injuries, with incidence or prevalence rate ratios of male to female from two to over five (Dandona *et al.*, 2000; Khatry *et al.*, 2004; Krishnaiah *et al.*, 2006; Nirmalan *et al.*, 2004); (Brain, 2010, Dannenberg *et al.*, 1992; Glynn, 1988; Jafari, 2010, Kanoff, 2010; Karlson, 1986; Klopfer *et al.*, 1992; MacEwen, 1989; Morris *et al.*, 1987; Schein *et al.*, 1988; Wong, 1999). Again, the higher risk in males reflects either the placement of male workers in more hazardous jobs or a lack of regard for safety practices compared to females. One study in the military found that males had a consistently higher risk of injury compared to females with the same specific occupation and job tasks (Smith, 2005). It is also interesting to note that differences between the genders disappear in older workers, perhaps related to changing risk behaviors in older males.

There are ethnic variations reported as well. However, the key variable is probably the socioeconomic status rather than ethnicity per se. In Baker's study in California, the highest risk of hospitalized work-related ocular injury occurred in young men of Hispanic origin (Baker *et al.*, 1996). In Singapore, half of the work-related injuries seen in the emergency setting were in non-resident foreign workers from Bangladesh, China and India (Voon *et al.*, 1998). Direct evidence for the role of socioeconomic status has also been identified in some population-based studies. In the urban population of the Andhra Pradesh Eye Disease Study (Dandona *et al.*, 2000), lower socioeconomic status was a risk factor for ocular injury, while alcohol consumption was identified as a risk factor in the Singapore Malay Eye Study.

Industry-specific rates

There is a wealth of data on industry-specific rates of ocular injury. In one study, Schein and associates at the Massachusetts Eye and Ear Infirmary observed that 63% of occupationally related injuries occurred among workers in the construction industry and 18% among auto repair workers (Schein, 1988).

A survey of 1552 firemen in the United Kingdom fire service indicated an annual incidence of 3500 ocular injuries per 100,000 firefighters (Owen, 1995). In Finland, industry-specific data showed that iron and steel, fabricated metal manufacturing and excavating and foundation industries have the highest annual incidence of ocular injuries at 680 per 100,000 workers (Saari, 1984). In a study of the chemical industry, an incidence of 2300 per 100,000 worker-years was observed, which reflects the high risks in this occupational group (Jones, 1992). In Australia, automotive industry workers had the highest relative incidence of open globe injuries compared to other occupations but these workers were also the least likely to wear safety eyewear (Fong, 1995). Another study in a large US automotive corporation estimated an annual incidence rate of 1500 eye injuries per 100,000 employees (Wong *et al.*, 1998).

Other high-risk occupations highlighted in recent years include professional sports such as basketball, baseball and boxing (Vinger, 1994). However, almost any professional sport can benefit from primary prevention with simple eye protection equipment. A classic and often cited example is the 90% decline in the incidence of ice-hockey-related ocular injury in Canada following the introduction of mandatory usage of appropriate helmets and eye protection (Pashby, 1985; Pashby *et al.*, 1975). Similarly, the military is a special occupational group at high risk of ocular injury both during wartime (Wong, 1997; Zhang, 2009) as well as in peacetime (Wong, 1999), but these injuries are likewise eminently preventable with proper eye protection. In the Israeli Defense Forces, not a single eye injury occurred amongst soldiers wearing proper goggles (Belkin, 1984).

In the rural developing world context, agricultural labor is one of the commonest causes of work-related ocular trauma. In Nepal, 25.9% of injuries occurred in farmers, and 27.4% of injuries took place in the fields and farms (Khatry *et al.*, 2004). Vegetable matter was the commonest instrument of injury in Andhra Pradesh (45.3%) (Krishnaiah *et al.*, 2006), and 66.8% of those reporting ocular trauma in the Aravind Comprehensive Eye Survey were agricultural laborers (Nirmalan *et al.*, 2004). In Nigeria, 37.2% of ocular injuries in geriatric subjects occurred on the farm, with 41.1% due to sticks or twigs (Onakpoya, 2010).

Types and Causes of Injuries

The types and causes of injuries vary depending on the severity of injury. For severe work-related trauma requiring hospitalization, one study found that the most common types were open globe injury (46%), adnexal wounds (20%), orbital fractures (11%) and traumatic hyphema (11%) (Baker *et al.*, 1999). The most common causes of these injuries were foreign-body or projectile objects (19%), transport vehicles (18%), cutting or piercing objects (17%) and assault (9%).

The spectrum is slightly different for less severe trauma not requiring hospital admission. For example, in the emergency department setting, the commonest types in one study were superficial foreign bodies (58.2%), corneal abrasion (25.1%) and blunt trauma (12.5%). The commonest causes were grinding (31%), foreign objects from cutting metal or drilling (21%) or construction-related activities (12%) (Voon *et al.*, 1998).

Economic impact

Beyond acute medical care, work-related ocular injuries may cause both short-term and long-term morbidity. (Schein *et al.*, 1988) observed that patients with open globe injuries had an average of 70 days of medical leave from work. In another study in the automotive industry, almost one-third of the injuries resulted in an inability of the worker to resume his normal duties (Wong, 1999). In terms of disability, nearly 10% of hospitalized injuries require long-term nursing or rehabilitation services (Baker *et al.*, 1999).

The overall economic impact of eye injuries has been difficult to estimate (Munoz, 1984). Less severe injuries are usually not reported, although they can account for enormous indirect costs (time off work). For severe injuries, Baker's study on hospitalized work-related injury estimated annual hospital charges (excluding professional fees) of $14.6 million in the US when work-related ocular trauma was the principal admitting diagnosis and $40 million when ocular trauma was either a principal or secondary diagnosis (Baker *et al.*, 1999). In addition, up to 40% of those with open globe injuries sustained at work could be pursuing costly legal action against their employers (Schein *et al.*, 1988). Work-related trauma in underdeveloped countries, where agricultural labor is the main occupation, may lead to lower absolute costs, but the individual economic burden is arguably greater as the visual outcome is frequently poorer and alternative sheltered employment is usually not readily available.

Assessment

Clinical Presentation

From a clinical management perspective, no two eyes are traumatized in an identical manner. There may be extreme variability and unpredictability. However, there are several specific features that distinguish work-related eye injuries from non-work-related injuries. First, work-related injuries tend to be more severe. For example, blunt trauma may be associated with blow-out fractures (fractures involving the orbital walls without involvement of the rim), traumatic hyphema (hemorrhage in the anterior chamber), angle damage (leading subsequently to glaucoma, sometimes decades later), lens dislocation (Fig. 3) and vitreous hemorrhage. Second, metallic intraocular foreign

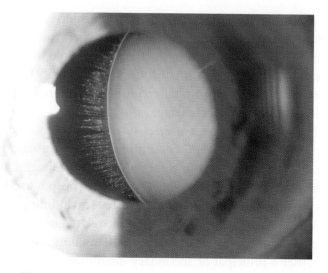

Fig. 3.   Dislocated lens from blunt trauma.

bodies (IOFBs) are common and have to be excluded in any work-related open globe injuries. Third, thermal, chemical and radiation injuries, rarely seen in non-occupational settings, are fairly important etiological agents in work-related injuries. Lastly, injuries from contaminated work-related instruments, vegetative matter in particular, are frequently complicated by severe infections by bacteria (e.g. *Bacillus cereus*) and fungi that may be more blinding than the initial injury.

Clinically, work-related ocular trauma can be classified according to the type of injury (e.g. blunt versus open globe), location of injury (e.g. anterior versus posterior segment of the eye) and etiology of injury (e.g. mechanical versus chemical or thermal). The Birmingham Eye Trauma Terminology (BETT) has been introduced to standardize ocular trauma reporting and has gained general acceptance (Kuhn, 2002b). Ocular injuries are classified into closed or open globe injuries. Closed globe injuries in turn are subclassified into contusions and lamellar (partial thickness) lacerations. Open globe injuries may be ruptures, in which a full thickness breach occurs secondary to blunt trauma, or lacerations due to a sharp object. Lacerations may take one of three forms — penetrating injuries without an exit wound, perforations with entry and exit wounds, or retained IOFBs.

Most open globe or penetrating injuries occur directly at the site of impact when secondary to a sharp instrument and opposite the site of impact when secondary to blunt trauma. The clinical features and complications vary. The more severe open globe injuries are usually easy to visualize and are accompanied by reduced visual acuity, a shallow anterior chamber, hyphema, a change in the shape of the pupil and an open wound in either the cornea or sclera.

In blunt injuries, compression and deformation of the eye are unusual occurrences because of the protection afforded to the eye by the surrounding bones of the orbit, particularly the orbital rim. However, even though no actual tissue loss occurs, the force of the blow may cause extensive injury to many of the delicate structures of the eye. These same structures usually have a limited ability to recover and repair the damage.

Surgical management is targeted at primary repair for even the most severe injuries, with enucleation (removal of the globe) indicated only if the globe is totally disorganized with loss of retinal tissue and if preoperative written consent has been obtained from an alert, sober patient. Frequently, secondary surgical procedures are required on an elective basis after the initial acute management.

History

A detailed history is extremely important in all work-related ocular injuries in the assessment of the extent of damage, potential for foreign bodies and complications (e.g. infection), and in the determination of appropriate investigative studies. The circumstances surrounding the injury are often important in future medico-legal actions. When, where and how the injury occurred should be reported in the patient's own words. A note should be made concerning whether the patient was wearing any type of ocular protection and the names of any witnesses should be recorded. A detailed description of the mechanism of injury (blunt or sharp), details about the size, composition and velocity of the object (e.g. nail) and activities (e.g. hammering) producing the injury is important, because radiologic studies are indicated if there is any possibility of an IOFB. An account of the events that occurred in the time interval between the injury and examination may suggest that additional damage or complication (e.g. infection) has occurred.

The patient's pre-injury ocular status should be documented. Pertinent information includes a history of previous eye injury, surgery or amblyopia. This is especially important in work-related eye injuries when disability compensation may become an issue later on.

Clinical Examination

Visual acuity should be measured in both eyes before any therapy is initiated. Pupil reactions to light (which may indicate optic nerve damage) should be elicited. The extent of injury (with drawings and photographs if possible) should be documented. If possible, maximal dilation of the pupil and ophthalmoscopy is indicated at the time of the initial examination because cataractous opacification of the lens or progressive vitreous hemorrhage may obscure fundus details within hours of the injury, precluding further examination. Ocular ultrasound is another alternative to evaluate eyes with opaque media. However, in patients with penetrating globe injuries, clinical maneuvers during physical examination may lead to further extrusion of intraocular contents. In these circumstances, the physical examination should be confined to measuring acuity only. If the vitreous cavity and retina cannot be visualized, radiologic studies are indicated to rule out an IOFB. Plain orbital X-rays with look-up and look-down views may reveal the presence of a radio-opaque orbital or IOFB. If an IOFB is suspected but the radiological or ultrasound investigations are negative, a CT scan of the orbit may be indicated.

In subjects where no injury is immediately apparent, certain signs mandate a high index of suspicion. These include an unusually deep or shallow anterior chamber, bullous subconjunctival hemorrhage in which the posterior extent is not visualized, gross hyphema, afferent pupillary defect, irregular pupil, and poor ocular motility.

Preoperative Management

Once the decision to operate has been made, the injured globe should immediately be protected with a hard shield that is supported by the bony parts of the face. Analgesia may reduce the patient's anxiety, thereby relieving lid blepharospasm and further pressure on the globe. The instillation of prophylactic antibiotic drops should probably be deferred until wound closure has been achieved to reduce manipulation of the globe as well as potential preservative toxicity. As cultures of the wound would involve additional manipulation, they are probably best performed in the operating room. Depending on the severity of the injury, surgery should probably be scheduled within 12 hours of the patient's admission to the hospital, when an operating room team can be assembled, because progressive wound edema and inflammation make identification of anatomical landmarks and wound closure increasingly difficult. Broad-spectrum prophylactic systemic antibiotic coverage is recommended in wounds caused by contaminated material or if the possibility of an IOFB exists. The timing of the surgery will be related to the patient's history of last known food or fluid intake because general anesthesia is preferred. The anesthetist should be informed of the nature of the injury and a request to avoid depolarizing neuromuscular-blocking agents like succinylcholine made as there is a theoretical risk of extrusion of globe contents. Although no documented cases of systemic tetanus following injury to the globe are present in the literature, this possibility must always be considered and prophylactic tetanus treatment is preferred.

Informed Consent

Since even the simplest open globe injuries may be associated with severe intraocular damage, a serious discussion with the patient and employer with regard to prognosis is extremely important preoperatively and a full informed consent taken. This is again of particular importance in work-related injuries when medico-legal compensation may be a future issue. The Ocular Trauma Score (OTS) is a clinical instrument that may be used in prognostication and counseling (Kuhn *et al.*, 2002a). The OTS is calculated from the following variables: initial vision, the presence of globe rupture, perforating injury, endophthalmitis, retinal detachment, and afferent pupillary defect. Based on the raw score, the patient may then be assigned to a prognostic category that gives estimates of the likelihood of achieving a certain level of final visual acuity. For example, a patient in category 1, the most severe category, has a 74% chance of no light perception acuity and only a 1% chance of achieving a final acuity of $\geq 6/12$. In contrast, a patient in the best prognostic category has a 0% chance of no light perception vision and a 94% chance of $\geq 6/12$ vision. In a recent publication from Mexico, the OTS has been shown to be ascertainable in 98.9% of ocular injuries. (LimaGomez, 2010). Recent studies from both caucasian and Asian populations have confirmed the utility of the OTS. A study on 31 open-globe injuries seen over 3 years in Hungary found the final visual outcome to be correlated with the initial OTS with a high degree of statistical significance ($p = 0.000095$), (Maneschg, 2010) and similar outcomes have been noted in Korea (Han, 2010).

Appropriate translation to the native language of the worker is necessary. Both the patient and employer must understand that 1) the goal of surgery is adequate wound closure with restoration of the integrity of the globe, 2) vision will be affected, complications such as bleeding and infection may occur and removal of the eye may be needed, 3) the healing period may be long and that additional operations to maximize visual potential may be indicated, and 4) long-term follow-up, for years after the injury, is required because of the risk of late glaucoma and retinal detachment. It is worth emphasizing to the employer that the injured worker may be unable to return quickly to his or her present job.

Management

Injuries to the Cornea and Sclera

The primary goal in repairing corneal and scleral lacerations is to achieve a watertight globe with structural integrity. Secondary goals include removing any disrupted lens fragments and vitreous, repositioning any uveal tissue, relieving vitreous incarceration, removing any IOFB, and restoring normal anatomic relationships with minimal globe distortion. A methodical surgical strategy is essential for injury repair.

Partial-thickness corneal injuries usually result in a shelved flap of edematous cornea that is in relatively good apposition with the surrounding tissue. Firm patching will often lead to re-epithelialization and complications are rare. If the visual axis is involved, secondary scarring may reduce visual acuity, but surgery is only indicated if the tissue is irregular and poorly opposed. Occasionally, a soft contact lens (bandage contact lens) may be used to reduce irritation and promote re-epithelialization of the area.

Full-thickness corneal lacerations can be in the form of puncture wounds or linear, irregular or avulsing lacerations. These injuries may be self-sealing or associated with a shallow or flat anterior chamber. Incarceration or prolapse of intraocular tissue further complicates management. Full-thickness corneal lacerations are at risk of endophthalmitis and patients should be routinely admitted for management. For small, self-sealing full-thickness corneal lacerations, a bandage contact lens may be sufficient to protect and support the wound as it heals. Corneal glue (cyanoacrylate surgical adhesive) can also be applied under topical anesthesia. If leakage persists for more than 24 hours or there is progressive shallowing of the anterior chamber, more definitive surgical treatment should be undertaken. On the other hand, large, non-shelving lacerations associated with a flat anterior chamber or incarcerated tissue usually require surgery to close the wound, to remove all incarcerated tissue and to re-form the anterior chamber (Fig. 4).

Injuries to the Lens

It is often difficult to diagnose lens damage or disruption in association with a corneal laceration, especially if the pupil is not maximally dilated and if blood and fibrin are present in the anterior chamber. In principle, removal of a damaged or cataractous lens rarely needs to be done in the emergency setting. However, in certain scenarios, mainly where a large breach in the anterior or posterior lens capsule has

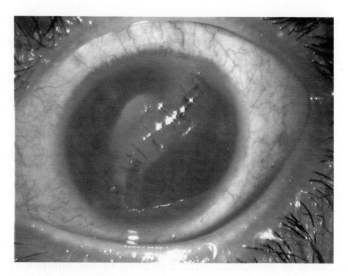

Fig. 4.   Surgical repair of full-thickness corneal laceration in a 25-year-old shipyard worker who was hit by a flying metal piece while drilling.

occurred, primary lens removal may be advantageous. If the anterior lens capsule is clearly damaged with flocculent lens material in the anterior chamber, or if the posterior capsule is disrupted and there is vitreous presenting in the anterior chamber, it may be preferable to complete all surgical interventions in one sitting. On the other hand, a small lens opacity with an intact capsule and no liberated material may be removed at a later date. If any doubt regarding lens clarity exists, however, the lens should be left in place in the acute setting. Various surgical techniques are available for the removal of the lens. Intraocular lens implantation in the primary trauma setting is controversial because of the risk of endophthalmitis. The patient's age, the visual and refractive status of the fellow eye, and the ability to use an aphakic contact lens postoperatively are factors in the decision.

Hyphema

Blood in the anterior chamber (hyphema) may lead to a number of secondary complications (Fig. 5). Even a small amount of blood in

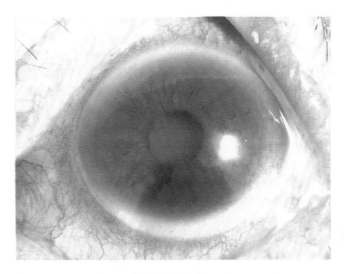

Fig. 5. Traumatic gross hyphema, sustained by a 21-year-old construction worker while hammering. A globe rupture must be excluded in all cases of severe blunt trauma.

the anterior chamber is significant because it indicates the possibility of serious intraocular damage.

Secondary (delayed) hemorrhage may occur at the time of clot retraction. If the hemorrhage is extensive, the blood may totally fill the anterior chamber and completely replace the aqueous (8-ball or blackball hyphema). The extravasated blood will turn from bright red to black as the aqueous circulation ceases and the hemoglobin becomes deoxygenated.

The main complications are glaucoma and corneal blood staining. Multiple mechanisms may lead to secondary glaucoma, which are usually difficult to manage. Blood breakdown products from hyphaema may diffuse into the cornea, causing corneal blood staining (reddish-orange opacification of the stroma). Blood staining may eventually clear; however, permanent staining is not uncommon, and may be severe enough to require subsequent corneal transplantation. Medical management is directed at controlling the intraocular pressure while waiting for spontaneous resolution. Surgical intervention is sometimes needed when this does not occur and optic nerve damage from glaucoma is likely.

Intraocular Foreign Body (IOFB)

An IOFB should always be excluded in work-related eye injuries as they are particularly common after activities involving striking metal on metal. Typically, the foreign body is small and the eye may not show obvious signs of trauma. Entry wounds through the cornea may be small and self-sealing, and subconjunctival bleeding or edema may cover those through the sclera. The entry site and intraocular site of damage may help delineate the trajectory and resting place of an IOFB. The IOFB is usually in one of the following locations: anterior chamber, lens (creating a focal cataract) (Fig. 6), vitreous cavity (Fig. 7) or embedded in the retina.

The composition of the foreign body involved determines the urgency of its removal. Some materials (e.g. iron and copper) may be toxic and stimulate inflammation and/or siderosis bulbi with long-term loss of vision, while others (e.g. vegetable matter) may pose a risk for severe infection. Contamination with *Bacillus cereus* in particular is well-known for causing a fulminant endophthalmitis

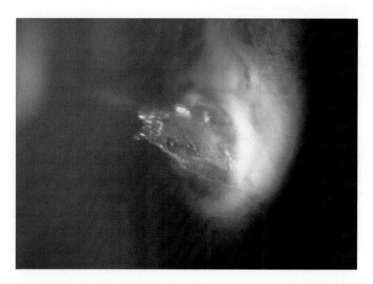

Fig. 6. Intraocular foreign body located in the lens. The surrounding lens usually turns cataractous within hours. In this instance, both the foreign body and the lens should be removed.

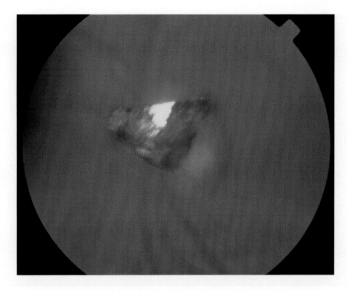

Fig. 7.   Intraocular foreign body located within the vitreous cavity. Removal of the foreign body may involve a complex posterior segment surgery (vitrectomy).

that may cause blindness in a matter of hours. These items should be removed promptly. On the other hand, inert substances such as plastic and glass may be well tolerated and left in place in certain situations. Surgery to remove IOFBs generally involves intraocular surgery with vitrectomy techniques, in which various grasping and cutting instruments, and occasionally intraocular magnets, are used to extract the IOFB and clear debris and inflammatory material.

Injuries to the Retina

Severe work-related blunt trauma commonly produces posterior segment injuries including retinal edema (known as Berlin's edema or commotio retinae), retinal hemorrhage, vitreous hemorrhage, retinal tears, choroidal tears and retinal detachment (Fig. 8). Even for mild blunt posterior segment trauma such as retinal edema, visual acuity is often affected and late pigmentary scarring may occur in the macular area, while peripheral areas of involvement may be the sites of future

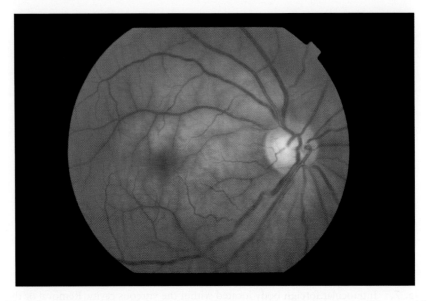

Fig. 8. Retinal photograph showing edema (commotio retinae) in a 21-year-old construction worker who sustained severe blunt trauma while hammering.

retinal tears. Choroidal tears may lead to the development of choroidal neovascular membranes that cause retinal scarring.

Penetrating injuries involving the posterior segment carry a less favorable prognosis than blunt trauma. The primary mechanical damage of vital structures by such injuries may be so great that useful vision is instantly destroyed. Major advances in the management of all posterior segment injuries are the development of microsurgery and vitrectomy. The latter, a closed intraocular procedure in which the surgeon can remove blood, debris or IOFB and repair retinal tears or detachment, has lead to an improvement in the prognosis of previously untreatable posterior segment injuries.

Enucleation

In all trauma cases, repair of the globe should be attempted. However, there are some severe work-related injuries (e.g. industrial accidents involving trauma from heavy machinery) which are beyond repair. Enucleation (removal of the globe) at the time of the original surgical procedure (primary enucleation) should be considered only in the event of total disruption of the globe; this includes those patients in whom large amounts of intraocular contents have been extruded or who have large scleral lacerations or ruptures associated with tissue loss that are completely irreparable. Initial primary repair permits evaluation of the total ocular status in the immediate postoperative period, with possible secondary enucleation at a later date. Thus, the patient is allowed a period of mental recovery to a more alert and oriented state. Also, both the patient and the employer recognize that the surgeon is making all possible efforts to salvage the injured globe. Should primary enucleation be considered, appropriate informed consent must be obtained. However, in cases where enucleation is delayed, the patient should be advised on the small but well-recognized risk of sympathetic ophthalmia, a condition in which an autoimmune reaction triggered by the trauma causes severe and blinding inflammation in the fellow uninjured eye.

Postoperative Management

The goals of postoperative management are to control infection, suppress inflammation, and visual rehabilitation.

To prevent infection, postoperatively, the eye should be protected by an eye shield and a topical broad-spectrum antibiotic should be prescribed. A combination of a cephalosporin (e.g. cefazolin) or vancomycin for gram-positive bacteria and an aminoglycoside (e.g. gentamicin) for gram-negative prophylaxis is appropriate. Vancomycin may be preferable to a cephalosporin because it has a better coverage of the *Bacillus* species and resistant *Staphylococcus epidermidis*. Clindamycin is added to this regimen if an intraocular foreign body is present, especially if the wound has been contaminated with vegetable matter, since such patients are prone to devastating *Bacillus* infections. Patients admitted to the hospital should receive 4–5 days of treatment with intravenous antibiotics, usually a cephalosporin or vancomycin and an aminoglycoside. Most cases of bacterial endophthalmitis present by the fifth postoperative day.

One must weigh the anti-inflammatory advantages against the risk of infection with corticosteroid use. Intensive corticosteroid use in early wound healing may also diminish the rate of stromal healing as well as the tensile strength of the wound. Topical corticosteroids should therefore be used cautiously to control inflammation only once infection is ruled out, usually 48 hours after the operation and continued until the eye is white and quiet.

Visual rehabilitation depends on the severity of the trauma. In certain cases, secondary operations such as corneal grafts may be indicated to improve vision when the eye is quiet and free from infection.

Chemical, Thermal, Electrical and Radiation Injuries

Chemical Injuries

Chemical injuries are common in a wide array of occupational settings, involving workers not just in the chemical industry (Bulbulia *et al.*, 1995; Griffith, 1994; Jones, 1992) but in other industries as well (Hong, 2010; Wong, 2009). The spectrum of ocular damage can be minor or severe, depending on the type of chemical, quantity, concentration, duration of exposure, directness of exposure, lipid solubility, anionic affinity and, most importantly, pH of the chemical.

For acid injuries, an instantaneous coagulative necrosis and precipitation of protein in the epithelium helps neutralize the acid and acts as a barrier to further penetration of the acid, limiting the intraocular damage. In addition, the tear film can act as a buffer against acids (unless the amount of acid is excessive or the pH is less than 3.0). Explosions of car batteries due to spark ignition of oxygen and hydrogen gas mixtures released by sulfuric acid have become one of the commonest types of acid injuries in mechanics and other workers involved in the automotive industry, and add an element of thermal injury (charring). While usually only superficial injuries occur, severe cases may result in corneal scarring, cataracts and glaucoma.

On the other hand, alkali injuries are extremely dangerous. Alkali denatures proteins and saponifies lipids, producing an immediate swelling of the epithelium followed by desquamation (rather than precipitation of protein as in the acid burn). Thus, the alkali is allowed direct access to the corneal stroma, through which it can penetrate rapidly via the corneal endothelium into the eye. In addition, alkali coagulates conjunctival and scleral blood vessels, which causes ischemic damage. When alkali gains access to the interior of the eye, it destroys lens and ciliary epithelial cells and causes extensive inflammation. Clinically, the conjunctiva has a porcelain-white appearance due to coagulation of the blood vessels. Later in the course of the injury, the inflammatory process further destroys corneal tissues, leading to extensive corneal ulceration and perforation. Alkali injury to the conjunctiva and lids also leads to scarring, dry eyes and other deformities.

Chemical injuries are one of few true ocular emergencies and should be treated immediately without delay to prevent blindness. Ideally, employers should have a protocol for dealing with these types of injury at the worksite. The single most important form of management is extensive and continuous eye irrigation at the time of injury. This could even be in the form of an eye wash with clean running tap water at the site of the accident prior to medical evacuation. Cement injuries are a special case of alkali injuries, as the particulate matter is difficult to remove by simple irrigation, and require meticulous forniceal sweeping and removal of all cement particles. Further management is directed at preventing complications (e.g. infection and glaucoma) and promoting re-epithelialization.

Thermal and Electrical Burns

The blink reflex usually protects the eye from most burn injuries. The cornea and conjunctiva may suffer extensive effects of secondary exposure when the lids and face are burned severely. The management of thermal burns is similar in many respects to chemical injuries from acids, with the primary aim to promote epithelial healing of the ocular surface.

Electrical injuries, especially if in the area of the head, can cause cataracts. Industrial accidents affect mainly the anterior superficial lens cortex whereas non-industrial electrical burns (e.g. lightning strikes) affect both the anterior and posterior parts of the lens. In extreme cases, there may be anterior uveitis or even anterior tissue necrosis.

Radiation Injuries

Radiation injuries are uncommon in non-occupational settings. The spectrum of ocular injuries depends on the type of radiation. Radiation may be either non-ionizing or ionizing. Ocular injuries from ionizing radiation are less common and are only applicable to workers in the medical profession of radiology. On the other hand, many more workers are exposed to different types of non-ionizing radiation, including long-wave radiation in the broadcast radio industry, microwave radiation in radar and communication industries, infrared radiation emitted from furnaces in glass and metal industries, visible radiation from sunlight in agricultural and construction industries and ultraviolet radiation from sunlight and welding in metal industries. Ultraviolet light sources in laboratories may also cause corneal burns. In addition, injuries from industrial lasers (either ultraviolet, visible or infrared radiation) are becoming increasingly important.

Microwave radiation causes thermal injuries to various ocular structures. Infrared waves can cause true exfoliation of the lens capsule (glassblowers' cataracts) as well as other effects. Visible light of sufficient intensity can cause chorioretinal burns, and is potentially sight-threatening if the burns involve the macula. Ocular effects of ionizing radiation include conjunctival and corneal telangiectasis and keratinization. Retinal microvasculopathy, vitreous hemorrhage and optic atrophy have also been reported in severe cases, and usually present many years after exposure. Ultraviolet radiation exposure has been implicated in many ocular conditions, such as conjunctivitis, keratitis and even macular damage. Welder's arc eye is a common condition and refers to an acute, painful, but frequently transient keratoconjunctivitis from ultraviolet radiation exposure in welders without adequate eye protection (Chou, 1996; Davies, 2007).

Other Occupational Eye Disorders

Non-trauma-related occupational eye disorders usually result from long-term exposure to various chemicals, infectious agents or radiation. Almost all industrial chemicals (including halides, solvents, insecticides, fungicides, herbicides and fertilizers) have been implicated in allergic conjunctivitis, keratitis, photophobia and other non-specific ocular irritation (Ansari, 1997; Ireland *et al.*, 1994; Marshall, 1995; Yokota *et al.*, 1999).

In addition to acute radiation eye injuries, long-term exposure to radiation can lead to chronic ocular conditions such as corneal diseases, cataracts and age-related macular degeneration (Milacic, 2009; Vano *et al.*, 1998). Microwaves have been shown to produce cataracts in animals experimentally but this has not been demonstrated convincingly in humans (Appleton *et al.*, 1975; Kurz, 1968). However, the evidence for ultraviolet radiation as a risk factor for ocular diseases is strong. Among the many different effects of this type of radiation, the two most important are cataracts and pterygium (Dolin, 1994; Moran, 1984). Taylor and colleagues effectively demonstrated the association between cortical cataracts and pterygium among Chesapeake Bay watermen (Taylor, 1982; Taylor *et al.*, 1989). A high prevalence of pterygium has been reported in postmen (Tang *et al.*, 1999) and welders (Karai, 1984; Norn, 1991) and patients engaged in outdoor activities (Viso, 2010). In the Tanjong Pagar Study in Singapore, participants who were outdoor workers, or laborers or agricultural workers were more likely to have pterygium and nuclear cataracts, respectively (Foster *et al.*, 2003; Wong *et al.*, 2001). These studies suggest that cataracts and pterygium can be considered work-related disorders in persons with long-term direct exposure to ultraviolet light (e.g. welders) (Davies, 2007; Okuno, 2010) or indirect exposure via sunlight (e.g. occupations requiring extensive outdoor work). There is also emerging evidence of a relationship between sunlight and ultraviolet radiation exposure and an increased risk of age-related macular degeneration (Peate, 2007; Plestina-Borjan, 2007).

Adult-onset myopia has been linked to occupations associated with an increased frequency of "near-work activities" (Simensen, 1994). For example, one study documented the onset and progression of adult myopia among clinical microscopists (McBrien, 1997). A population-based survey of refractive errors observed a higher prevalence of myopia among professionals and clerks relative to other occupations (Wensor, 1999). Similarly, in the Tanjong Pagar Study in

Singapore, higher levels of education, near-work-related occupations and higher income were associated with myopic refractive errors (Wong *et al.*, 2002).

Other occupations are associated with higher risks of specific ocular disorders. For example, a higher risk of fungal infection of the cornea has long been associated with agricultural occupations (Lin *et al.*, 1999). Another example is the "ocular discomfort" and "eyestrain" among operators working long hours in front of video display terminals or computer monitors (Acosta, 1999; Nakaishi, 1999; Piccoli *et al.*, 1996).

Eye Protection

Modern injury prevention theory does not support the claim that injuries are "accidents" or "bad luck" (Baker *et al.*, 1992). Most work-related ocular injuries occur in well-defined, predictable and consistent settings and are hence potentially preventable.

There are a number of preventive strategies available. First, the exposure itself may be altered. For example, toxic chemicals can be redesigned or substituted by less toxic alternatives. Radiation doses may be reduced to decrease the risk of radiation injuries. Second, the work environment may be modified to reduce ocular hazards. Static shielding equipment like transparent plastic boards may prevent foreign body and other mechanical injuries. Similarly, radiation barrier shields will decrease the risk of radiation injuries. Efficient exhaust systems that draw toxic fumes from the work area will help prevent chemical injuries. Appropriate provisions for first aid such as irrigating solutions and eye shields should also be in place at the workplace to reduce the morbidity from ocular injuries.

Third, personal ocular protective equipment should be available to prevent nearly all types of injury. This may range from general head and face protectors to goggles designed to prevent specific types of injury (e.g. laser protective goggles) (Davies, 2007; Okuno, 2010). Multiple studies have shown that adequate eye protection equipment in the workplace can prevent many serious eye injuries and makes economic sense (Wong, 2009). However, the awareness of workers concerning the use of eye protection equipment has not changed in recent years.

A major problem is compliance among workers. This is partly related to poorly designed and uncomfortable eyewear as well as a lack of organizational emphasis on ocular safety, as typified in the military (Belkin, 1984; Morley, 2010; Scott, 2011; Wong, 1997). Interestingly, a survey on the depiction of protective eyewear use in the mass media showed that adequate protective eyewear was shown in only 12% of exposure scenes. (Glazier, 2010) More attention should be directed to the development of ergonomic protective eyewear for use in occupational settings. Specific criteria for protective eyewear must be developed. Polycarbonate plastic lenses and frames which are sturdy and impact-resistant provide optimal protection while lensless goggles, streetwear and spectacle correction glasses do not provide adequate eye protection (Simmons, 1984). Other important design features include appropriate venting (indirect) and side shields (Peate, 2007). There must be increasingly active participation from all ophthalmologists and occupational physicians in the prevention of work-related eye injuries, including addressing particular industrial needs, identifying high-risk workers and continued education of the public on the need for protective eyewear.

References

Acosta MC, Gallar J, Belmonte C. (1999) The influence of eye solutions on blinking and ocular comfort at rest and during work at video display terminals. *Exp Eye Res* **68**: 663–669.

Ansari EA. (1997) Ocular injury with xylene — a report of two cases. *Hum Exp Toxicol* **16**: 273–275.

Appleton B, Hirsch S, Kinion RO, *et al.* (1975) Microwave lens effects in humans. II. Results of five-year survey. *Arch Ophthalmol* **93**: 257–258.

Baker RS, Wilson MR, Flowers CW Jr, *et al.* (1996) Demographic factors in a population-based survey of hospitalized, work-related, ocular injury. *Am J Ophthalmol* **122**: 213–219.

Baker RS, Wilson RM, Flowers CW Jr, *et al.* (1999) A population-based survey of hospitalized work-related ocular injury: Diagnoses, cause of injury, resource utilization, and hospitalization outcome. *Ophthalmic Epidemiol* **6**: 159–169.

Baker SP, O'Neill B, Ginsburg MJ, Li G. (1992). Occupational injury. In: *The Injury Fact Book*, pp. 114–133. New York: Oxford University Press.

Belkin M, Treister G, Dotan S. (1984). Eye injuries and ocular protection in the Lebanon War, 1982. *Isr J Med Sci* **20**: 333–338.

Brian G, du TR, Ramke J, Szetu J. (2010) Population-based study of self-reported ocular trauma in Fiji. *Clin Experiment Ophthalmol.*

Bulbulia A, Shaik R, Khan N, *et al.* (1995) Ocular health status of chemical industrial workers. *Optom Vis Sci* **72**: 233–240.

Centers for Disease Control. (1984) Leading work-related diseases and injuries — United States. *MMWR* **33**: 213–215.

Chou BR, Cullen AP. (1996) Ocular hazards of industrial spot welding. *Optom Vis Sci* **73**: 424–427.

Cruciani F, Lucchetta F, Regine F, *et al.* (1997) Work-related accidents of ophthalmologic interest in Italy during 1986–1991. *Ophthalmologica* **211**: 251–255.

Dandona L, Dandona R, Srinivas M, *et al.* (2000). Ocular trauma in an urban population in southern India: The Andhra Pradesh Eye Disease Study. *Clin Experiment Ophthalmol* **28**: 350–356.

Dannenberg AL, Parver LM, Brechner RJ, Khoo L. (1992) Penetration eye injuries in the workplace. The National Eye Trauma System Registry. *Arch Ophthalmol* **110**: 843–848.

Davies KG, Asanga U, Nku CO, Osim EE. (2007) Effect of chronic exposure to welding light on Calabar welders. *Niger J Physiol Sci* **22**: 55–58.

Desai P, MacEwen CJ, Baines P, Minassian DC. (1996) Incidence of cases of ocular trauma admitted to hospital and incidence of blinding outcome. *Br J Ophthalmol* **80**: 592–596.

Dolin PJ, Johnson GJ. (1994) Solar ultraviolet radiation and ocular disease: A review of the epidemiological and experimental evidence. *Ophthalmic Epidemiol* **1**: 155–164.

Fong LP, Taouk Y. (1995) The role of eye protection in work-related eye injuries. *Aust N Z J Ophthalmol* **23**: 101–106.

Foster PJ, Wong TY, Machin D, *et al.* (2003) Risk factors for nuclear, cortical and posterior subcapsular cataracts in the Chinese population of Singapore: The Tanjong Pagar Survey. *Br J Ophthalmol* **87**: 1112–1120.

Glazier R, Slade M, Mayer H. (2010) The depiction of protective eyewear use in popular television programs. *J Trauma.*

Glynn RJ, Seddon JM, Berlin BM. (1988) The incidence of eye injuries in New England adults. *Arch Ophthalmol* **106**: 785–789.

Griffith GA, Jones NP. (1994) Eye injury and eye protection: A survey of the chemical industry. *Occup Med (Lond)* **44**: 37–40.

Han SB, Yu HG. (2010) Visual outcome after open globe injury and its predictive factors in Korea. *J Trauma* **69**: E66–E72.

Hong J, Qiu T, Wei A, Sun X, Xu J. (2010) Clinical characteristics and visual outcome of severe ocular chemical injuries in Shanghai. *Ophthalmology* **117**: 2268–2272.

Ireland B, Acquavella J, Farrell T, *et al.* (1994) Evaluation of ocular health among alachlor manufacturing workers. *J Occup Med* **36**: 738–742.

Jafari AK, Anvari F, Ameri A, Bozorgui S, Shahverdi N. (2010) Epidemiology and sociodemographic aspects of ocular traumatic injuries in Iran. *Int Ophthalmol* **30**: 691–696.

Jones NP, Griffith GA. (1992) Eye injuries at work: A prospective population-based survey within the chemical industry. *Eye* **6**(4): 381–385.

Kanoff JM, Turalba AV, Andreoli MT, Andreoli CM. (2010) Characteristics and outcomes of work-related open globe injuries. *Am J Ophthalmol* **150**: 265–269.

Karai I, Horiguchi S. (1984) Pterygium in welders. *Br J Ophthalmol* **68**: 347–349.

Karlson TA, Klein BE. (1986) The incidence of acute hospital-treated eye injuries. *Arch Ophthalmol* **104**: 1473–1476.

Khatry SK, Lewis AE, Schein OD, *et al.* (2004) The epidemiology of ocular trauma in rural Nepal. *Br J Ophthalmol* **88**: 456–460.

Klopfer J, Tielsch JM, Vitale S, *et al.* (1992) Ocular trauma in the United States. Eye injuries resulting in hospitalization, 1984 through 1987. *Arch Ophthalmol* **110**: 838–842.

Krishnaiah S, Nirmalan PK, Shamanna BR, *et al.* (2006) Ocular trauma in a rural population of southern India: The Andhra Pradesh Eye Disease Study. *Ophthalmology* **113**: 1159–1164.

Kuhn F, Maisiak R, Mann L, *et al.* (2002) The Ocular Trauma Score (OTS). *Ophthalmol Clin North Am* **15**: 163–165.

Kuhn F, Morris R, Witherspoon CD. (2002) Birmingham Eye Trauma Terminology (BETT): Terminology and classification of mechanical eye injuries. *Ophthalmol Clin North Am* **15**: 139–143.

Kurz GH, Einaugler RB. (1968) Cataract secondary to microwave radiation. *Am J Ophthalmol* **66**: 866–869.

Lima-Gomez V, Blanco-Hernandez DM, Rojas-Dosal JA. (2010) Ocular trauma score at the initial evaluation of ocular trauma. *Cir Cir* **78**: 209–213.

Lin SH, Lin CP, Wang HZ, *et al.* (1999) Fungal corneal ulcers of onion harvesters in southern Taiwan. *Occup Environ Med* **56**: 423–425.

MacEwen CJ. (1989) Eye injuries: A prospective survey of 5671 cases. *Br J Ophthalmol* **73**: 888–894.

Maneschg OA, Resch M, Papp A, Nemeth J. (2010) Prognostic factors and visual outcome for open globe injuries with intraocular foreign bodies. *Klin Monbl Augenheilkd.*

Marshall EC, Meetz RE. (1995) Ocular health status of chemical industrial workers. *Optom Vis Sci* **72**: 686–687.

McBrien NA, Adams DW. (1997) A longitudinal investigation of adult-onset and adult-progression of myopia in an occupational group. Refractive and biometric findings. *Invest Ophthalmol Vis Sci* **38**: 321–333.

Milacic S. (2009) Risk of occupational radiation-induced cataract in medical workers. *Med Lav* **100**: 178–186.

Moran DJ, Hollows FC. (1984) Pterygium and ultraviolet radiation: A positive correlation. *Br J Ophthalmol* **68**: 343–346.

Morley MG, Nguyen JK, Heier JS, Shingleton BJ. (2010) Blast eye injuries: A review for first responders. *Disaster Med Public Health Prep* **4**: 154–160.

Morris RE, Witherspoon CD, Helms HA Jr, *et al.* (1987) Eye Injury Registry of Alabama (preliminary report): Demographics and prognosis of severe eye injury. *South Med J* **80**: 810–816.

Munoz E. (1984) Economic costs of trauma, United States, 1982. *J Trauma* **24**: 237–244.

Nakaishi H, Yamada Y. (1999) Abnormal tear dynamics and symptoms of eyestrain in operators of visual display terminals. *Occup Environ Med* **56**: 6–9.

National Society to Prevent Blindness. (1980) Fact Sheet. New York: National Society to Prevent Blindness.

Negrel AD, Thylefors B. (1998) The global impact of eye injuries. *Ophthalmic Epidem* **5**: 143–169.

Nirmalan PK, Katz J, Tielsch JM, *et al.* (2004) Ocular trauma in a rural south Indian population: The Aravind Comprehensive Eye Survey. *Ophthalmology* **111**: 1778–1781.

Norn M, Franck C. (1991) Long-term changes in the outer part of the eye in welders. Prevalence of spheroid degeneration, pinguecula, pterygium, and corneal cicatrices. *Acta Ophthalmol (Copenh)* **69**: 382–386.

Okuno T, Ojima J, Saito H. (2010) Blue-light hazard from CO_2 arc welding of mild steel. *Ann Occup Hyg* **54**: 293–298.

Onakpoya OH, Adeoye A, Adeoti CO, Ajite K. (2010) Epidemiology of ocular trauma among the elderly in a developing country. *Ophthalmic Epidemiol* **17**: 315–320.

Owen CG, Margrain TH, Woodward EG. (1995) Aetiology and prevalence of eye injuries within the United Kingdom fire service. *Eye* **9**(6 Su.): 54–58.

Pashby T. (1985) Eye injuries in Canadian amateur hockey. *Can J Ophthalmol* **20**: 2–4.

Pashby TJ, Pashby RC, Chisholm LD, Crawford JS. (1975) Eye injuries in Canadian hockey. *Can Med Assoc J* **113**: 663–6, 674.

Peate WF. (2007) Work-related eye injuries and illnesses. *Am Fam Physician* **75**: 1017–1022.

Piccoli B, Braga M, Zambelli PL, Bergamaschi A. (1996) Viewing distance variation and related ophthalmological changes in office activities with and without VDUs. *Ergonomics* **39**: 719–728.

Plestina-Borjan I, Klinger-Lasic M. (2007) Long-term exposure to solar ultraviolet radiation as a risk factor for age-related macular degeneration. *Coll Antropol* **31**(Suppl 1): 33–38.

Saari KM, Parvi V. (1984) Occupational eye injuries in Finland. *Acta Ophthalmol Suppl* **161**: 17–28.

Schein OD, Hibberd PL, Shingleton BJ, *et al.* (1988) The spectrum and burden of ocular injury. *Ophthalmology* **95**: 300–305.

See J, Wong TY, Khan C, Chuah CT. (1998) Profile of ocular diseases presenting to the eye casualty service of the Singapore General Hospital. *Invest Ophthalmol Vis Sci* **39**: S1008.

Simensen B, Thorud LO. (1994) Adult-onset myopia and occupation. *Acta Ophthalmol (Copenh)* **72**: 469–471.

Simmons ST, Krohel GB, Hay PB. (1984) Prevention of ocular gunshot injuries using polycarbonate lenses. *Ophthalmology* **91**: 977–983.

Smith GS, Lincoln AE, Wong TY, Bell NS. (2005) Does occupation explain gender and other differences in work-related eye injury hospitalization rates? *J Occup Environ Med* **47**(6): 640–648.

Tang FC, Chen SC, Lee HS, *et al.* (1999) Relationship between pterygium/pinguecula and sunlight exposure among postmen in central Taiwan. *Zhonghua Yi Xue Za Zhi (Taipei)* **62**: 496–502.

Taylor HR. (1982). Ultraviolet radiation and pterygium. *JAMA* **247**: 1698.

Taylor HR, West SK, Rosenthal FS *et al.* (1989) Corneal changes associated with chronic UV irradiation. *Arch Ophthalmol* **107**: 1481–1484.

Tielsch JM. (1995) Frequency and consequences of ocular trauma. A population perspective. *Ophthalmol Clin North Am* **8**: 559–567.

Tielsch JM, Parver L, Shankar B. (1989) Time trends in the incidence of hospitalized ocular trauma. *Arch Ophthalmol* **107**: 519–523.

Vano E, Gonzalez L, Beneytez F, Moreno F. (1998) Lens injuries induced by occupational exposure in non-optimized interventional radiology laboratories. *Br J Radiol* **71**: 728–733.

Vinger PF. (1994) The eye and sports medicine. In: Tasman W, Jaeger EA (eds). *Duane's Clinical Ophthalmology*, pp. 1–103. Philadelphia: J.B. Lippincott.

Viso E, Gude F, Rodriguez-Ares MT. (2010) Prevalence of pinguecula and pterygium in a general population in Spain. *Eye (Lond)*.

Voon LW, Wong TY, See J, Tan DT. (1998) Epidemiology of eye trauma in Singapore: Perspective from a major eye casualty center. *Invest Ophthalmol Vis Sci* **39**: 637.

Wensor M, McCarty CA, Taylor HR. (1999) Prevalence and risk factors of myopia in Victoria, Australia. *Arch Ophthalmol* **117**: 658–663.

White MF Jr, Morris R, Feist RM, *et al.* (1989) Eye injury: Prevalence and prognosis by setting. *South Med J* **82**: 151–158.

Wong TY, Foster PJ, Johnson GJ, Seah SK. (2002) Education, socioeconomic status, and ocular dimensions in Chinese adults: The Tanjong Pagar survey. *Br J Ophthalmol* **86**: 963–968.

Wong TY, Foster PJ, Johnson GJ, *et al.* (2001) The prevalence and risk factors for pterygium in an adult Chinese population in Singapore: The Tanjong Pagar survey. *Am J Ophthalmol* **131**: 176–183.

Wong TY, Lincoln A, Tielsch JM, Baker SP. (1998) The epidemiology of ocular injury in a major US automobile corporation. *Eye* **12**(5): 870–874.

Wong TY, Seet B. (1997) A behavioral analysis of eye protection use by soldiers. *Mil Med* **162**: 744–748.

Wong TY, Tielsch JM. (1999) A population-based study on the incidence of severe ocular trauma in Singapore. *Am J Ophthalmol* **128**: 345–351.

Wong TY, Tielsch JM. (2009) Epidemiology of ocular trauma. In: Tasman W, Jaeger EA (eds). *Duane's Foundations of Clinical Ophthalmology*, pp. 1–13. Philadelphia: J.B. Lippincott.

Yokota K, Johyama Y, Yamaguchi K, *et al.* (1999) Exposure-response relationships in rhinitis and conjunctivitis caused by methyltetrahydrophthalic anhydride. *Int Arch Occup Environ Health* **72**: 14–18.

Zhang Y, Zhang MN, Qiu HY. (2009) Epidemiological characteristics of eye injury among soldiers in 15 military hospitals. *Zhonghua Liu Xing Bing Xue Za Zhi* **30**: 740–742.

Chapter 13

Occupational Infections

Iain Blair* and Tar-Ching Aw*,†

Introduction

Occupational infections are diseases caused by pathogenic micro-organisms that are associated with work activity. The infections are varied, and many are not confined to occupational situations alone. For an infection to be labeled as occupational, the particular occupational activity is required to carry with it a recognized risk of acquiring the specified infection.

Occupational infections can be classified in several ways:

— By mode of transmission, e.g. blood-borne infections, zoonoses, vector-borne infections, and those transmitted by droplet infection;
— By etiological agent, e.g. viruses, bacteria, rickettsia, fungi; and
— By occupational groups at risk, e.g. healthcare workers, farmers, forestry workers, vets, zoo staff.

This chapter will consider selected common and important occupational infections.

*Department of Community Medicine, Faculty of Medicine and Health Sciences, UAE University, Al-Ain, United Arab Emirates.
†Corresponding author. E-mail: tcaw@uaeu.ac.ae

Blood-borne Infections

Infections transmitted through contact with blood and body fluids are a major concern for occupational health departments in the healthcare industry. This is because of the risk of disease to the healthcare workers (HCWs) themselves and the risk of transmission from HCWs to patients. In many countries healthcare is one of the biggest employers of labor and therefore there are large numbers of HCWs with regular patient contact. Preventing occupational blood-borne infections in this industry is of considerable public health importance. The main blood-borne infections are human immunodeficiency virus (HIV), hepatitis B (HBV) and hepatitis C (HCV).

Human Immunodeficiency Virus

HIV is the retrovirus that causes acquired immune deficiency syndrome (AIDS). The main modes of spread are sexual contact, injecting drug use and mother-to-infant vertical transmission, with only a small proportion of cases acquired through occupational transmission. However, such occupational transmission attracts a disproportionate amount of media and public attention. Evidence of HIV transmission from HCWs to patients is limited to three incidents involving transmission to eight patients. The first involved a dentist in Florida where poor infection control may have contributed to five patients becoming infected (Ciesielski *et al.*, 1994). The second involved a French orthopedic surgeon with HIV who sustained a sharps injury while operating and bled into the wound of the patient (Lot *et al.*, 1999; Dorozynski, 1997). This resulted in HIV seroconversion in the patient. The link between the source and the resulting cases was confirmed by DNA sequencing. The third case involved a gynecologist practising in Barcelona who passed on HIV to a woman during a Cesarean section (Bosch, 2003).

HIV transmission from patients to HCWs is more common, with over 100 confirmed cases of occupational spread and many more probable cases (Heptonstall *et al.*, 1993). In the UK, confirmed occupational transmission of HIV is becoming less common because of post-exposure prophylaxis (Health Protection Agency, 2008). Since 1997, there has been only one documented case of HIV sero-conversion following a significant occupational exposure (Hawkins *et al.*, 2001).

National practice with respect to HIV testing of HCWs and HIV testing of patients before surgery varies. Such testing has limitations, including a possible window period when an infected person may be seronegative and the fact that a single negative result at one point in time does not guarantee that infection will not occur at some future time as a result of occupational or community exposure. Regular HIV testing of HCWs is not practical. Nevertheless, in the UK, pre-employment HIV testing is now required for HCWs who will perform exposure-prone procedures (Department of Health, 2007). Exposure-prone procedures (EPP) have been defined as procedures

> where there is a risk that injury to the worker may result in exposure of the patient's open tissues to the blood of the worker. These procedures include those where the worker's gloved hands may be in contact with sharp instruments, needle tips or sharp tissues (spicules of bone or teeth) inside a patient's open body cavity, wound or confined anatomical space where the hands or fingertips may not be completely visible at all times (UK Health Departments, 1998).

This change in policy is designed to maintain public confidence in health services and reduce the need for look-back patient notification exercises. The logic of one-off testing has been questioned, given the ongoing risk of exposure, but professional codes require HCWs who may have been exposed to infection in whatever circumstance to seek professional advice. This applies to HCWs already in post and is considered to obviate the need for repeat testing.

Following needlestick injuries involving a HIV source, the prompt administration of combination antiviral drug therapy may reduce the chances of seroconversion (Department of Health, 2008). Seroconversion is more likely when the injury is from a hollow-bore needle containing infected blood. The volume of infected blood involved also determines the risk. It has been estimated that there is a 0.3% chance of seroconversion following a single percutaneous exposure to HIV-infected blood. In comparison, the risk of infection following a sharps injury from a HBeAg-positive source is 33% and the risk for HCV is around 3% (Health Protection Agency, 2008).

Needlestick injuries in HCWs are common and attempts at reducing such injuries will reduce the occupational transmission of blood-borne infections. Occupational health and safety measures include provision and use of approved secure containers for containing sharps, proper disposal of sharps, avoiding resheathing needles, and information, instruction and training for all HCWs (BMA, 1990). A further approach to reducing exposure is to assume that all blood, tissues and some body fluids are a potential source of infection, and to comply with "standard precautions" at all times (UK Health Departments, 1998; World Health Organization, 2007).

Hepatitis B

The hepatitis B virus (HBV) belongs to the hepadnavirus family of DNA viruses. It has an outer lipoprotein coat which is detectable as hepatitis B surface antigen (HBsAg) and an internal hepatitis B core antigen (HBcAg) (Lee, 1997). A further marker is hepatitis B e antigen (HbeAg) which is a marker of high infectivity. HBV is transmitted through sexual contact, injecting drug use, from mother to infant and through contact with infected blood and body fluids. Following infection, there is either a complete clearance of the virus or a chronic carrier state develops. The carrier state manifests as the persistence of HBsAg and/or HBeAg. Carriers have an increased lifetime risk of chronic liver disease, hepatocellular carcinoma and are a continuing source of transmission of infection to others.

An antibody to surface antigen is produced following successful immunization with a serum-derived or a genetically engineered yeast-derived vaccine (Salisbury, Ramsay and Noakes, 2006). An accelerated schedule should be used, with the vaccine given at zero, one and two months; for those who are at continued risk, a fourth dose is recommended at 12 months. In HCWs, anti-HBs titers should be checked 1–4 months after the primary course of vaccine. Individual workers should be told their result so that they know if they are protected and what to do if they are subsequently exposed.

Ideally anti-HBs levels above 100 mIU/ml should be achieved although levels of 10 mIU/ml or more are accepted as protective. In immunocompetent HCWs with anti-HBs above 100 mIU/ml, further measurement of levels is not required but a reinforcing dose of vaccine should be given at five years. Some HCWs, particularly those over the age of 40, may not develop a satisfactory antibody response. Those with anti-HBs levels of 10–100 mIU/ml should receive one additional dose of vaccine but otherwise, if they are immunocompetent, no additional action is required.

Vaccine non-responders (anti-HBs below 10 mIU/ml) should be tested for markers of current or past infection and should receive a repeat course of vaccine. Those who still have anti-HBs levels below 10 mIU/ml and who have no markers of current or past infection should be counseled about their reduced immunity to infection if they are involved in exposure-prone procedures or if they are likely to come into contact with blood and body fluids in the course of their work. They will require hepatitis B immune globulin (HBIG) for protection if exposed to the virus.

Occupational health departments should make a note of laboratory documentation on antibody levels in HCWs' occupational health records. It is also useful to reinforce the advice that immunization against hepatitis B does not protect against other forms of hepatitis or other blood-borne infections.

Worldwide, 48 HBV infected HCWs were involved in 50 reported outbreaks between 1972 and 2000. These incidents have resulted in the transmission of HBV to approximately 500 patients (United Kingdom Advisory Panel, 2009). In the UK new healthcare employees who will perform EPPs should be tested for HBsAg which indicates current hepatitis B infection. If they are positive for HBsAg, they should be tested for hepatitis B e-markers. If they are HbeAg-positive, they should not be allowed to perform EPPs. If they are HbeAg-negative, they should have their hepatitis B viral load (HBV DNA) tested. If the HBV DNA is greater than 10^3 genome equivalents/ml, they should not perform EPPs.

Hepatitis C

In recent years incidents involving transmission of hepatitis C (HCV) from patient to HCW and from HCW to patient have been reported more frequently. Of the 2296 percutaneous exposures reported to the UK surveillance scheme between 2000 and 2007, nearly half (48%, 1113) involved HCV-positive source patients and 14 seroconversions were reported (Health Protection Agency, 2008). Only those source patients who are HCV-RNA-positive pose a risk of HCV transmission to HCWs following exposure but many exposed HCWs who have not been followed up with the appropriate HCV tests remain unaware of the outcome of their exposure.

There have been five cases reported in the world literature of transmission of HCV from HCWs, resulting in infection in 13 patients. In the UK between 1994 and 2003 there were five incidents of HCV transmission from infected surgeons involving 15 patients (United Kingdom Advisory Panel, 2009). While effective interventions are available for HBV and HIV, this is not the case with hepatitis C. In the UK newly employed staff who perform EPPs must test negative for HCV antibody or, if positive, must test negative for HCV RNA (Department of Health, 2007).

Case Study 1: Occupational Exposure to a Blood-borne Virus

As a nurse is taking a sample from an arterial line of a patient in the intensive therapy unit, blood splashes into his eyes. He is not wearing protective eyewear.

Occupational exposures to blood-borne viruses (HIV, HBV, HCV) are common and usually result from a failure to handle sharp items safely or to wear protective eyewear when indicated. The risk of infection following a percutaneous injury has been estimated at 1:3 for HBV, 1:30 for HCV and 1:300 for HIV (Health Protection Agency, 2008). Mucocutaneous exposures carry a lower risk of infection, estimated at 1:1000 for HIV. There is currently no evidence on the risk of transmission for HBV and HCV following mucocutaneous exposure.

Following an exposure, all HCWs should have immediate, 24-hour access to an expert service including a designated doctor. Such a service is best delivered by an occupational health department but out-of-hours cover may be provided by the emergency room. The importance of preventing blood-borne viruses exposure should not be overlooked but healthcare providers must also ensure there are robust post-exposure arrangements including policies, services and staff training.

After such exposures, the wound should be washed liberally with soap and water and free bleeding should be encouraged. Exposed mucous membranes including conjunctivae should be irrigated and contact lenses should be removed. The injury should be reported promptly.

The designated doctor should assess the risk of transmission of HIV, HBV and HCV and the need for post-exposure management. The risk assessment is based on the type of body fluid involved and the route and severity of the exposure. Injuries from sharp objects that break the skin, exposure of broken skin and exposure of mucous membranes including the eye are significant injuries. Most body fluids pose a risk of transmission. The exceptions are urine, vomit, feces and saliva unless visibly bloodstained. Saliva associated with dentistry is considered bloodstained.

As a routine, the designated doctor or member of the clinical team (not the exposed worker) should approach the source patient (if known) and obtain informed consent, after pre-test discussion, to test for anti-HIV, HBsAg, anti-HCV and HCV RNA. Testing of the source patients should be completed within 8–24 hours.

If there is an HIV risk, post-exposure prophylaxis (PEP) should be started within one hour. Subsequently PEP may be discontinued if it is established that the source patient is HIV-negative.

Zidovudine is the only drug which has been shown to reduce the risk of HIV transmission following occupational exposure (Cardo, 1997) but newer, better-tolerated drugs are now preferred although none are licensed for PEP and therefore must be used "off-label". Various PEP regimens have been recommended. In the United Kingdom, on the basis of acceptability and shelf life, the following

PEP starter packs are used: one Truvada tablet (245 mg tenofovir and 200 mg emtricitabine (FTC)) once a day plus two Kaletra film-coated tablets (200 mg lopinavir and 50 mg ritonavir) twice a day.

PEP should be started within hours and certainly within 48–72 hours of exposure and continued for at least 28 days. If the HCW is pregnant, has an existing medical condition, is taking other medication or if there is the possibility of viral resistance, then expert advice should be obtained. The HCW should be followed up weekly during the period of PEP, to monitor treatment side effects and ensure compliance.

The HBV immunity of the HCW should be assessed and if necessary blood should be taken for urgent anti-HBs testing. An accelerated course of vaccine, a booster dose of vaccine and/or HBIG may be given according to published algorithms (Salisbury, Ramsay and Noakes, 2006). For HCV no immunization or prophylaxis is available.

A baseline blood sample should be obtained from the exposed worker and stored for two years. If the source is HIV-infected, the worker should be tested for anti-HIV at least 12 weeks after the exposure or after HIV PEP is stopped, whichever is later. Testing for anti-HIV at six weeks and six months is no longer recommended. If the source is HCV-infected, the worker should be tested for HCV RNA at six and 12 weeks and for anti-HCV at 12 and 24 weeks.

In the absence of seroconversion, modification of working practices is not necessary but infection control measures, safer sex practices and avoiding blood donation should be observed during the follow-up period. Generally, management of workers exposed to a potential source of blood-borne virus whose status is unknown or a source that is unavailable for testing will depend upon a risk assessment and a discussion of the benefits of intervention.

Zoonoses

Zoonotic infections are those that normally affect animals, but can occasionally be transmitted to man. Some of these infections occur because of close associations between animals and man in certain occupations, such as farming, veterinary practice, forestry, and zoo work.

Anthrax

This is caused by *Bacillus anthracis*, a gram-positive, sporing bacterium. The spores may remain dormant for several years and are present in soil and animal hide, horn, bone and bone meal. Anthrax can present as "malignant pustules" on the skin, localized effects on the respiratory system, or septicemia. The skin lesions are characteristic black pustules or eschars on the skin at the site of primary infection (Snashall, 1996). The pulmonary effects include bronchitis and bronchiolitis, and pleural effusion. The septicemic form may lead to meningitis as a complication, and like the pulmonary form is potentially fatal. Pulmonary anthrax was termed "woolsorter's disease" after recognition of the increased risk in workers exposed to the spores present in untreated wool. Cleaning, preparation and treatment of wool and hides originating from endemic areas before export has helped to reduce the incidence of anthrax. In Europe the infection occurs sporadically in animals and humans (Safe Food International, 2010) but is more common in Asia and Africa. Human cases occurred in the United States in 2001, associated with the deliberate release of spores, and recently three fatal cases were reported from the United States, Scotland and England in drum makers who handled animal hides (Anaraki *et al.*, 2008).

Orf

This zoonotic infection is often included in chapters on occupational infections because of its odd-sounding name rather than the severity of the infection. Orf is a self-limiting localized blister lesion, usually on the hands, caused by a parapoxvirus. It affects communities involved in farming sheep and goats. A third of Welsh farmers responding to a questionnaire reported having suffered from orf (Buchan, 1996). 20% of the 251 respondents reported more than one previous episode. The infection was also common amongst family members. Complications reported include rash and blisters on the face, body or mouth.

Q Fever

Q fever is caused by a spore-forming rickettsia, *Coxiella burnetii*. It is transmitted by droplet infection, and through contact with infected meat. It may present with anorexia, nausea, headache and fever and a raised gamma-glutamyl transferase level on laboratory investigation. A definitive diagnosis depends on demonstrating a rise in specific antibody titers. Animal handlers including veterinarians and abattoir workers are at risk of occupational acquisition (Aw and Ratti, 1997). Vaccination of abattoir workers will reduce the risk in this occupational group but vaccinating farm animals is less effective and therefore is not generally performed. Sporadic cases occur throughout the year in the UK. A study of North Dakota sheep farmers showed a prevalence of 3.5% with increased risk in those involved in lambing outdoors. Q fever is now a reportable disease in that state (Guo *et al.*, 1998).

Nipah Virus

This is an interesting "new" virus with a high case-fatality rate that affected several hundred individuals in Malaysia in 1998/1999. Amongst the occupational groups affected were pig farmers, abbatoir workers (also reported in Singapore), pork vendors, and healthcare workers. The causative agent is a paramyxovirus, with transmission following contact with pigs and/or infected individuals. The presenting clinical features include fever, headache, dizziness, vomiting, reduced consciousness, non-productive cough, myalgia and focal neurological signs. Laboratory investigations show thrombocytopenia and raised serum aminotransferases in about a third of the cases (Goh *et al.*, 2000).

Public health measures taken to limit the spread of the outbreak included restricting the movement of pigs and destroying affected herds. Adverse media attention contributed to unwarranted public concerns in regard to the risk of acquiring infection. For a period there was a considerable reduction in the consumption of pork by the public, even though there was no evidence that this was a food-borne infection. The epidemic reinforced the importance of risk communication in occupational and public health. The epidemic peaked and cases declined towards the end of 1999. However, there have been recent reports of re-emergence of the infection in countries such as Bangladesh (Hsu *et al.*, 2004). This stresses the need for continuing vigilance regarding such infections.

Vector-borne Occupational Infections

These are infections transmitted by insect vectors and affect workers in occupations that expose them to the risk of such insect bites (Aw and Harrison, 1998).

These occupations include forestry workers and those working in rural areas.

Malaria

Malaria is an endemic infection in many tropical areas in Asia, Africa and South America. It is caused by different strains of *Plasmodia* (e.g. *falciparum, vivax, ovale* and *malariae*), and is transmitted by the bite of *Anopheles* mosquitoes. These vectors breed in pools of stagnant water. *Plasmodium falciparum* causes cerebral malaria and a severe hemolysis which can present as blackwater fever which describes the resulting hamoglobinuria causing the urine to have a characteristic dark discoloration. Malaria also presents as hepatomegaly and splenomegaly. Malaria is diagnosed by identifying the malaria parasite in red blood cells from a thick blood film stained with Giemsa stain.

Workers from temperate areas sent to rural and forested areas in the tropics appear to be particularly susceptible, and are advised to take anti-malarial medication before, during and after working in such areas. Occupational health departments and websites are sources of up-to-date advice on the need for malaria prophylaxis when traveling to different countries (The National Travel Health Network and Centre, 2010).

Other personal preventive measures include the use of anti-mosquito sprays, repellents, and long-sleeved shirts and long trousers to protect against mosquito bites. Public health preventive measures include the use of fish or introduction of a layer of oil on stagnant water to destroy mosquito larvae, removal of receptacles that may trap water which facilitates mosquito breeding, and fogging operations with pesticides against adult mosquitoes.

Dengue Hemorrhagic Fever

The causative agent of dengue hemorrhagic fever is a group of flaviviruses, transmitted by *Aedes* mosquitoes. As the name suggests, the characteristic clinical manifestation is a petechial rash, accompanying a febrile illness. Other symptoms and signs include severe headache, retro-orbital pain, joint and muscle aches, hepatomegaly and circulatory collapse. As with malaria, the occupational link is in regard to workers traveling to dengue endemic areas for work. Unlike malaria, there is no specific effective medication for dengue hemorrhagic fever. No effective vaccines are available for both mosquito-borne infections, although there have been considerable efforts over the years to develop such vaccines. The main approach to prevention remains control of the vector population, and provision of advice on measures to reduce the likelihood of mosquito bites.

Lyme Disease

This is caused by a spirochete *Borrelia burgdorferi*, and named after the area in the United States where a cluster of cases was first reported in 1997. Deer and rodents are natural hosts, and humans are infected by bites of ixodid ticks which are the vectors for the disease. A papule appears at the site of the tick bite, and this then spreads to cause itching, pain and discomfort. Complications include polyarthritis, myocarditis and neurological complications. These may be prevented by the prompt administration of antibiotics. Penicillin, cephalosporins and tetracyclines are effective, and the choice of antibiotic depends on the form and severity of the disease (Pancewicz and Zajkowska, 1999).

Occupational Infections Spread Mainly by Aerosols or Droplet Infection

Tuberculosis

Tuberculosis (TB) is an infection of the lungs and/or other organs, usually with *Mycobacterium tuberculosis* (MTB). TB is typically spread by inhalation of droplets from an infectious case and this depends on the presence of cough and MTB in the sputum together with the proximity and duration of contact. Droplet aerosols may also be generated in healthcare settings from autopsy, bronchoscopy and intubation. Only about 5% of those who are infected develop clinically apparent primary disease. In most, the primary TB focus heals spontaneously but MTB may survive within the lesion, giving rise to latent TB infection (LTBI). LTBI may reactivate later in life and this has important implications for global TB control. The lifetime risk of reactivation is usually estimated at 5–10% (Horsburgh, 2004) and depends on age, chronic disease and immunosuppression, particularly the presence of HIV/AIDS.

The incidence of active clinical TB varies greatly between and within countries. The highest rates are seen in South Asia and Sub-Saharan Africa. Risk factors for TB are exposure to MTB and immunosuppression, and these particularly affect immigrants and travelers from high-incidence countries, the elderly, close contacts of infectious cases, those living in poor housing conditions and those with poor health and nutrition because of homelessness, drug abuse or alcoholism.

The gold standard for diagnosing active TB is culture of MTB but no such standard is available for diagnosing LTBI. Until recently, the century-old tuberculin skin test (TST) was the only diagnostic tool available. However, blood tests that measure T-cell interferon-gamma release in response to unique TB antigens are now widely used. These tests are known collectively as interferon-gamma release assays (IGRA). Generally, IGRA tests have good validity and can replace TSTs such as the Mantoux test where resources allow (Nienhaus, Schablon and Diel, 2008).

TB has important occupational health dimensions. HCWs, including mortuary staff, have twice the expected incidence of TB, allowing for age, sex and ethnic factors (Meredith *et al.*, 1996). There may also be an excess risk of TB in other occupations such as prison staff although studies that show this are subject to reporting bias and confounding factors such as country of birth and social, economic and lifestyle factors (Seidler, Nienhaus and Diel, 2005). TB incidents in institutions and other community settings are an increasing problem. For example, in England in 2008, 301 incidents were reported from healthcare, educational and custodial premises involving potential exposure of staff or residents (Tuberculosis Incident and Outbreak Surveillance, 2010). Typical scenarios include a patient who is admitted to hospital with tuberculosis but not appropriately isolated, leading to potential exposure of other patients, or a HCW recruited from a high-TB-incidence country who later develops TB and exposes his/her patients to TB.

Evidence-based guidelines for managing the occupational health aspects of TB have been published (National Collaborating Centre for Chronic Conditions, 2006). Most countries implement pre-employment screening for HCWs because of the public health implications of infectious TB in a HCW. HCWs who will have contact with patients or clinical specimens should be screened for LTBI before employment. Screening should comprise a health questionnaire and documentary evidence of BCG status, TST or IGRA in the preceding five years. If documentary evidence is not available, a TST or IGRA test should be carried out. Those who are TST/IGRA-negative are offered BCG immunization (after risk assessment for HIV infection) while those who are positive are evaluated clinically and may be offered a course of anti-TB treatment to prevent later reactivation of disease.

HCWs and laboratory staff who have contact with patients and/or clinical materials are more likely than the general population to be exposed to MTB. They should be offered BCG immunization (after HIV risk assessment) if they are not immunized and are TST/IGRA-negative. There are other occupational groups who may be at increased risk of TB and who may also benefit from BCG vaccination: veterinary staff and others such as abattoir workers who handle animal species known to be susceptible to TB, such as simians; prison staff working directly with prisoners; staff of care homes for elderly people; staff of hostels for homeless people and facilities accommodating refugees and asylum seekers; and people going to work with local people for more than one month in a high-incidence country.

Case Study 2: Healthcare Worker with Tuberculosis

A healthcare assistant (HCA) attends the employee health clinic with a seven-month history of cough, sputum, weight loss and night sweats. She has acid-fast bacilli in her sputum and changes on her chest X-ray typical of pulmonary tuberculosis. Originally from Zimbabwe, she has been working in the local health services for five years. She was initially employed by a neighboring hospital where she underwent pre-employment screening. She then left to work in a community nursing home. To supplement her income, through a staffing agency, she works extra shifts in local hospitals.

She should be seen urgently by the local TB service so that treatment can be initiated under the supervision of a respiratory specialist with TB experience. The specialist should be mindful of the possibility of drug-resistant TB and the possibility of HIV co-infection. The HCA should be isolated at home until deemed no longer infectious and her close household contacts should be identified for screening according to best practice.

Her patients and work colleagues have been exposed to a risk of TB infection. An incident meeting should be convened involving the local occupational health services, public health authorities, the TB service and managers of the healthcare premises where she has worked. A risk assessment should be made based on the degree and duration of infectivity; which patients she has cared for; the nature of the care provided and the care environment; and whether any of the patients are unusually susceptible to infection because of age, immunosuppression, etc. A similar risk assessment should be made for her work colleagues. Patients and staff who are deemed to have been exposed for long enough to be equivalent to *household contacts* or if they are particularly susceptible to infection should be managed as equivalent to household contacts, traced and offered testing for TB. Tracing and testing contacts with lesser degrees of exposure is generally not beneficial; however, the exposure should be documented in the contact's clinical notes and his/her medical attendant should be informed. The contact should receive information on the symptoms of TB and advice to seek medical consultation if necessary.

When the HCW was recruited from overseas and first employed in the health services she would have undergone TB screening appropriate for a newly employed HCW. Because she had documentary evidence of having had BCG in the past, no testing was carried out. However, she should have been screened to the higher standard advised for new entrants from high-incidence settings (Department of Health, 2007). New employees who are from countries of high TB incidence should always have a chest X-ray and a TST/IGRA test. The HCW was symptomatic for several months before she sought medical attention.

Reminders of the symptoms of TB and the need for prompt reporting should be sent annually to staff who may be exposed to TB. When a staff member changes jobs, documentary evidence of the results of past screening should be reviewed. If this is not available then rescreening should be carried out. The same standards for pre-employment checks should apply to providers of temporary staff. Health clearance appropriate to the HCW's duties should be verified before the individual undertakes any clinical work. This also applies to agency staff. Agencies should be responsible for supplying staff who are fit to practise but the managers of the healthcare setting in which the temporary workers are based should satisfy themselves that the staff they receive have the necessary clearance.

Rubella

Rubella infection in a pregnant woman can result in congenital abnormalities in the newborn. These abnormalities may vary in severity, but are in any case preventable by ensuring that all pregnant women are immune to rubella. Rubella vaccination or infection in childhood will confer immunity. However, where this has not occurred, an additional preventive procedure is to ensure that all HCWs, regardless of sex, are immunized against rubella (Salisbury, Ramsay and Noakes, 2006). This will further reduce the likelihood of HCWs transmitting the infection to non-immune pregnant women through contact in the occupational setting.

At pre-employment assessment of both male and female healthcare staff, hospital occupational health services can check whether there is a history of rubella infection. If there has not been previous infection, or if there is uncertainty regarding this, then the presence of rubella antibodies can be checked for. In the absence of rubella antibodies, the individual should be immunized and this recorded in the occupational health records.

Legionnaires' Disease

Legionnaires' disease is caused by *Legionella pneumophila*, and is spread by inhalation of aerosols. The organism was first identified in 1976 after a number of attendees at an American Legion convention at the Bellevue-Stratford hotel in Philadelphia became ill with a flu-like illness. Clinical features included high fever, chills, cough, headache and mental confusion. Some patients developed diarrhea, vomiting and delirium. There were a number of fatalities (the case-fatality rate is around 10%), and epidemiological and laboratory investigations led to isolation of the causative organism. *Legionella pneumophila* has been classified as part of the Legionellaceae family with several serogroups. Occupational groups or members of the public can be affected. Elderly male smokers with pre-existing respiratory illness or other serious illness appear to be more susceptible to *Legionella* infection.

While the organism is ubiquitous, it has been responsible for outbreaks associated with hot water and air-conditioning systems in large buildings such as office blocks, hotels and hospitals. Well-publicized outbreaks include those linked to hospital cooling towers in the UK, the BBC building in London, and an aquarium in Melbourne, Australia. Outbreaks can be prevented by ensuring that the temperature of water supplied to hospitals and large buildings is maintained below 20°C or above 60°C. At these temperature extremes, the organism is unable to flourish (Department of Health and Social Security, 1988). For delivery of hot water to users, the temperature at delivery should be reduced to prevent scalding. Refrigerated food display units with humidifiers have recently been identified as a source of *Legionella,* causing two deaths from Legionnaires' disease (CDSC, 2000). Preventive measures include proper maintenance of these machines with antibacterial treatment and regular testing of the ultraviolet lamps which are part of these units.

Severe Acute Respiratory Syndrome

On March 12, 2003, the World Health Organization issued a global health alert stating that a new, unrecognizable, flu-like disease might spread to HCWs. We now know this illness as severe acute respiratory syndrome (SARS). The disease is caused by a novel SARS coronavirus. By August 2003, there were 8422 SARS cases and 916 deaths reported from 29 countries across the globe. This emerging respiratory infection galvanized the world's attention to the threat of emerging infectious diseases, and provided a dress rehearsal for subsequent challenges such as H5N1 and H1N1 influenza.

Several insights were gained from the SARS epidemic (Koh and Sng, 2010). SARS reminded us that healthcare work can be hazardous to health, as HCWs comprised around 40% of SARS patients in countries such as Canada and Singapore. The effects of SARS extended beyond the infection, and included psychosocial impacts which affected HCWs as well as their families. General principles of prevention and control, such as early detection and isolation of cases, were effective against SARS. SARS posed both a public as well as an occupational health threat. Besides HCWs, other occupational groups such as food handlers, transport workers and laboratory workers were affected. SARS also demonstrated that emerging infectious diseases will continue to pose threats to the world.

Influenza (H5N1 and H1N1)

In recent years influenza viruses have circulated in seasonal (H3N2, H1N1) and avian (e.g. H5N1) forms. There has been concern that influenza A (H5N1), a worldwide cause of large poultry outbreaks, which by December 2009 had affected 467 persons (282 deaths), would drift or shift to become the next pandemic strain. However, in April 2009 "swine flu" caused by a new strain of influenza A, "Pandemic (H1N1) 2009", emerged. This has now become the dominant strain, producing an illness that is transmitted in the same way as seasonal influenza, which in most cases is mild, can be effectively treated with antivirals and for which a vaccine is now available.

By the end of 2009 many countries were still reporting disease activity and an impact on healthcare services (World Health Organization, 2010). When pandemic influenza is widespread in a community there is a risk of spread from patient to HCW and from HCW to patient within the healthcare environment. The former carries a greater risk, usually as a result of an unprotected HCW undertaking aerosol-generating procedures on an infected patient. Community spread also occurs following hand-to-hand contact. Hand-washing, covering the nose and mouth when sneezing, and remaining at home when unwell with flu-like symptoms may be relatively simple measures that can limit transmission.

Case Study 3: Healthcare Worker with Pandemic (H1N1) 2009 Influenza

During the current influenza pandemic a pediatric resident faints during a hectic ward round. While she recovers in the staff room the occupational health department is telephoned for advice.

During a pandemic, clinicians will diagnose influenza cases on the basis of symptoms. The clinical diagnostic criteria are fever ($\geq 38°C$) or a history of fever and two or more symptoms of an influenza-like illness (cough, sore throat, headache, etc). Staff members who satisfy this case definition should be sent home and advised not to work until fully recovered. Ideally they should receive sick pay. A risk assessment should be carried out. The possible risk of transmission from the HCW to patients and other staff members should be considered in terms of the excess risk compared to acquiring the infection from other community sources.

Even if infectious, clinicians who practise good respiratory and hand hygiene will limit the risk of transmission to others. Standard and droplet precautions should be in place (World Health Organization, 2009). Standard precautions minimize exposure to potentially infected blood and body fluids and include hand hygiene and the use of appropriate personal protective equipment.

Droplet precautions require that a medical mask is worn when working within one metre of the patient. When performing aerosol-generating activities, further measures are taken, including the use of particulate respirators and eye protection. In addition, respiratory or cough etiquette should be observed so that all persons cover their mouth and nose with a disposable tissue when coughing or sneezing. Within the healthcare setting administrative, environmental and engineering controls such as frequent cleaning should also be in place.

Generally it will not be appropriate to conduct contact tracing of patients or to provide antiviral prophylaxis. However, if there has been a particular type of contact between HCW and patient (for example intubation) or if a patient is at high risk of severe or complicated infection, then further risk assessment is indicated with a view to offering prophylaxis. An alternative approach, if practical, is to monitor exposed persons and administer antiviral treatment if symptoms develop. When vaccine is available, first priority should be given to immunizing HCWs.

Finally, Table 1 provides other examples of occupational infections.

Table 1. Other Examples of Occupational Infections

Occupation at Risk	Mode of Transmission	Disease	Organism
Laboratory staff and other healthcare workers	Needlestick injuries	Malaria Syphilis	*Plasmodium spp* *Treponema pallidum*
Clinical staff and other healthcare workers	Droplet infection and contact with infected material	Cytomegalovirus infection Hemorrhagic fever Salmonellosis	Cytomegalovirus Marburg & Ebola viruses *Salmonella spp*
Bird breeders	Aerosols Droplet infection from chickens	Psittacosis/ornithosis Conjunctivitis	*Chlamydia psittaci* Newcastle virus
Farmers	Close contact Close contact/droplet infection	Brucellosis Meningitis	*Brucella abortus* *Streptococcus suis*
Hairdressers	Close contact	Ringworm	*Microsporum audouini*
Sewage workers	Contact with rat urine	Leptospirosis	*Leptospira interrogans*
Gardeners	Injury from thorny plants	Sporotrichosis	*Sporothrix schenckii*

References

Anaraki S, Addiman S, Nixon G, *et al.* (2008) Investigations and control measures following a case of inhalation anthrax in East London in a drum maker and drummer. *Euro Surveill* **13**(51): 733–735.

Aw TC, Ratti N. (1997) Occupational infection in an offal porter: A case of Q fever. *Occup Med* **47**(7): 432–434.

Aw TC, Harrison J. (1998) Exposure-based hazards: Biological. In: Herzstein JA, Bunn WB, Fleming LE, *et al.* (eds). *International Occupational and Environmental Medicine*. St. Louis: Mosby.

Bosch X. (2003) Second case of doctor-to-patient HIV transmission. *Lancet Inf Dis* **3**: 261.

BMA. (1990) *A Code of Practice for the Safe Use and Disposal of Sharps.* London: British Medical Association.

Buchan J. (1996) Characteristics of orf in a farming community in mid-Wales. *Brit Med J* **313**(7051): 203–205.

Cardo D, Culver DH, Ciesielski CA, *et al.* (1997) A case control study of HIV seroconversion in health care workers after percutaneous exposure. *N Engl J Med* **337**: 1485–1490.

Ciesielski CA, Marianos DW, Schochetman G, *et al.* (1994) The 1990 Florida dental investigation. The press and the science. *Ann Intern Med* **121**: 886–888.

Communicable Disease Surveillance Centre. (2000) Legionella from guests of Welsh hotel indistinguishable from humidifier isolates. *Commun Dis Rep CDR Wkly* **10**(16): 141.

Department of Health and Social Security. (1988) *The Control of Legionellae in Health Care Premises: A Code of Practice.* London: HMSO.

Department of Health. (2007) *Health Clearance for Tuberculosis, Hepatitis B, Hepatitis C and HIV: New Healthcare Workers.* London: Department of Health. http://www.dh.gov.uk/prod_consum_dh/groups/dh_digitalassets/@dh/@en/documents/digitalasset/dh_074981.pdf (accessed January 2010).

Department of Health. (2008) *HIV Post-exposure Prophylaxis: Guidance from the UK Chief Medical Officers' Expert Advisory Group on AIDS.* London: Department of Health.

Dorozynski A. (1997) French patient contracts AIDS from surgeon. *Brit Med J* **314**: 250.

Guo HR, Gilmore R, Waag DM, *et al.* (1998) Prevalence of *Coxiella burnetii* infections among North Dakota sheep producers. *J Occ Env Med* **40**(11): 999–1006.

Goh KJ, Tan CT, Chew NK, *et al.* (2000) Clinical features of Nipah virus encephalitis among pig farmers in Malaysia. *New Engl J Med* **342**(17): 1229–1235.

Hawkins DA, Asboe D, Barlow K, Evans B. (2001) Seroconversion to HIV-1 following needle stick injury despite combination post exposure prophylaxis. *J Infect* **43**: 12–15.

Health and Safety Executive. (1997) *Anthrax: Safe Working and the Prevention of Infection.* Sudbury: HSE Books.

Health Protection Agency. (2008) *Eye of the Needle. Surveillance of Significant Occupational Exposure to Blood Borne Viruses in Healthcare Workers.* London: Health Protection Agency.

Heptonstall J, Gill ON, Porter K, *et al.* (1993) Health care workers and HIV: Surveillance of occupationally acquired infection in the UK. *CDR Review* **3**: 147.

Horsburgh CR Jr. (2004) Priorities for the treatment of latent tuberculosis infection in the United States. *N Engl J Med* **350**: 2060–2067.

Hsu VP, Hossain MJ, Parashar UD, *et al.* (2004) Nipah virus encephalitis re-emergence, Bangladesh. *Emerg Infect Dis* **10**(12): 2062–2087.

Koh D, Sng J. (2010) Lessons from the past: Perspectives on severe acute respiratory syndrome. *Asia Pacific J Public Health* **22**(3): 132S–136S.

Lee WM. (1997) Hepatitis B virus infection. *New Engl J Med* **337**: 1733–1745.

Lot F, Sigeur JC, Fergueux S, *et al.* (1999) Probable transmission of HIV from an orthopaedic surgeon to a patient in France. *Ann Intern Med* **130**: 1–6.

Meredith S, Watson JM, Citron KM, *et al.* (1996) Are healthcare workers in England and Wales at increased risk of tuberculosis? *Brit Med J* **313**(7056): 522–525.

National Collaborating Centre for Chronic Conditions. (2006). *Tuberculosis: Clinical Diagnosis and Management of Tuberculosis, and Measures for Its Prevention and Control.* London: Royal College of Physicians. http://www.nice.org.uk/nicemedia/pdf/CG033Full-Guideline.pdf (accessed January 2010).

Nienhaus A, Schablon A, Diel R. (2008) Interferon-gamma release assay for the diagnosis of latent TB infection — analysis of discordant results, when compared to the tuberculin skin test. *PLoS ONE* **3**(7): e2665.

Pancewicz SA, Zajkowska J. (1999) Treatment of Lyme borreliosis. *Medycyna Pracy* **50**(5): 439–442.

Safe Food International. (2010) [webpage on the Internet] *Europe: Anthrax Reports 2008.* http://regionalnews.safefoodinternational.org/page/Europe%3A+Anthrax+Reports+2008 (accessed January 2010).

Salisbury D, Ramsay M, Noakes K. (2006) *Immunisation Against Infectious Disease.* London: Department of Health. http://www.dh.gov.uk/prod_consum_dh/groups/dh_digitalassets/@dh/@en/documents/digitalasset/dh_108820.pdf (accessed January 2010).

Seidler A, Nienhaus A, Diel R. (2005) Review of epidemiological studies on the occupational risk of tuberculosis in low-incidence areas. *Respiration* **72**: 431–446.

Snashall D. (1996) Occupational infections. *Brit Med J* **313**: 551–554.

The National Travel Health Network and Centre. (2010) [webpage on the Internet] http://www.nathnac.org/ (accessed January 2010).

Tuberculosis Incident and Outbreak Surveillance. (2010) [webpage on the Internet] http://www.hpa.org.uk/web/HPAweb&HPAwebStandard/ HPAweb_C/1195733751639 (accessed January 2010).

UK Health Departments. (1998) *Guidance for Clinical Healthcare Workers: Protection Against Infection with Blood-borne Viruses.* London: Department of Health. http://www.dh.gov.uk/prod_consum_dh/ groups/dh_digitalassets/@dh/@en/documents/digitalasset/dh_4014 474.pdf (accessed January 2010).

United Kingdom Advisory Panel for Healthcare Workers Infected with Bloodborne Viruses. (2009) *Second Report. 1st April 2004 to 31st December 2006.* London: Health Protection Agency. http:// www.hpa.org.uk/web/HPAwebFile/HPAweb_C/1228291495165 (accessed January 2010).

World Health Organization. (2007) *Standard Precautions in Health Care.* Geneva: World Health Organization. http://www.who.int/csr/ resources/publications/EPR_AM2_E7.pdf (accessed January 2010).

World Health Organization. (2009) *Infection Prevention and Control in Health Care for Confirmed or Suspected Cases of Pandemic (H1N1) 2009 and Influenza-like Illnesses. Interim Guidance.* Geneva: World Health Organization. http://www.who.int/csr/resources/publications/ cp150_2009_1612_ipc_interim_guidance_h1n1.pdf (accessed January 2010).

World Health Organization. (2010) [webpage on the Internet] *Pandemic (H1N1) 2009 — update 83.* http://www.who.int/csr/don/2010_ 01_15/en/index.html (accessed January 2010).

Chapter 14

Metabolic Disorders: Obesity and Diabetes

See-Muah Lee[*,‡] *and Chee-Fang Sum*[†]

Introduction

Metabolic disorders encompass a wide variety of diseases, caused by problems with chemical processes in the body. Diabetes mellitus and obesity, two common metabolic disorders, will be considered here. The two are also closely intertwined, sharing places among the clustering of risk factors that comprise metabolic syndrome.

Kylin (1923) and Vague (1947) were among the first to provide insights into the clustering of metabolic disturbances as risk predictors. However, it was not until 1988 that this clustering was adopted into the common medical lexicon, first as "syndrome X", introduced by Reaven (1988) during his famous Banting lecture, and subsequently as the more chilling and alarming "deadly quartet", a term coined by Kaplan (1989). Over the years, the more prosaic term

*Department of Epidemiology and Public Health, Yong Loo Lin School of Medicine, National University of Singapore. Diabetes Clinic, Khoo Teck Puat Hospital, Singapore.

[†]Khoo Teck Puat Hospital, Singapore, Yong Loo Lin School of Medicine, National University of Singapore.

[‡]Corresponding author. E-mail: see_muah_lee@nuhs.edu.sg

"metabolic syndrome" gained wider usage and remains today the term describing the clustering of metabolically related cardiovascular risk factors which also predict a high risk of developing diabetes (if not already present).

Although there was broad agreement over the core components of the syndrome, various expert groups, including the World Health Organization and the European Group for the Study of Insulin Resistance (EGIR), were divided on the specific criteria for the identification of the syndrome.

The definition given in 2009 (Table 1) is a harmonized standard agreed between the International Diabetes Federation (IDF) and American Heart Association (AHA)/National Heart, Lung and Blood Institute (NHLBI) (Alberti, Eckel and Grundy, 2009). The presence of any three out of the five risk factors constitutes a diagnosis of metabolic syndrome.

Table 1.   Criteria for Clinical Diagnosis of Metabolic Syndrome

Measure	Categorical Cut-off Points
Elevated waist circumference	Population- and country-specific definitions
Elevated triglycerides (TG) (drug treatment for elevated triglycerides is an alternate indicator)	≥ 1.7 mmol/l
Reduced high-density lipoprotein cholesterol (HDL-C) (drug treatment for reduced HDL-C is an alternate indicator)	<1.0 mmol/l for males <1.3 mmol/l for females
Elevated blood pressure (antihypertensive drug treatment in a patient with a history of hypertension is an alternate indicator)	Systolic ≥ 130 and/or diastolic ≥ 85 mmHg
Elevated fasting glucose (drug treatment of elevated glucose is an alternate indicator)	≥ 5.5 mmol/l

Obesity

Obesity is a well-established risk for insulin resistance and contributes significantly to the development of type 2 diabetes mellitus and cardiovascular morbidity and mortality.

Obesity is a global health threat. The Royal College of Physicians has defined obesity as "a disorder in which excess fat has accumulated to an extent that health may be adversely affected" (Royal College of Physicians, 2003). This definition is based on the body mass index (BMI), or Quetelet index, which is the weight divided by the square of the height.

The World Health Organization (WHO) defines "overweight" as a BMI equal to or more than 25 kg/m², and "obesity" as a BMI equal to or more than 30 kg/m². These cut-off points provide a benchmark for individual assessment, but there is evidence that risk of chronic disease in populations increases progressively from a BMI of 21 kg/m² (WHO, 2009). The cut-off point for observed risk varies from 22 kg/m² to 25 kg/m² in different Asian populations; for high risk it varies from 26 kg/m² to 31 kg/m². The WHO consultation team further recommends public health action points at 23.0, 27.5, 32.5 and 37.5 along the continuum of BMI (WHO Expert Consultation, 2004).

Ethnic variations, mostly explained by body composition and build, can occur. Asian groups who have a lower critical threshold for the development of cardiometabolic risks generally have lower skeletal muscle mass and volume, lower mineral bone content and, unfortunately, more body fat for the same BMI, compared to Europids and Americans, indicating the role of ethnicity as a determinant (Deurenberg *et al.*, 1999).

The cut-off for Asian populations based on risk equivalence has been set at 23 kg/m² for being overweight and 27.5 kg/m² for obesity.

The converse, of a BMI above the set criteria and yet not reflecting excess body fat, must also be borne in mind for muscular individuals. Thus some authorities have further advocated the percentage of body fat for measuring overweight and obesity.

Another predictor of cardiometabolic risk is the waist circumference. The intra-abdominal adipose tissue is metabolically active. Its surrogate measurement by means of the waist circumference, as an indicator of central obesity, is also another useful indicator. Waist circumference should be measured in a horizontal plane, midway between the inferior margin of the ribs and the superior border of the iliac crest. The waist circumference threshold differs for different ethnic groups (Table 2) (Misra and Wasir, 2005; Wells, 2009; Janssen, Katzmarzyk and Ross, 2002, 2004).

Facts about Overweight and Obesity

The World Health Organization estimated in 2005 that 1.6 billion adults above the age of 15 years were overweight and at least 400 million

Table 2.   Ethnic-specific Values for Waist Circumference

Country/Ethnic Group	Waist Circumference	
Europids	Males	≥94 cm
(In the USA, the ATP III values (102 cm male; 88 cm female) are likely to continue to be used for clinical purposes)	Females	≥80 cm
South Asians	Male	≥90 cm
(Based on a Chinese, Malay and Asian-Indian population)	Female	≥80 cm
Chinese	Male	≥90 cm
	Female	≥80 cm
Japanese	Male	≥90 cm
	Female	≥80 cm
Ethnic South and Central Americans	Use South Asian recommendations until more specific data are available	
Sub-Saharan Africans	Use European data until more specific data are available	
Eastern Mediterranean and Middle East (Arab) populations	Use European data until more specific data are available	

Table 3.   Rising Prevalence of Obesity in Singapore

Year	1992	1998	2004
% overweight	n.a.	30.4	32.5
% obese[1]	5.1	6.0	6.9
% obese[2]	5.3	6.2	6.8

Source: [National Health Survey 1998 & 2004, Ministry of Health Singapore, Age 18 to 74 Years]. Classification used at time of survey: Overweight: BMI > 25. Obese: BMI > 30.
[1] Crude prevalence.
[2] Age-standardized prevalence.

adults were obese. The WHO further projects that by 2015, approximately 2.3 billion adults will be overweight and more than 700 million will be obese.

Once considered a problem only in high-income countries, being overweight or obese is now dramatically on the rise in low- and middle-income countries, particularly in urban settings. Singapore, a small nation state with a population of 6 million, is no exception, as seen in Table 3.

Medical Consequences of Being Overweight and Obese

Besides being a major risk factor for cardiovascular diseases and diabetes, obesity is also highly associated with osteoarthritis, respiratory disorders and sleep apnea. Certain cancers, like breast, colon and endometrial cancers, are also more common among the obese. Sometimes grave and profound emotional and psychological sequelae of body dysmorphism also occur.

Implications of Obesity in the Workplace

Are there jobs for which being overweight or obese is potentially a medical disqualifier?

A central consideration would be whether the workplace poses unacceptable risk to the health of the overweight or obese workers.

In the investigation of occupational health hazards and obesity, five models were proposed (Schulte *et al.*, 2008). The examples in models A and B are based on known associations; others describe hypothetical situations for which further research is required.

Model A: Obesity affects occupational exposure disease associations

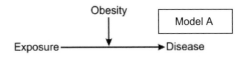

There is already a known risk of certain diseases inherent in the occupational exposures. Being overweight and obese in increasing levels increases the risk significantly.

A case in point would be occupations like vocational diving. Nitrogen is more soluble in fat tissues. Therefore, the risk of diving-related disorders like "bends" might be increased with increased body fat composition. A body fat content in excess of 30% may be considered a reason for rejection until the weight has been satisfactorily reduced (Norwegian Guidelines, 2000).

Another consideration is the increased likelihood of biomagnification and accumulation of environment xenobiotic compounds, like pesticides, e.g. aldrin, dichlorodiphenyltrichloroethane (DDT), chlordane and others. Many of these compounds, collectively known as persistent organic pollutants (POPs), have an affinity for bioaccumulation in adipose tissues (Li *et al.*, 2006).

Other specific workplace factors that might pose additional health risks for the obese worker include physical hazards like those related to heat disorders, e.g. in military operations or outdoor work in the tropics.

Model B: Workplace factors leading to obesity

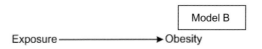

Labor-saving devices in the workplace, the increasing use of technology to save the need for physical activity and to improve safety and productivity are some aspects of modern employment life that conflict with weight-reducing behavior. However, few would recommend this as grounds for disqualifying an obese person from the job.

Model C: Obesity and occupational exposure are independent risk factors for the same disease

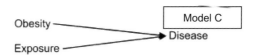

A case in point would be carpal tunnel syndrome where both obesity and repetitive work at the computer are known risk factors whose biological interaction in the causation of the syndrome is not known.

Arguably, a job that requires frequent entertainment on an expense account may be cited as an additional risk to the causation of cardiometabolic problems in the overweight or obese employee.

Model D: Work or workplace exposures affect obesity-disease relationships

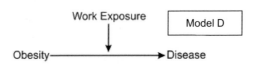

In this model, workplace exposures may affect the relationship between obesity and disease. For example, obesity has been identified in epidemiological studies as a possible risk factor for asthma, but the mechanism is not known. Do obese workers have an innate airway responsiveness that make them more susceptible to workplace asthmatogens?

Model E: Occupational exposures cause one disease and
obesity causes another and the two diseases interact

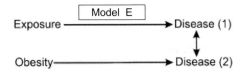

This model illustrates that obesity may cause one disease and occupational exposure may cause another disease and there may be some interaction between the two diseases. For example, work-related vibration can cause vibration-induced injury (Bernard, 1997). Obesity can lead to diabetes. The effect of diabetes on the micro-capillary circulation as well as other vascular damage is well-known (Ngo *et al.*, 2005). How will these two effects then interact with one another?

When slimness is a condition of work

What are the jobs for which slimness and weight limits are fundamental to competent performance? An interesting example would be the race jockey, who for the purpose of the job, has to maintain a weight usually not exceeding 130 pounds. This is no beauty contest, but few would dispute that the race jockey's competitive excellence, all things being equal, may be decided by a difference of a few pounds. The same might apply to competitive car racing.

Many other considerations are related to esthetic appeal and may have little to do with ability or unacceptable health risk increments to the obese worker. Considerations related to co-morbidities will have to be assessed from that perspective.

Discrimination, stigmatization and ability to do the job

Unfortunately, it is a fact borne from research evidence that obese people suffer stigmatization, discrimination and prejudice (Puhl and Hyuer, 2009). Compared to normal weight people, they face more difficulty being hired; and when hired, they are less likely to be promoted and more likely to be fired (Puhl and Brownell, 2001). Obesity incurs a wage penalty. Not surprisingly, the severely obese were the most severely affected (Baum and Ford, 2004). Obese workers are often stereotyped as being lazier, less conscientious and less agreeable than their normal weight counterparts.

One reason for this is the profusion of research studies on obesity. Many such studies, based on populations, fairly or unfairly, have been applied to individual persons. Such studies inform us of the increased accidents (Pollack and Cheskin, 2007; Schmier, Jones and Halpern, 2006), sickness absence (Ferrie *et al.*, 2007), increased medical costs and increased compensation claims incurred by overweight and obese workers (Ostbye, Dement and Krause, 2007). However, what population studies yield is evidence in terms of probability.

Research of the kind that accepts obesity, as race or gender has been, as an element of workplace diversity, and as a sign of a compassionate and tolerant workplace, is practically non-existent.

Is there any legal protection against discrimination of the obese worker or job applicant? Anti-discrimination laws are probably well-established for protection against race, gender and age discrimination. Disability discrimination laws may also be in place, but whether obesity, much less being overweight, falls within the legal definition, thereby entitling the condition to legal protection, remains doubtful. Legal disability is defined as a "physical or mental impairment which has a substantial and long-term adverse effect on his ability to carry out normal day to day activities". Furthermore, even if the obese worker succeeds in qualifying his obesity as a legal disability (such as having severe osteoarthritis affecting mobility), it remains to be successfully argued that this disability does not affect his capacity to do the job or to do so with the employer making reasonable accommodations. He also has to argue his case of less favorable treatment compared to an appropriately selected comparator worker who does not have the disability in question (DDA, 2005).

In all cases, while doctors have to be aware of the evidence and risks based on population studies, it is still necessary for the fitness-to-work assessment to be made on an individual basis. An objective evaluation should be based on the demands of the job and the suitability of the individual. Even for manual jobs, it is important to remind ourselves that there are overweight, perhaps even obese people, who are physically active and far better at coping with physically demanding jobs than the slim sedentary person. Such objective evaluations take time, but can be undertaken together with the work supervisors. A refinery recruiting operators has been known to bring the prospective applicants on a site tour with hands-on testing, such as opening valves, handling stretchers and water hoses. Unsurprisingly, a few of the overweight workers have demonstrated acceptable agility and more than adequate lifting strength.

It is still within the law in most countries and in most instances for employers to be free to employ and reject applicants, sometimes for the most biased or capricious reasons.

Accommodations and adjustments in the workplace

The overweight worker probably does not face many issues at work. But for the obese, especially those who are morbidly so, ergonomic issues may come to the fore (Box 1). In these cases, adjustments may range from the relatively simple, such as ordering special size uniforms, to the more complex, such as special furniture and special fittings for other personal protective equipment like face masks, respirators, boots and gloves.

Many of the workplaces were designed in an earlier era when people's sizes were smaller. Many parts of such workplaces, for example,

Box 1. Sensitive Human Resource Management

"I was extremely delighted to get the job, even more so when I reported for work, and noticed that my chair was extra large. That's what I call a good HR manager."

— A person with a BMI of 40

"Not to employ someone because of pre-conceived stereotyping about obesity might mean losing out on real talent. Some accommodations are really very simple to make."

— HR Manager

escape hatches, confined space entry points in industrial areas, may have to be re-designed to fit larger sizes.

However, thought and care must go into the planning. A space designed to fit a larger person may result in a misfit for the smaller-sized worker, who may have difficulty with reach. This is relevant in shared workplaces, like in control rooms.

Health Promotion Program

Obesity has been classified as a disease in the International Statistical Classification of Diseases and Related Health Problems, 10th Revision, Chapter IV, E65–68. It is highly visible and instantly recognizable, unlike many other conditions like hypertension and diabetes.

It is a popular ground whenever companies and employers wish to start a health promotion program. It also lends itself as a perennial favorite for the ubiquitous employee assistance program of modern times. There has been no lack of enthusiasm for workplaces to conduct such programs. Reasons commonly cited are that the workplace is captive, there could be ready access to occupational health services, and workplace factors such as food in the staff canteen can be manipulated.

Finally, it is always enthusiastically and warmly believed that investments in such programs can translate into lower healthcare costs. Some corporate leaders seem to need this kind of economic assurance; the intrinsic and altruistic worth in helping workers does not seem to be a strong enough motivation by itself.

One also hears of employers of big organizations conducting highly publicized health campaigns sporadically, usually at the end of the financial year when extra funds are discovered. Healthy lifestyle promotion is also often a theme in such campaigns, and because of its highly publicized nature, brings a lot of discomfiting attention to the obese workers.

One popular view held equates obesity with lifestyle choice. It views obesity as a consequence of laziness, lack of self-control and gluttony. Failing to appreciate that the etiology is complex, with many causal factors beyond the individual's control, can lead to further "blame" and deepening of stigmatization when such well-intentioned health programs, which of course target the obese, fail to achieve successful performance indicators.

Employers should be mindful of the ethical dimension of obesity intervention programs. If an obese employee does not desire to lose weight, is hard paternalism in the form of compulsory or even subtly coerced participation in such programs justified (Holm, 2007)? Losing weight is good for health and is well and good if it can be achieved voluntarily and enthusiastically. But what if such programs cause anxiety, depression and lowered self-esteem, thereby negatively affecting a person's emotional and mental well-being? Does the program provide for a sensitive and holistic approach? Box 2 lists some reactions to such programs.

Summary Points

- Obesity is a risk factor for many morbid conditions.
- Is there an additional risk created for the obese person at work compared to when he is not at work? Is this risk acceptable? If not, can this risk be reduced?
- Employers can help to promote a healthy lifestyle. However, this should be done in a supportive and sensitive manner.

Box 2.   Quotable Quotes: What Works and What Does Not

"We were given a half hour off to listen to an exercise trainer and a dietician. He told us to walk 10,000 steps a day. The dietician told us to eat less. I am already way beyond that. It was a total waste of time. Who are these people?"

"Leave me alone, I can take care of my health, and I am happy being fat. My unhappiness comes from you telling me to lose weight."

"I love the idea of the company gym. I do a half-hour work-out, bathe and change and am ready for a hard day's work. I wonder why so few make use of it. It has always been there for as long as I can remember."

"I work in a hospital. I know it is bad for the image of a health-care worker to be overweight. The manager in my unit looks at me and I can sense her pity and contempt. There is a weight loss program, where all the big-size staff are encouraged to sign up. We have to attend work half an hour earlier in order to attend the gym class. I am still unable to lose weight. It is all so depressing."

"I eat all the fruits I need daily at the staff canteen. I am too lazy to shop for them. It is great."

"Strange, but I am getting used to the idea of fruit at meetings, rather than all the sticky sweet confectionary."

"My colleagues and managers were supportive. There was no pressure. I walk more; I try to diet, even though it is not successful all the time. I have not lost weight, but I have not lost hope."

"I am a marketing executive. I travel a lot to the Far East. There is a culture of eating and drinking in business entertainment. It is considered rude in certain places to refuse the offer of food. How you behave can affect client relations. Worst part is, I put on weight very easily."

Diabetes Mellitus

Prevalence of Type 1 and Type 2 Diabetes Mellitus

There is evidence that both type 1 and type 2 diabetes mellitus are increasing in incidence (Box 3) (Wild, Roglic and Green, 2004; Patterson *et al.*, 2009). In the case of type 1, environmental factors related to immunogenicity have sometimes been blamed (Gillespie, 2006; van der Werf *et al.*, 2007). Type 2 diabetes mellitus is largely due to physical inactivity, over-nutrition and obesity. Genetics also plays a role and it is entirely possible to be slim and diabetic (Barroso, 2005). Beta-cell failure and insulin resistance underlie the pathogenesis of diabetes.

The vicious cycle of diabetogenesis is also further aggravated by uterine exposure to maternal hyperglycemia and obesity, as indicated by such offspring who, independent of other factors, are also at higher risk of developing diabetes, compared to those who are not similarly exposed *in utero* (Dabalea, 2007).

Box 3.   World Health Organization Diabetes Facts (WHO, 2006)

The World Health Organization estimates that more than 180 million people worldwide have diabetes. This number is likely to more than double by 2030.

In 2005, an estimated 1.1 million people died from diabetes.

Almost 80% of diabetes deaths occur in low- and middle-income countries.

Almost half of diabetes deaths occur in people under the age of 70 years; 55% of diabetes deaths are in women.

WHO projects that diabetes deaths will increase by more than 50% in the next 10 years without urgent action. Most notably, diabetes deaths are projected to increase by over 80% in upper-middle-income countries between 2006 and 2015.

Table 4. Values for Diagnosis of Diabetes Mellitus and Other Categories of Hyperglycemia (WHO, 2006)

	Glucose Concentration, mmol^{-1} (mg dl^{-1})		
	Venous (Whole Blood)	Capillary	Venous (Plasma)
Diabetes Mellitus			
Fasting *or*	≥6.1 (≥110)	≥6.1 (≥110)	≥7.0 (≥126)
2 h post-glucose load	≥10.0 (≥180)	≥11.1 (≥200)	≥11.1 (≥200)
Impaired Glucose Tolerance (IGT)			
Fasting (if measured) *and*	<6.1 (<110) and	<6.1 (<110) and	<7.0 (<126) and
2 h post-glucose load	≥6.7 (≥120)	≥7.8 (≥140)	≥7.8 (≥140)
Impaired Fasting Glycemia (IFG)			
Fasting	≥5.6 (≥100) and <6.1 (<110)	≥5.6 (≥100) and <6.1 (<110)	≥6.1 (≥110) and <7.0 (<126)
and (if measured)			
2 h post-glucose load	<6.7 (<120)	<7.8 (<140)	<7.8 (<140)

The term "diabetes mellitus" (WHO diagnostic values given in Table 4) has been described by the World Health Organization as a metabolic disorder of multiple etiology, characterized by chronic hyperglycemia with disturbances of carbohydrate, fat and protein metabolism resulting from defects in insulin secretion, insulin action, or both.

Treatment has made possible the increased survival of people with diabetes and this has also contributed significantly to its increasing prevalence. A condition once considered a corollary to old age is now affecting young people. Besides, many countries, especially those in the developed world, partly because of economic expediency, are raising their retirement age. It follows to reason that many in the workplace will be affected by this condition.

Diabetes Management and Employment

One objective of managing diabetic patients, like in all other illnesses, would be to, as far as possible, enable their rehabilitation and help them attain maximal normal functioning. This would certainly apply to all workers with diabetes.

Following the landmark Diabetes Control and Complications Trial (DCCT) studies on type 1 diabetes, and the Kumamoto study on type 2 diabetes, it is now established that ideal management to prevent microvascular and, to some extent, macrovascular complications requires good control (DCCT, 1993; UKPDS 33, 1998; Kumamoto, 2000), preferably with HbA1c targets at non-diabetic levels or less than 6.5%. In all cases, of course, targets should be individualized according to the circumstances of the patient.

Hypoglycemia

Tight control of diabetes often comes at the cost of hypoglycemia (Cryer, Davies and Shamoon, 2003; Cryer *et al.*, 2009), which can be disabling and, if severe, alarming to both the patient and his colleagues at work. The neurogenic symptoms and the accompanying neuroglycopenia which causes cognitive impairment are often cited as reasons for impaired work ability (Briscoe and Davis, 2006).

Physicians taking care of such workers must also be familiar with the concept of hypoglycemic unawareness. This is a condition in which the patient loses neurogenic perception, because of an altered hypoglycemic threshold, due to repeated, uncorrected hypoglycemic exposures. The danger is that the patient so afflicted can plunge into neuroglycopenia, when the brain is already in a fuel-deficient state.

Hypoglycemia can be avoided. Its management involves discussion with the workers, the triggers which mainly center on food intake, medication and physical activity (Cryer *et al.*, 2009). The last aspect is of particular relevance to work which may have a high manual content. Planning of meal times and medication, e.g. insulin injections, in relation to work takes on special challenges in circumstances like shift work and driving over long distances.

Case Study 1

Mr. X, who is 32 years old, has type 2 diabetes mellitus and has newly started on twice-daily insulin injections. He works in a dispatch company, where he packs and transfers loads of varying weights. He is required to do this for most of his working day, although up to one quarter of his time may be spent on documentation work. Overtime work of two additional hours is required at least twice a week.

Since starting on insulin, he has been experiencing late-morning giddiness, sweating and tremors. His doctor however has insisted that he copes with it, because in the long run, a "low HbA1c is good for him".

Mr. X needs advice on how he can manage his hypoglycemia. In the immediate short term, he must be instructed on how to respond appropriately to his hypoglycemia by consuming rapidly absorbable carbohydrates. If necessary, he should be referred to a diabetologist, who can then make adjustments to his treatment. Meals, timing, dosage, choice of insulin and self-monitoring of blood glucose all have a role to play.

Physical activity is always to be encouraged, both aerobic and anaerobic. It improves insulin sensitivity. However, it has to be done safely. A further aspect for consideration is that he may be operating heavy machinery at work, such as lifting aids. Depending on the severity and the extent to which the hypoglycemia can be immediately remedied, Mr. X's job may have to be modified in the interim. An individualized risk assessment, with periodic reviews, has to be made before establishing any opinion on fitness.

Hyperglycemia

The harms of insulin resistance and hyperglycemia are well-documented. Hyperglycemia is also considered a pro-inflammatory state associated with oxidative stress, harmful advanced glycation end products and endothelial damage (Zozulinska and Wysocka, 2006). It causes retinopathy, nephropathy and neuropathy.

Lifestyle changes are often necessary for good control. Beyond that, the progressive nature of the disease, adherence to therapy, willingness to accept additional therapeutic measures such as daily insulin injections — itself a life-changing event — are all challenges that the patient has to face constantly.

Case Study 2

Ms. Y is a copyeditor. She has poorly controlled diabetes. Her HbA1c on the few occasions when it was measured has been in the unacceptable range above 9%. She is now 45 years old and lately has experienced some blurring of vision. She is now worried about how it might affect her career.

The implication of diabetic retinopathy on someone who works as a copyeditor is obvious. Early ophthalmological intervention can help to arrest its progression, as would optimal glycemic control. However, clinical trials have demonstrated that approximately eight years are needed before the benefits of glycemic control are reflected in a reduction of microvascular complications, which is why the message has to be sent and sent early (Goddijn *et al.*, 1999). In the event that visual impairment has taken place, Ms. Y should be referred to specialized centers for retraining to maximize her use of her remaining vision.

Diabetes management

In some settings, occupational physicians are also responsible for the primary healthcare of workers. If that is the case, then the duty of care to the worker includes informing the worker of the need for good diabetes management, and apprising her of the consequences of good control in order to minimize the risk of metabolic complications.

Concerns about the side effects of treatments, especially those related to hypoglycemia caused by insulins and insulin secretagogues, are of special relevance to workers. It is therefore not surprising that much energy is devoted to addressing this issue in therapeutics. In this respect, the insulin analogs, such as glargine, levemir, aspart, lispro and glulisine, may be offered as viable alternatives to the traditional human insulins when hypoglycemia is a troubling side effect (Tibaldi, 2008; DeWitt and Dugdale, 2003).

Incretin enhancers, in the class of gliptins, and incretin mimetics, in the class of exenatides, also show salubrious effects with regard to glycemic controls that can avoid or minimize the side effect of hypoglycemia (Lovshin and Drucker, 2009).

The therapeutic armamentarium used in the control of hyperglycemia is an ever-evolving field. Its judicious use can be of considerable assistance to suit the needs of the individual. The fear of hypoglycemia is no excuse for poor control that allows blood sugar to rise unchecked. The standard of care in diabetes management includes regular monitoring and screening for diabetic retinopathy, diabetic kidney disease, dyslipidemia and podiatry. Regular dietetic counseling is also necessary, as would be self-monitoring of blood glucose, especially among type 1 diabetics.

Psychoeducational intervention training programs such as Blood Glucose Awareness Training have also been proven to be effective in reducing unfavorable events, notably driving mishaps among patients with diabetes (Cox *et al.*, 2001). Techniques such as self-estimation of blood glucose levels based on internal cues, matched against self-monitoring of blood glucose, plotted on a grid, along with descriptive data, enable patients to have a better awareness of their glycemic situation.

Are there jobs from which a diabetic person should be disqualified?

A worker with diabetes who is motivated and is able to manage his diabetes meticulously should have no difficulty doing his job like any other healthy person. Public interest and safety issues arising from poor control have to be considered, but should be done in perspective. Thus, in this context, different considerations would apply for a heavy goods vehicle driver as compared to a sales manager or a bank executive.

It seems that hypoglycemia is an inevitable complication in the lifetime of many diabetic patients. The American Diabetes Association Workgroup has proposed a classification of hypoglycemia (see Box 4) (ADA, 2005).

Box 4.   American Diabetes Association Workgroup on Hypoglycemia Classification, 2005

Severe hypoglycemia

An event requiring the assistance of another person to actively administer carbohydrate, glucagon or other resuscitative actions. These episodes may be associated with sufficient neuroglycopenia to induce seizure or coma. Plasma glucose measurements may not be available during such an event, but neurological recovery attributable to the restoration of plasma glucose to normal levels is considered sufficient evidence that the event was induced by a low plasma glucose concentration.

Documented symptomatic hypoglycemia

An event during which typical symptoms of hypoglycemia are accompanied by a measured plasma glucose concentration ≤3.9 mmol/l.

Asymptomatic hypoglycemia

An event not accompanied by typical symptoms of hypoglycemia but with a measured plasma glucose concentration ≤3.9 mmol/l.

Probable symptomatic hypoglycemia

An event during which symptoms of hypoglycemia are not accompanied by a plasma glucose determination (but that was presumably caused by a plasma glucose concentration ≤3.9 mmol/). Since many people with diabetes choose to treat symptoms with oral carbohydrate without a plasma glucose test, it is important to recognize these events as "probable" hypoglycemia.

(Continued)

> *(Continued)*
>
> **Relative hypoglycemia**
>
> An event during which the person with diabetes reports any of the typical symptoms of hypoglycemia, and interprets those as indicative of hypoglycemia, but with a measured plasma glucose concentration >3.9 mmol/l. This category reflects the fact that patients with chronically poor glycemic control can experience symptoms of hypoglycemia at plasma glucose levels >70 mg/dl (3.9 mmol/l) as plasma glucose concentrations decline toward that level. Though causing distress and interfering with the patient's sense of well-being, and potentially limiting the achievement of optimal glycemic control, such episodes probably pose no direct harm.

Hypoglycemia can be minimized, but its complete avoidance is mostly impossible, especially among those receiving insulin and whose control is satisfactory. The risk and its implications of this on public interest and safety must be assessed in perspective. In some countries, this is deemed important enough for their exclusion, as a matter of regulation, from work such as driving heavy goods vehicles and public transport (DVLA, 2009).

On the other hand, for most jobs, even when their emergency nature is a given, such considerations may be, on closer look, not as critical as they are assumed to be. An example would be the unarmed condominium guard, whose job is not necessarily to give chase to armed robbers and put himself at risk, but to call for help when needed. Any number of contentious job situations can be imagined: a croupier working in a casino, a clerk in a bank, an airport baggage handler, a dispatch driver (motorbike or car or van?), or a safety inspector required to check confined spaces; the list goes on.

In all such cases, an individual risk assessment has to be applied (ADA, 2009). This risk assessment includes an evaluation of how well the individual has controlled his diabetes as well as an appraisal of the surrounding factors, such as availability of accompanying colleagues, accommodating of affected employees, proximity and access to medical help. A task analysis of the job would also be useful to examine which parts of the job are at high risk and therefore require special attention. There has to be a balance between what is sometimes seen as a recommended overindulgence of the diabetic worker, public safety, and protection of the economic interests of the employers.

Practical considerations in the workplace

The worker who has diabetes also needs to negotiate with the employer on meal flexibility, breaks as required for self-monitoring of blood glucose, hygienic disposal of sharps and refrigerator storage space for insulin vials.

Disclosure of medical information

It would be noted from the above that, ideally, an employee should have an open, honest and transparent relationship with his employer and colleagues. The challenges confronting the diabetic worker, as would be with any worker with chronic medical problems, can then be overcome.

However, not all workers with diabetes are forthcoming and willing to let their employers know. There is still much confusion and ignorance about the illness, not only in the general community, but even within the medical community itself. Disclosure should be encouraged, especially to specified colleagues, who can help to respond appropriately in case of emergencies. Veiling the condition in secrecy can only aggravate the stigmatization of such workers. Understandably, there are good reasons for affected workers to want to keep their condition confidential. Employers may perceive their condition to be a danger at work. Healthcare costs are another concern.

Disclosure of medical conditions, as a condition for employment, is a matter for negotiation between the employer and the employee.

How the employer and the employee wish the physician to play a role in this has to be clarified from the very start, and should not compromise the doctor's ethical position. Doctors have a role as health advocates for the workers whose health they have been entrusted with. Employers also have legitimate economic interests to protect.

Disclosure by the physician in the absence of consent by the worker is a breach of patient confidentiality. It can be sanctioned only if legislatively driven or if the physician can show justification based on public interest, e.g. the case of a patient with erratic diabetic control who is required to handle firearms at work.

Healthcare Costs in Diabetes Care

Healthcare costs in diabetes are an increasing concern to be reckoned with by employers (see Box 5) (Kleinfield, 2006). In the United States, it is estimated that the yearly medical costs of a diabetic patient is around US$13,243. This probably represents the high end of medical care costs, but it cannot be unsubstantial even in less developed countries using cheaper medicine for a disease we know to be progressive and chronic. There are also additional, indirect costs of productivity losses, such as those incurred by time off for doctor's visits and other consultations.

Box 5.   Diabetes Healthcare Claims

"When I first joined the company, they reassured me that all medical care would be taken care of. Over the next three months, after I submitted my claims, the human resource manager called me and said that they could no longer afford to pay for my care."

— 32-year-old man with type 1 diabetes, on daily multi-dose insulin and attending regular care at a Singapore public hospital

Good control of diabetes will enable the patient to stave off many complications associated with the disease. But the economic cost of companies getting involved is difficult to assess. Personnel turnover may be high, medical technologies become increasingly sophisticated and expensive, patients of course have a legitimate claim to competent care and doctors are ever cautious about negligence claims. All these factors should warn health promotion enthusiasts and human resource personnel alike not to put too much emphasis on motivations based on economic savings. Being able to assist employees when companies are financially able to do so should be reason enough. There should be other ways to control healthcare costs.

Summary Points

- Diabetes is a chronic and progressive condition. Its multidimensional nature requires a multi-faceted approach in its medical management. Risks associated with hypoglycemia, hyperglycemia and its cardiovascular risk and complications such as retinopathy, neuropathy and nephropathy have to be regularly monitored and managed.
- Are there any legislations pertaining to the employment of diabetic people for the work being considered?
- Is there an additional risk created for the diabetic worker at work compared to when he is not at work? Is this risk acceptable? If not, can this risk be reduced and managed?
- Is there a risk created for other colleagues or the public when a worker with diabetes is employed? Have there been reported incidents? What is the magnitude of the risk? Can this risk be reduced and managed?
- Healthcare costs for such workers have to be managed in a rational way.

Further Reading

Williams N. (2008) *Managing Obesity in the Workplace*. Oxford: Radcliffe Publishing.

References

ADA. (2005) American Diabetes Association workgroup report: Defining and reporting hypoglycemia in diabetes. *Diabetes Care* **28**: 1245–1249.

ADA. (2009) American Diabetes Association position statement: Diabetes and employment. *Diabetes Care* **32**(Suppl 1): S80–84.

Alberti KGMM, Eckel RH, Grundy SM. (2009) Harmonizing the metabolic syndrome: A joint interim statement of the International Diabetes Federation Task Force on Epidemiology and Prevention; National Heart, Lung, and Blood Institute; American Heart Association; World Heart Federation; International Atherosclerosis Society; and International Association for the Study of Obesity. *Circulation* **120**: 1640–1645.

Barroso I. (2005) Genetics of type 2 diabetes. *Diabetic Med* **22**: 517–535.

Baum CL, Ford WF. (2004) The wage effects of obesity: A longitudinal study. *Health Econ* **13**: 885–899.

Bernard B. (1997) *Musculoskeletal Disorders and Workplace Factors: A Critical Review of Epidemiologic Evidence for Work-related Musculoskeletal Disorders of the Neck, Upper Extremities and Low Back.* Cincinnati, Ohio: National Institute for Occupational Safety and Health. Centers for Disease Control and Prevention.

Briscoe VJ, Davis SN. (2006) Hypoglycemia in type 1 and type 2 diabetes: Physiology, pathophysiology, and management. *Clin Diabetes* **24**(3): 115–121.

Cox DJ, Gonder-Frederick L, Polonsky W, *et al.* (2001) Blood glucose awareness training (BGAT-2): Long-term benefits. *Diabetes Care* **24**(4): 637–642.

Cryer PE, Axelrod L, Grossman AB, *et al.* (2009) Evaluation and management of adult hypoglycemic disorders: An endocrine society clinical practice guideline. *J Clin Endocrinol Metab* **94**(3): 709–728.

Cryer PE, Davies SN, Shamoon H. (2003). Hypoglycemia in diabetes. *Diabetes Care* **26**: 1902–1912.

Dabalea D. (2007). The predisposition to obesity and diabetes in offspring of diabetic mothers. *Diabetes Care* **30**(Suppl 2): 169–174.

DCCT. (1993) The effect of intensive treatment of diabetes on the development and progression of long-term complications in insulin-dependent diabetes mellitus. The Diabetes Control and Complications Trial Research Group. *N Engl J Med* **329**: 977–986.

DDA. (2005) Disability Discrimination Act, UK.

Deurenberg P, Deurenberg-Yap M, Wang J *et al.* (1999) The impact of body build on the relationship between body mass index and percent body fat. *Int J Obesity* **23**: 537–542.

DeWitt DE, Dugdale DC. (2003) Using new insulin strategies in the outpatient treatment of DM. *JAMA* **289**: 2265–2269.

Driver and Vehicle Licensing Agency. (2009) http://www.dvla.gov.uk/medical.aspx.

Ferrie JE, Head J, Shipley MJ, *et al.* (2007) BMI, obesity, and sickness absence in the Whitehall II study. *Obesity (Silver Spring)* **15**(6): 1554–1564.

Gillespie KM. (2006) Type 1 diabetes: Pathogenesis and prevention. *CMAJ* **175**(2): 165–170.

Goddijn PP, Bilo HJ, Feskens EJ, *et al.* (1999) Longitudinal study on glycaemic control and quality of life in patients with type 2 diabetes mellitus referred for intensified control. *Diabetic Med* **16**: 23–30.

Holm S. (2007) Obesity interventions and ethics. *Obes Rev* **8**(Suppl 1): 207–210.

International Diabetes Federation. (2006) http://www.idf.org/webdata/docs/IDF_Meta_def_final.pdf.

Janssen I, Katzmarzyk PT, Ross R. (2002) Body mass index, waist circumference, and health risk: Evidence in support of current National Institutes of Health guidelines. *Arch Intern Med* **162**(18): 2074–2079.

Janssen I, Katzmarzyk PT, Ross R. (2004) Waist circumference and not body mass index explains obesity-related health risk. *Am J Clin Nutr* **79**(3): 379–384.

Kaplan NM. (1989) The deadly quartet. Upper-body obesity, glucose intolerance, hypertriglyceridemia, and hypertension. *Arch Intern Med* **149**(7): 1514–1520.

Kleinfield NR. (2006) Diabetics in the workplace confront a tangle of laws. *The New York Times*, December 26.

Kylin E. (1923) Studien ueber das hypertonie-hyperglykämie-hyperurikämie syndrom. *Zentralblatt Fuer Innere Med* **44**: 105–127.

Kumamoto Study. Shichiri M, Kishikawa H, Ohkubo Y, Wake N. (2000) Long-term results of the Kumamoto Study on optimal diabetes control in Type 2 diabetic patients. *Diabetes care* **23**(Suppl 2): B21–B29.

Li QQ, Loganath A, Yap SC, *et al.* (2006) Persistent organic pollutants and adverse health effects in humans. *J Toxicol Environ Health* **69**(Part A): 1987–2005.

Lovshin JA, Drucker DJ. (2009) Incretin-based therapies for type 2 diabetes mellitus. *Nat Rev Endocrinol* **5**(5): 262–269.

Misra A, Wasir JS. (2005) Waist circumference criteria for the diagnosis of abdominal obesity are not applicable uniformly to all populations and ethnic groups. *Nutrition* **21**: 969–976.

Ngo BT, Hayes KD, DiMiao DJ, *et al.* (2005) Manifestations of cutaneous diabetic microangiopathy. *Am J Clin Dermatol* **6**(4): 225–237.

Norwegian Guidelines for Occupational Divers. (2000).

Ohkubo Y, Kishikawa H, Araki E, *et al.* (1995) Intensive insulin therapy prevents the progression of diabetic microvascular complications in Japanese patients with non-insulin-dependent diabetes mellitus: A randomized prospective 6-year study. *Diabetes Res Clin Pract* **28**: 103–117.

Ostbye T, Dement JM, Krause KM. (2007) Obesity and workers' compensation: Results from the Duke Health and Safety Surveillance System. *Arch Intern Med* **167**(8): 766–773.

Patterson CC, Dahlquist GG, Gyürüs E, *et al.* (2009) Incidence trends for childhood type 1 diabetes in Europe during 1989–2003 and predicted new cases 2005–20: A multicentre prospective registration study. *Lancet* **373**: 2027–2033.

Pollack KM, Cheskin LJ. (2007) Links obesity and workplace traumatic injury: Does the science support the link? *Inj Prev* **13**(5): 297–302.

Puhl RM, Hyuer CA. (2009) The stigma of obesity: A review and update. *Obesity (Silver Spring)* **17**(5): 941–964.

Puhl RM, Brownell KD. (2001) Bias, discrimination, and obesity. *Obes Res* **9**: 788–905.

Reaven GM. (1988) Banting lecture 1988. Role of insulin resistance in human disease. *Diabetes* **37**: 1595–1607.

Royal College of Physicians. (2003) Storing up problems. Report of a Working Party.

Schmier JK, Jones ML, Halpern MT. (2006) Cost of obesity in the workplace. *Scand J Work Environ Health* **32**(1): 5–11.

Schulte PA, Wagner GR, Downes A, Millera DB. (2008) Framework for the concurrent consideration of occupational hazards and obesity. *Ann Occup Hyg* **52**(7): 555–566.

Tibaldi J. (2008) Initiating and intensifying insulin therapy in type 2 diabetes mellitus. *Am J Med* **121**(6 Suppl): S20–S29.

UKPDS 33. (1998) UK Prospective Diabetes Study Group: Intensive blood-glucose control with sulphonylureas or insulin compared with conventional treatment and risk of complications in patients with type 2 diabetes. *Lancet* **352**: 837–853.

Vague J. (1947) La différentiation sexuelle. Facteur determinant des formes de l'obesité. *Presse Medl* **53**: 339–340.

van der Werf N, Kroese FG, Rozing J, Hillebrands JL. (2007) Viral infections as potential triggers of type 1 diabetes. *Diabetes Metab Res Rev* **23**(3): 169–183.

Wells JCK. (2009) Ethnic variability in adiposity and cardiovascular risk: The variable disease selection hypothesis. *Int J Epidemiology* **38**: 63–71.

WHO. (2009) http://www.who.int/topics/obesity/en/.

WHO Expert Consultation. (2004) Appropriate body-mass index for Asian populations and its implications for policy and intervention strategies. *Lancet* **363**: 157–163.

Wild S, Roglic G, Green A. (2004) Global prevalence of diabetes: Estimates for the year 2000 and projections for 2030. *Diabetes Care* **27**: 1047–1053.

Zozulinska D, Wysocka BW. (2006) Type 2 diabetes as inflammatory disease. *Diabetes Res Clin Pract* **74**: S12–S16.

Chapter 15

Female Reproductive Disorders

Helena Taskinen, Marja-Liisa Lindbohm†
and Sin-Eng Chia‡,§*

Introduction

Women are increasingly participating in the workforce; women with paid employment outside the home make up 49% of the workforce of the developed economies and European Union (International Labour Office, 2008). More women are also entering the workforce in developing countries. Specific health issues of women at work are therefore increasingly important. Among the issues are the reproductive health of women and the development of fetuses.

Reproductive Health Impacts in Adult Females

Occupational and environmental exposure to a reproductive toxicant can have adverse impacts on the reproductive health of an adult female. These effects may appear as delayed menarche, alterations in

*Finnish Institute of Occupational Health, Hjelt Institute, Faculty of Medicine, University of Helsinki, Helsinki, Finland.
†Finnish Institute of Occupational Health, Helsinki, Finland.
‡Department of Epidemiology and Public Health, Yong Loo Lin School of Medicine, National University of Singapore.
§Corresponding author. E-mail: ephcse@nus.edu.sg

sex hormones, menstrual disorders, ovarian dysfunction and earlier age at menopause (Table 1). Menstrual symptoms are among the most common disorders of women. Severe menstrual symptoms have been associated with regular absence from work in 3–10% of all fertile women (Lemasters, 1996). Several processes involved in the maturation of oocytes may be sensitive to chemical disturbances, especially through interference with hormone regulation in the hypothalamic-pituitary-gonadal axis (Mattison, 1985). Irregularities of the menstrual cycle are often caused by disturbances of follicular maturation or hormonal disturbances, whereas early onset of menopause has been interpreted as a marker of damage to the follicular pool. Disorders of menstruation may express as a decrease in individual fertility potential or a very early pregnancy loss.

Exposure to lead has been related to menstrual disorders among lead battery plant workers (Tang and Zhu, 2003). Lead is accumulated in the bone and increased endogenous lead exposure has been demonstrated in women during periods of increased bone turnover,

Table 1.   Occupational Exposures Associated with Menstrual Function and Menopause

Exposure	Effects
Dichlorodiphenyltrichloroethane (DDT)	Menstrual disorders, earlier age at menopause
Dichlorodiphenyldichloroethylene (DDE)	Changes in ovarian hormone patterns, earlier age at menopause
Polychlorinated biphenyls (PCBs)	Menstrual disorders, endometriosis
Pesticides	Menstrual disorders
Lead	Menstrual disorders, delayed menarche
Mercury	Menstrual disorders
Organic solvents	Menstrual disorders
Phthalates	Endometriosis
Environmental tobacco smoke	Menstrual disorders, earlier age at menopause
Shift/night work	Menstrual disorders, endometriosis
Work stress	Menstrual disorders

Source: Adapted from Mendola, Messer and Rappazzo (2008).

such as menopause. This may constitute a potential health issue to the woman in old age (Vahter *et al.*, 2002).

Dichlorodiphenyltrichloroethane (DDT), its metabolite dichloro-diphenyldichloroethylene (DDE) and polychlorinated biphenyls (PCBs) are widespread organochlorines in the environment and human tissue. Menstrual disorders have been observed in women exposed to DDT and PCBs (Mendola, Messer and Rappazzo, 2008). Changes in ovarian hormone patterns (progesterone, estrogens) have been associated with DDE. Use of hormonally active pesticides (lindane, atrazine, mancozeb or maneb) has also been related to long menstrual cycles, intermenstrual bleeding and missed periods (Farr *et al.*, 2004). Several studies have found increased serum PCB values among endometriosis patients (Mendola, Messer and Rappazzo, 2008). While many of these pesticides have been banned in the developed countries they could be or are still being used in the developing countries.

Organic solvents are used widely in various fields of industries. Exposure to some solvents has been associated with menstrual disorders (Cho *et al.*, 2001). Women exposed to phthalates have in some studies had an increased risk of endometriosis (Mendola, Messer and Rappazzo, 2008).

Working shifts or at night appears to increase the risk of menstrual disorders (Hatch, Figa-Talamanca and Salerno, 1999; Su *et al.*, 2008) and endometriosis (Marino *et al.*, 2008). Work stress has also been related to menstrual disorders (Hatch, Figa-Talamanca and Salerno, 1999) and dysmenorrhea (László and Kopp, 2009).

Reproductive Health Impacts on Pregnancy

Occupational or environmental exposure to hazardous agents during pregnancy may disturb the development of the fetus, thereby leading to adverse pregnancy outcomes. The exposure may affect the fetus directly or indirectly by interfering with the maternal, placental or fetal membrane functions. Developmental toxicity may appear as infertility, spontaneous abortion, stillbirth, intrauterine growth retardation, preterm birth, low birth weight, malformation, postnatal death, functional disturbances or childhood cancer.

Exposure may be associated with one or many reproductive outcomes, depending on both the time and duration of the exposure and the dose of the agent received.

Occupational Hazards

Organic Solvents

Organic solvents are among the most important occupational reproductive hazards for women. Most of them are volatile and are absorbed via inhalation and through the skin. The passage of several solvents through the placenta has been demonstrated in humans and animals. Organic solvents have also induced malformations, retarded growth and produced lethal effects to embryos in experiments on mammals.

Exposure to high levels of solvents has been related to increased risk of miscarriage, congenital malformation and reduced fertility (Table 2; Lindbohm and Taskinen, 2000). Exposure has also been linked with central nervous system defects, oral clefts and cardiac defects (Chevrier *et al.*, 2006; Wennborg *et al.*, 2005). In some studies an increased risk of stillbirth, perinatal death and low birth weight, as well as leukemia and brain tumor have been noted in the children of exposed women (Ha *et al.*, 2002; Infante-Rivard *et al.*, 2005).

Particular solvents associated with adverse effects include some glycol ethers and their acetates, tetrachloroethylene, toluene and benzene (Lindbohm and Taskinen, 2000). The study's findings on individual solvents must be interpreted with caution, because coincident exposure to multiple solvents is common among workers, making it difficult to ascribe an adverse effect to an individual agent. As such, the occupational physician who has to deal with solvent exposure and pregnancy will need to evaluate each worker on a case-by-case basis.

Workers may be highly exposed to solvents in manufacturing, dry cleaning, painting and lacquering, shoe, pharmaceutical, semiconductor and laboratory industries. Some solvents have been labeled in the European Union with these risk phrases: "May cause harm to the

Table 2. Chemical Occupational Exposures Associated with Adverse Reproductive Effects

Hazard	Reported Effects	Industry or Occupational Group
Anesthetic gases	Reduced fertility, fetal loss, birth defects[a]	Hospital, dental and veterinary personnel
Nitrous oxide	Reduced fertility, fetal loss[a]	Hospital, dental and veterinary personnel
Antineoplastic drugs	Reduced fertility,[a] fetal loss, birth defects[a]	Hospital personnel, pharmaceutical industry, laboratory personnel
Ethylene oxide	Fetal loss[a]	Hospital personnel, chemical industry
Metals		
Inorganic mercury	Reduced fertility,[a] fetal loss[a]	Lamp industry, chlor-alkali industry, dental personnel
Lead	Reduced fertility,[a] fetal loss,[a] preterm birth,[a] low birth weight,[a] impaired cognitive development[a]	Battery industry, lead smelting, foundries, pottery industry, ammunition industry and some other metal industries
Solvents	Reduced fertility, fetal loss, birth defects	Painting, several other fields of industry
Some ethylene glycol ethers and their acetates	Reduced fertility, fetal loss	Electronics industry, silk screen printing, photography and dyeing, other industries
Formaldehyde	Reduced fertility,[a] fetal loss[a]	Mechanical wood industry, pathology laboratories
Tetrachloroethylene	Reduced fertility,[a] fetal loss	Dry cleaning, degreasing
Toluene	Reduced fertility,[a] fetal loss	Shoe industry, painting, laboratory work
Aliphatic hydrocarbons	Fetal loss[a]	Graphic and shoe industries, painting
Estrogens	Fetal loss[a]	Pharmaceutical industry
Pesticides	Reduced fertility,[a] fetal loss,[a] birth defects, preterm birth[a]	Agriculture, gardening, greenhouse work

[a]Inconclusive evidence.

unborn child" (R61) or "Possible risk of harm to the unborn child" (R63). The solvents include formamide, N,N-dimethylformamide, carbon disulphide, toluene and some glycol ethers. Exposure to the solvents labeled with these risk phrases and to solvents classified as carcinogens should be avoided during pregnancy. It would also be prudent to minimize exposure to other organic solvents during pregnancy. Practically, how can this measure be implemented? The following case study illustrates some aspect of the measures to be taken.

Case Study 1

A 30-year-old woman in the 10th week of pregnancy works in a dry cleaning shop. She fills up the washing machines and irons the clothes. She is not a dry cleaning operator, but she works in the same room, where dry cleaning and spot removing is done with tetrachloroethylene. According to hygienic measurements the concentration of tetrachloroethylene is 2.3 ppm beside the dry cleaning machine and 2.6 ppm in spot removing. The threshold limit value (TLV) of tetrachloroethylene is 10 ppm in Nordic countries (70 mg/m^3) and 25 ppm in the USA (ACGIH). Hygienic measurements in other dry cleaning shops have shown high levels of tetrachloroethylene in ironing of heavy dry-cleaned clothes. This substance is probably carcinogenic to humans.

What are the issues the attending physician needs to tackle?

1. Are the solvents that she is exposed to known to affect pregnancy and what is the level of exposure?
2. If harmful effects are possible or exposure level is high, can she be transferred to another section where there is no solvent exposure?
3. If transfer is not possible, can her exposure be minimized?

Inorganic Lead

Lead and lead compounds are used, for instance, in pigments, paints, accumulators, crystal glass, as stabilizers in PVC plastics, in brass, soldering metal, bullets and gun powder. Lead exposure is possible in the industrial processes of the production, repair or demolishing of lead-containing goods or materials. Also, in indoor shooting ranges there may be exposure to lead. Many of the lead compounds are classified as carcinogens or suspected carcinogens.

Lead is transferred across the placenta, and at birth the blood lead concentration in the umbilical cord is close to that of the mother. Rather low concentrations of lead in the maternal blood have been associated with miscarriages (blood lead concentration, B-Pb > 0.24 μmol/L; Borja-Aburto *et al.*, 1999), preterm births and small for gestational age babies (B-Pb = 0.24–0.5 μmol/L; Torres-Sánchez *et al.*, 1999; Jelliffe-Pawlowski *et al.*, 2006). Maternal exposure to lead may also affect the child's mental development (Bellinger *et al.*, 2005).

The level of B-Pb among pregnant women should not exceed the level of the unexposed population (in many countries the B-Pb level of the unexposed is 0.3 μmol/L or 6.2 μg/dL). Exposed workers should be followed-up regularly and they should be informed about the harmful effects. Women planning pregnancy should best be withdrawn from excess exposure before the start of pregnancy, but at the latest at the beginning of the pregnancy. Exposure to carcinogenic lead compounds should be avoided during pregnancy. Occupational health personnel and employers should negotiate and find good solutions in such a situation.

Inorganic Mercury

It is possible to be exposed to inorganic mercury in the chlor-alkali industry, in waste management and in the recovery of mercury. Smaller degrees of exposure may occur in healthcare and dental care.

Inorganic mercury is transferred to the fetus and accumulates in the placenta. Animal data gives support to the existence of harmful effects on the development of the fetus. Inorganic mercury is toxic to the nervous system and to the kidneys, thus exposure during pregnancy should be avoided.

The level of the actual exposure can be traced by measuring the concentration of inorganic mercury in the blood (B-Hg); it should not exceed the level of the non-exposed population ($\leq$ 25 nmol/L). The concentration in the urine (U-Hg) reflects the long-term body burden of exposure, and a U-Hg level of 50 nmol/L should not be exceeded during pregnancy.

The effects of methyl mercury are well-known as far as fetal effects are concerned; the exposure comes mainly from polluted fish in the diet. In the follow-up of the exposure, organic and inorganic mercury should be analyzed separately in the blood.

Welding Fumes

Welding fumes may contain various metals and other compounds; some metals may be carcinogenic (e.g. hexavalent chromium, nickel) or suspected reproductive toxicants (e.g. cadmium, manganese). In the welding of stainless steel there may be exposure to carcinogenic compounds (hexavalent chromium, nickel), and therefore the exposure, measured as biological monitoring values, for the unexposed population should not be exceeded (hexavalent chromium in urine, U-Cr $\leq$ 0.01 μmol/L; nickel in urine, U-Ni $\leq$ 0.06 μmol/L).

Carbon Monoxide

Exposure to carbon monoxide may occur in smoke-producing operations in various industries, e.g. iron foundries, welding, production of smoked foods, and in locations where combustion engines produce exhaust gases (e.g., car garages). There is also some exposure to carbon monoxide from traffic in the general environment of big cities.

Carbon monoxide is transported through the placenta and in the fetus the blood carboxyhemoglobin concentration is 10–15% higher than in the mother's blood. In connection to maternal carbon monoxide intoxications, intrauterine death and brain injury of the child have been reported. Disturbances in the pregnancy, neurological defects and small birth weight of the child have been reported after maternal exposure to 100 ppm of carbon monoxide for four hours (Norman and Halton, 1990).

The concentration of carbon monoxide in the working environment of pregnant woman should not exceed 9 ppm (10 mg/m^3).

Pesticides

In agricultural work, greenhouse work and in pesticide production, exposure to pesticides is possible. Pesticides enter the body through the skin, from inhaled air or from ingested food and drink. In warm environments it is also difficult to get and use proper protective clothing, so higher exposure through the skin is more likely. In greenhouses the exposure levels are usually higher than in outdoor cultivation. Many pesticide formulations contain organic solvents, which may be toxic to reproduction too. Various organophosphates, carbaryl, atrazine, endosulfan, mancozeb and maneb have been suggested to decrease fecundity (Fuortes *et al.*, 1997). Some pesticides have shown reproductive and/or developmental toxicity (e.g. benomyl, carbaryl, dibromochloropropane, ethylenethiourea, maneb, zineb, thiram) in animals or humans (Nurminen, 1995).

The risk of infertility was increased among women who had worked in industries associated with agriculture and if the woman resided on a farm (Fuortes *et al.*, 1997). In another study a slightly elevated risk of prolonged time to pregnancy was observed among primigravid women working in greenhouses and the risk of spontaneous abortions was elevated (Bretveld *et al.*, 2008). An increased risk of spontaneous abortion has been found among women in agricultural occupations, and among gardeners who sprayed pesticides during pregnancy (Nurminen, 1995). In one study the increased risk of spontaneous abortion was seen only among those who used pesticides three to five days a week during the first trimester of pregnancy. The risk was not increased, however, when a proper respirator was used on its own or with protective clothing (Taskinen *et al.*, 1995). An increased risk of spontaneous abortions among farmers (Kristensen *et al.*, 1997) has also been associated with rainy summers, when molds and exposure to mycotoxins (from mold) might be possible explanations for the finding. Stillbirths without birth defects were increased among women who worked in agriculture or horticulture more than 30 h/week (McDonald *et al.*, 1987). Women exposed to pesticides had an increased risk of stillbirth (Goulet and Theriault, 1991; Pastore *et al.*, 1997). Environmental exposure to malathion, insecticides and herbicides was associated with stillbirths too (Nurminen, 1995). An increase in birth defects has been associated with some individual pesticides or with work in which pesticides or pesticide mixtures are used. Limb anomalies and orofacial clefts have been reported in several studies. Exposure to chlorophenoxy herbicides, e.g. 2,4-D, has been associated with central nervous system, circulatory/respiratory, urogenital, and musculoskeletal malformations. Exposure to pesticide combinations was associated with neural tube defects (Stillerman *et al.*, 2008).

Exposure to pesticides, like organophosphate pesticides, chlorpyrifos, triazine herbicides in combination with other pesticides, and atrazine in drinking water has been correlated with preterm birth and reduced fetal growth (Stillerman *et al.*, 2008).

Parental exposure to pesticides was in some studies associated with childhood cancer (all sites), leukemia, lymphomas, and tumors of the brain and nervous system (Gold and Sever, 1994), but conflicting results have also been presented.

The research results suggest that exposure to pesticides during pregnancy may be harmful. Thus, exposure to pesticides at work during pregnancy should be minimized or avoided. The exposure is highest during spraying in greenhouses or outside. Spraying should not be conducted by a pregnant worker. To avoid residues from earlier spraying, workers should wear long sleeves and gloves when handling sprayed plants.

Anesthetic Gases

Several studies, although not all, have shown an increased risk of miscarriage among women occupationally exposed to trace concentrations of anesthetic gases (Lindbohm and Taskinen, 2000). With the exception of nitrous oxide, the effects of individual anesthetic gases have not been examined in humans. Exposure to nitrous oxide has been related to an increased risk of miscarriage in dental personnel and reduced birth weight in midwives (Rowland *et al.*, 1995, Axelsson, Ahlborg and Bodin, 1996; Bodin, Axelsson and Ahlborg, 1999). Dental assistants exposed to high levels of unscavenged nitrous oxide and midwives assisting numerous nitrous oxide deliveries per month had also a lower fecundability as compared with unexposed women (Ahlborg, Axelsson and Bodin, 1996; Rowland *et al.*, 1995). Halothane and nitrous oxide have been found to be fetotoxic and teratogenic in animals. Concerning isoflurane and enflurane, an experts' committee concluded that a lack of human data precludes assessment of their effects, and sufficient animal data show that no classification "as a reproductive toxicant" is indicated (Committee for Compounds Toxic to Reproduction, 2002).

Hospital personnel in operating rooms, delivery wards, dental offices and veterinary surgeries may be exposed to anesthetic gases. Harmful exposure may occur especially when administering anesthesia to small children in arms and in operating rooms with poor ventilation or inefficient scavenging equipment.

Antineoplastic Agents

An increased risk of miscarriage has been observed in nurses who prepare injectable antineoplastic drug solutions for patients (Lindbohm and Taskinen, 2000). High occupational exposure to these drugs has also been related to reduced fertility and increased risk of premature delivery and low birth weight (Fransman *et al.*, 2007). An excess of congenital malformations has also been reported. There is, however, evidence indicating that safety measures can protect health personnel against the adverse effects of antineoplastic drugs on reproduction (Skov *et al.*, 1992).

Nurses and other hospital workers may be exposed to antineoplastic agents when handling the concentrated drugs (preparation, administration and disconnection of infusion system), nursing and during cleaning activities. Exposure can also occur in laundries, pharmaceutical industries and veterinary clinics. Exposure to these agents should be minimized by using protective garments and equipment (for example, closed infusion systems), good work practices and the

428 Textbook of Occupational Medicine Practice, 3rd Edition

workers' increasing awareness of the potential hazards. Current prevention measures may not, however, completely eliminate opportunities for exposure, and some countries have therefore adopted a policy of transferring pregnant workers who dilute and prepare antineoplastic drug solutions to other jobs.

Other Drugs

Some drugs have known adverse effects on the development of the fetus. Excess vitamin A is teratogenic in many species, although the teratogenic dose in humans is unknown. Diethylstilbestrol (DES) is a known human reproductive hazard. Congenital malformations have been observed in children of women exposed to DES during pregnancy. Daughters of DES-exposed mothers are at increased risk of developing cancer of the vagina and uterus after puberty. Some other sex hormones have induced masculinization of female fetuses and feminization of male fetuses in animal experiments (IARC, 1999). Occupational exposure has been related to symptoms of hyperestrogenism and increased risk of miscarriage in pharmaceutical factory workers (Taskinen, Lindbohm and Hemminki, 1986). Combined oral estrogen-progestogen contraceptives have been classified as carcinogens to humans by the IARC (Group 1).

Ribavirin, an antiviral agent, is administered to patients as an aerosol in a tent. It has been found to be teratogenic and embryolethal in animal experiments, but the absorbed doses among hospital staff are likely to be very small. Other antiviral agents, such as acyclovir, ganciclovir and zidovudine, have induced decreased implantation and embryolethality in animal experiments. Some adverse reproductive effects have also been observed in animals exposed to azathioprine and cyclosporin A (Frazier and Hage, 1998).

Aerosolized pentamidine is used to treat *Pneumocystis carinii (jiroveci)* pneumonia. An experimental study in rats indicated that the normal human parenteral doses of pentamidine caused pregnancy resorptions when given early in embryogenesis, but no significant increase in congenital abnormalities. Limited human experience with the use of pentamidine during pregnancy has not suggested adverse effects (Frazier and Hage, 1998).

Pregnant women should not be occupationally exposed to the aforementioned drugs.

Carcinogenic Chemicals

Carcinogenic agents, which may cause changes in the cells' genome, are considered potentially harmful to the fetus as they might cause changes also in the fetal cells. Pregnant women should not be exposed to carcinogens or strongly suspected carcinogens.

Contagious Diseases

Some infectious agents may be harmful to the pregnancy and the fetus (Table 3). A European Union directive identifies toxoplasmosis as such, and therefore pregnant women should not perform tasks with risk of infection. Also, pregnant women should be protected at work from contagious contact with listeria, rubella, cytomegalovirus, hepatitis B and C, and HI (HIV) viruses. Pregnant women are also at risk of having more severe disease from the influenza A (H1N1) pandemic viral infection ("swine flu"), and therefore should not work in close contact with patients suffering from that infection. Pregnant women are prioritized to be vaccinated against that virus.

Women in jobs where exposure to viral infections are common, e.g. in healthcare and child care occupations, can be asked at the preplacement examination by occupational health personnel about possible immunity, achieved "naturally" or from vaccinations, against common contagious diseases. Vaccinations may be recommended, if available, for workers in risky occupations.

Ionizing Radiation

Small doses of radiation are not expected to increase the risk of congenital malformations, but it may have effects on growth and increase the risk of childhood cancer. Ionizing radiation includes X-rays and radiation from radionuclides. X-rays penetrate tissues and reach the fetus. Radionuclides vary in their ability to reach the fetal tissues and

Table 3.   Physical and Biological Occupational Exposures Associated with Adverse Reproductive Effects

Hazard	Reported Effects	Industry or Occupation
Ionizing radiation	Fetal loss[a]	Healthcare personnel
Noise	Reduced fertility,[a] preterm birth,[a] growth retardation, low birth weight	Industrial manufacturing
Cosmic radiation	Fetal loss[a]	Flight attendants
Contagious diseases	Fetal loss, growth retardation, birth defects	Healthcare personnel, childcare workers
Mycotoxins in grain	Midpregnancy delivery[a]	Grain farming

[a] Inconclusive evidence.

the exposure assessment may require analysis of biological samples. Exposure to ionizing radiation may occur in nuclear power plants, healthcare professions (X-rays, radionuclides), and flying aircraft (Aspholm *et al.*, 1999).

A large cohort study among nuclear industry workers exposed to low-level ionizing radiation observed no evidence of a link between exposure and congenital malformations. Maternal preconception monitoring was related to an increased risk of fetal death, but the findings are equivocal and require further investigation. There was weak evidence of an association between exposure and primary infertility in women, but the relatively small number of monitored women prevented a detailed examination of the data (Doyle *et al.*, 2000; 2001).

Work where exposure to radiation is high (i.e. a yearly dose of 6 mSv or more or a local dose to the eyes, skin, hands or legs higher than 30% of the allowed limits for those areas) is not allowed for the pregnant worker. Such exposure may occur in giving regular isotope therapy, and also other work, where the fetal equivalent dose of ionizing radiation during pregnancy would exceed 1 mSv. For flying personnel the same limit is valid and the number of flights during pregnancy has to be planned accordingly. The radiation exposure in airplanes is dependent on the length and the height of the flight. It has been estimated that the mean cosmic radiation dose is 3.2 (range: 0–9.5) mSv per active work year among Finnish aircraft cabin attendants (Kojo, Aspholm and Auvinen, 2004).

Noise

Noise may have adverse reproductive effects through a stress reaction induced by an increase in maternal catecholamine secretion, which may further stimulate or retard uterine contractions and affect uteroplacental blood flow. Some studies have indicated that exposure to high noise levels (around 85 $dBL_{Aeq(8h)}$ or higher) is associated with fetal growth retardation (Lindbohm and Taskinen, 2000). Excesses of hormonal disturbances, delayed conception, infertility and miscarriage have also been reported for occupational noise exposure (Table 4).

Noise has been suspected to have adverse effects on the hearing of the fetus. Environmental noise penetrates the tissues and fluids surrounding the fetal head and stimulates the inner ear through a bone conduction route. The fetus hears predominately low-frequency sounds, and high-frequency sounds are greatly attenuated by the abdomen (Gerhardt and Abrams, 2000). Two early reports suggest

Table 4. Physical and Psychosocial Work Load Factors Associated with Adverse Reproductive Effects

Hazard	Reported Effects
Shift work, night work	Fetal loss,[a] preterm birth, low birth weight
Long working hours	Fetal loss,[a] low birth weight
Physical strain, including prolonged standing, physically demanding work	Reduced fertility,[a] fetal loss,[a] preterm birth, intrauterine growth retardation, low birth weight,[a] birth defects[a]
Psychosocial strain	Pre-eclampsia,[a] preterm births,[a] fetal loss[a]

[a] Inconclusive evidence.

that occupational noise exposure (85–95 $dBL_{Aeq(8h)}$ or >100 dB) may increase the risk of hearing deterioration in the children. The reports have been criticized because of their methodological limitations. No hearing impairment was observed in children of mothers exposed to occupational noise (>80 dB but <90 dB) during pregnancy when compared to the children of unexposed mothers (Rocha, Frasson de Azevedo and Ximenes Filho, 2007).

All in all, the current evidence suggests that high noise exposure should be considered a potential reproductive hazard. According to the European Union guidelines (COM, 2000), pregnant workers should not be exposed to noise levels exceeding the national limit value (for example, in Finland, 85 $dBL_{Aeq(8h)}$). A-weighted [L_{Aeq}] sound pressures, which are used in routine work place noise measurements, filter away the small frequencies that reach the fetus effectively. Therefore, fetal exposure assessment should be based on measurements of C-weighted sound pressure levels (dBL_{Ceq}) including also the small frequencies. Leaning against a vibrating device or machine should also be avoided during pregnancy, because vibrations on the external surface of the maternal abdomen can induce sounds inside the uterus.

Shift Work

Shift work has been considered potentially harmful for reproduction, because it may interfere with the circadian regulation of human metabolism. This may lead to changes in hormonal concentrations that may affect reproductive capability. A meta-analysis indicated that the risk of preterm birth is slightly increased among women in shift work whereas the evidence tends to favor no effect on the risk of having a small for gestational age baby (Bonzini, Coggon and Palmer, 2007). An elevated risk of miscarriage and reduced fertility has also been indicated for shift work, although not consistently so in all investigations. It has, however, remained unclear which forms of shift work — rotating or changing schedules, night work, irregular working hours or shift work in general — may be harmful to reproductive health.

Shift work is common in healthcare, manufacturing and transport and communication work. According to a European Union directive

(92/85/EEC), a pregnant or nursing woman should not be obliged to do night work, if a medical certificate declares it necessary for the safety or health of the worker. The woman should be transferred to daytime work or granted leave from work where such a transfer is not feasible.

Case Study 2

A 39-year-old pregnant nurse works full-time at a hospital. She was in gestational week 7 when referred and this is her fourth pregnancy. She had a transient bleeding episode of a few days in the eighth week of the current gestation. She was feeling a little tired, but otherwise she was healthy. She works in a forward-rotating three-shift schedule (0700–1500, 1500–2300 and 2300–0700) and has on average four night duties per month. Job tasks include administration of pharmaceuticals, assistance of physicians and care tasks such as transfer of disabled patients from bed to chair and vice versa, in particular during evening and night shifts. There are about 15 patient transfers during a shift — usually performed by two persons.

What options can the attending physician suggest to the worker and employer?

1. Can she be transferred to another department where she does not need to be on shift work, e.g. in outpatient clinics?
2. She should be advised not to lift heavy burdens which in this case would include transfer of patients. Some job adjustment may be needed, depending on her pregnancy status further into the gestation.

Physical Strain

Work entailing pronounced physical exertion may have harmful effects on the reproductive health of women, although moderate physical activity is safe both for the mother and fetus. Strong physical effort may alter the hormonal balance and increase intrauterine pressure, and thus decrease the nutritional blood flow to the fetus. In later pregnancy it may also promote uterine contractions and consequently increase the risk of early delivery.

Prolonged standing (>3 hours/day) or walking, long working hours and physically demanding work have been shown to increase the risk of preterm delivery and reduced fetal growth in several studies (Mozurkewich *et al.*, 2000; Bonzini, Coggon and Palmer, 2007). Some studies also suggest an association between physically demanding work and high blood pressure and pre-eclampsia. Use of preventive measures — reassignment to a safer job or preventive withdrawal from work — has been observed to decrease the risk of adverse outcomes (Croteau, Marcoux and Brisson, 2007).

Strenuous physical exertion should be considered in the assessment and prevention of occupational reproductive hazards. During the second and third trimesters the physical work load may need to be decreased, opportunities for rest organized, and continuous standing and walking avoided. The European Union has given guidance on the assessment of specific risks to pregnant employees and actions needed to ensure that she is not exposed to anything which will damage either her health or that of her developing child (COM, 2000). The employer must ensure that pregnant workers are not exposed, for example, to manual handling involving risk of injury, awkward movements and postures, especially in confined spaces, and work at heights. Where appropriate, work equipment and lifting gear should be adapted, storage arrangements altered, or workstations or job content redesigned. Long periods spent handling loads or spent standing or sitting without regular movement to maintain healthy circulation should also be avoided.

Pregnancy and Fitness for Work

If a pregnant woman is not exposed to any known reproductive hazard it is generally not an issue for her to continue work throughout the pregnancy. However, one needs to appreciate the physiological changes associated with each trimester of pregnancy and relate it to the working conditions and possible agents that she may be exposed to. For example, in the first trimester of pregnancy, some women may experience more nausea which could be aggravated by chemicals with strong, unpleasant odors. In the last trimester fatigue will increase which may pose a problem for the woman if the working conditions are inflexible or she is engaged in shift work, especially that involving night shifts.

Breastfeeding and Work

Chemical contamination of breast milk through exposure of mothers at work has become a matter of concern in recent years among women who have followed advice to breastfeed their infants. Maternal exposure at work to various pollutants may cause contamination of breast milk. Milk fat is excreted as fat globules, and chemicals may be bound to the surface of globules or trapped within the globules. The amount of chemicals in breast milk is determined by the extent of the exposure to the chemicals and the properties of the chemicals. Small lipophilic organic molecules, e.g. organic solvents, halocarbons and pesticides, are easily transferred from blood plasma to mammary gland cells, and are concentrated in the fat globules. The chemical exposure may be lifelong exposure (accumulated chemicals) or periodic high exposure. Many chemicals enter from industrial plants or from agricultural use into the general environment and the food chain. Therefore, the control of use and of pollution due to toxic chemicals in general is important to keep human milk safe for infants. The ban and restriction of use of such chemicals have in many cases led to lowered contamination of breast milk. A review of organic and inorganic chemicals in breast milk concludes that it is important to identify contaminant trends and highly exposed groups and take measures to improve the situation where possible (Massart *et al.*, 2008).

Many organochlorine pesticides and insecticides and other organohalogen chemicals have been banned or their use restricted in numerous countries. Many of them stay in the environment and in the fat tissue of exposed persons for a long time, from several years up to 20 years. They are also concentrated in the breast milk so that the concentration may be four to six times higher than that in the blood of the lactating mother (Massart *et al.*, 2008). Volatile organic compounds, e.g. many organic solvents, are in general short-lived in the body, thus reflecting recent exposure, although some solvents may persist longer, for a few days or weeks. Breast milk concentration levels may be slightly higher than in the blood, e.g. perchloroethylene levels in the milk are threefold higher than its blood levels (Massart *et al.*, 2008). The amount of toxic metals is smaller in breast milk than in the blood (about 20–50%) (Sharma and Pervez, 2005; Massart *et al.*, 2008).

Many chemicals could be excreted through breast milk. As a general guiding principle, women who are breastfeeding should not return to work with exposure to chemicals unless it can be ascertained that the chemicals cannot be excreted via breast milk. They should only be returned to their original work when their children have been weaned. The employer, wherever possible, should make available facilities for the women to express their milk and keep it refrigerated so their children can continue to have breast milk.

Legislation

The European Union has launched a directive (92/85/EEC) on the protection of pregnant, newly delivered and breastfeeding women, which binds the member states to adapt their national legislation accordingly.

The directive prohibits for pregnant women exposures including the following:

— Work in hyperbaric atmosphere, e.g. pressurized enclosures and underwater diving;
— Biological agents, e.g. toxoplasma, rubella virus, unless the pregnant workers are proved to be adequately protected against such agents by immunization;
— Chemical agents, e.g. lead and lead derivatives in so far as these agents are capable of being absorbed by the human organism;
— Unsuitable working conditions, e.g. underground mining work.

In addition, the European Commission has published guidelines for assessing risks to pregnancy and the child from several other work exposures. The Communication from the Commission provides guidelines on the assessment of the chemical, physical and biological agents and industrial processes considered hazardous to the safety or health of pregnant workers and workers who have recently given birth or are breastfeeding (COM 2000).

In some countries there are specific restrictions concerning occupational exposure to harmful agents (e.g. in Denmark; Finland; Sweden; Quebec, Canada). Evidence from scientific research is necessary for regulations at the international and national levels. It should be kept in mind that paternal exposure at work may also affect the fertility of the couple and the development of the child, and therefore the reproductive health of men should be protected from external exposures as well.

References

Ahlborg G Jr, Axelsson G, Bodin L. (1996) Shift work, nitrous oxide exposure and subfertility among Swedish midwives. *Int J Epidemiol* **25**: 783–790.

Aspholm R, Lindbohm ML, Paakkulainen H, *et al.* (1999) Spontaneous abortions among Finnish flight attendants. *J Occup Environ Med* **41**: 486–491.

Axelsson G, Ahlborg G Jr, Bodin L. (1996) Shift work, nitrous oxide exposure, and spontaneous abortion among Swedish midwives. *Occup Environ Med* **53**: 374–378.

Bellinger DC. (2005) Teratogen update: Lead and pregnancy. *Birth Defects Res A Clin Mol Teratol* **73**(6): 409–420.

Bodin L, Axelsson G, Ahlborg G. (1999) The association of shift work and nitrous oxide exposure in pregnancy with birth weight and gestational age. *Epidemiology* **10**: 429–436.

Bonzini M, Coggon D, Palmer KT. (2007) Risk of prematurity, low birth weight and pre-eclampsia in relation to working hours and physical activities: A systemic review. *Occup Environ Med* **64**: 228–243.

Borja-Aburto VH, Herz-Picciotto I, Rojas Lopes MR, *et al.* (1999) Blood lead levels measured prospectively and risk of spontaneous abortion. *Am J Epidemiol* **150**: 590–597.

Bretveld RW, Hooiveld M, Zielhuis GA, *et al.* (2008) Reproductive disorders among male and female greenhouse workers. *Reprod Toxicol* 1: 107–114.

Chevrier C, Dananché B, Bahuau M, *et al.* (2006) Occupational exposure to organic solvent mixtures during pregnancy and the risk of non-syndromic oral clefts. *Occup Environ Med* 63: 617–623.

Cho SI, Damokosh AI, Ryan LM, *et al.* (2001) Effects of exposure to organic solvents on menstrual cycle length. *J Occup Environ Med* 43: 567–575.

COM. (2000) *Guidelines on the Assessment of the Chemical, Physical and Biological Agents and Industrial Processes Considered Hazardous for the Safety or Health of Pregnant Workers and Workers Who Have Recently Given Birth or are Breastfeeding (Council Directive 92/85/EEC).* http://osha.europa.eu/fop/bulgaria/bg/legislation/directives/treatment/31992l0085en.doc (accessed 23 November 2009).

Committee for Compounds Toxic to Reproduction. (2002) *Enflurane. Evaluation of the Effects on Reproduction, Recommendation for Classification.* The Hague: Health Council of the Netherlands.

Croteau A, Marcoux S, Brisson C. (2007) Work activity in pregnancy, preventive measures, and the risk of preterm delivery. *Am J Epidemiol* 166: 951–965.

Doyle P, Maconochie N, Roman E, *et al.* (2000) Fetal death and congenital malformation in babies born to nuclear industry employees: Report from the nuclear industry family study. *Lancet* 356: 1293–1299.

Doyle P, Roman E, Maconochie N, *et al.* (2001) Primary infertility in nuclear industry employees: Report from the nuclear industry family study. *Occup Environ Med* 58: 535–539.

Farr SL, Cooper GS, Cai J, *et al.* (2004) Pesticide use and menstrual cycle characteristics among premenopausal women in the Agricultural Health Study. *Am J Epidemiol* 160: 1194–1204.

Fransman W, Roeleveld N, Peelen S, *et al.* (2007) Nurses with dermal exposure to antineoplastic drugs: Reproductive outcomes. *Epidemiology* 18: 112–119.

Frazier L, Hage M. (1998) *Reproductive Hazards of the Workplace.* New York: John Wiley & Sons Inc.

Fuortes L, Clark MK, Kirchner HL, Smith EM. (1997) Association between female infertility and agricultural work history. *Am J Ind Med* 31(4): 445–451.

Gerhardt KJ, Abrams RM. (2000) The fetus. Fetal exposures to sound and vibroacoustic stimulation. *J Perinatol* 20: S20–S29.

Gold EB, Sever LE. (1994) Childhood cancers associated with parental occupational exposures. *Occupational Medicine: State of the Art Reviews* **9**: 495–539.

Goulet L, Theriault G. (1991) Stillbirth and chemical exposure of pregnant workers. *Scand J Work Environ Health* **17**: 25–31.

Ha E, Cho SI, Chen D, *et al.* (2002) Parental exposure to organic solvents and reduced birth weight. *Arch Environ Health* **57**: 207–214.

Hatch MC, Figa-Talamanca I, Salerno S. (1999) Work stress and menstrual patterns among American and Italian nurses. *Scand J Work Environ Health* **25**: 144–150.

Infante-Rivard C, Weichenthal S. (2007) Pesticides and childhood cancer: An update of Zahm and Ward's 1998 review. *J Toxicol Environ Health*, Part B, **10**: 1–2, 81–99.

Infante-Rivard C, Siemiatycki J, Lakhani R, Nadon L. (2005) Maternal exposure to occupational solvents and childhood leukemia. *Environ Health Perspect* **113**: 787–792.

International Agency for Research on Cancer (IARC). (1999) IARC monographs on the evaluation of carcinogenic risks to humans. In: *Hormonal Contraception and Post-menopausal Hormonal Therapy*, Vol. 72. Lyon: IARC.

International Labour Office. (2008) *Global Employment Trends for Women.* http://www.ilo.org/wcmsp5/groups/public/---dgreports/---dcomm/documents/publication/wcms_091225.pdf (accessed 21 November 2009).

Jelliffe-Pawlowski LL, Miles SQ, Courtney JG, *et al.* (2006) Effect of magnitude and timing of maternal pregnancy blood lead (Pb) levels on birth outcomes. *J Perinatol* **26**(3): 154–162.

Kojo K, Aspholm R, Auvinen A. (2004) Occupational radiation dose estimation for Finnish aircraft cabin attendants. *Scand J Work Environ Health* **30**: 157–163.

Kristensen P, Irgens LM, Andersen A, *et al.* (1997) Gestational age, birth weight, and perinatal death among births to Norwegian farmers, 1967–1991. *Am J Epidemiol* **146**(4): 329–338.

László KD, Kopp MS. (2009) Effort-reward imbalance and overcommitment at work are associated with painful menstruation: Results from the Hungarostudy Epidemiological Panel 2006. *J Occup Environ Med* **51**: 157–163.

Lemasters GK. (1996) Epidemiology of reproductive hazards in the workplace. *Occup Med: State of the Art Reviews* **11**: 545–560.

Lindbohm ML, Taskinen H. (2000) Reproductive hazards in the workplace. In: Goldman MB, Hatch MC (eds). *Women and Health*, pp. 463–473. San Diego: Academic Press.

Marino JL, Holt VL, Chen C, Davis S. (2008) Shift work, hCLOCK T3111C polymorphism, and endometriosis risk. *Epidemiology* **19**: 477–484.

Massart F, Gherarducci G, Marchi B, Saggese G. (2008) Chemical biomarkers of human breast milk pollution. *Biomarker Insights* **3**: 159–169.

Mattison DR. (1985) Clinical manifestations of ovarian toxicity. In: Dixon RL (ed). *Reproductive Toxicology*, pp. 109–130. New York: Raven Press.

McDonald AD, McDonald JC, Armstrong B. (1987) Occupation and pregnancy outcome. *Br J Ind Med* **44**: 521–526.

Mendola P, Messer LC, Rappazzo K. (2008) Science linking environmental contaminant exposures with fertility and reproductive health impacts in the adult female. *Fertil Steril* **89**: 81–94.

Mozurkewich EL, Luke B, Avni M, Wolf FM. (2000) Working conditions and adverse pregnancy outcome: A meta-analysis. *Obstet Gynecol* **95**: 623–635.

Norman CA, Halton DM. (1990) Is carbon monoxide a workplace teratogen? A review and evaluation of literature. *Ann Occup Hygiene* **34**: 335–347.

Nurminen T. (1995) Maternal pesticide exposure and pregnancy outcome. *J Occup Environ Med* **37**: 935–940.

Pastore LM, Hertz-Picciotto, Beaumont JJ. (1997) Risk of stillbirth from occupational and residential exposures. *Occup Environ Med* **54**:511–518.

Rocha EB, Frasson de Azevedo M, Ximenes Filho JA. (2007). Study of the hearing in children born from pregnant women exposed to occupational noise: Assessment by distortion product otoacoustic emissions. *Braz J Otorhinolaryngol* **73**: 359–369.

Rowland AS, Baird DD, Shore DL, *et al.* (1995) Nitrous oxide and spontaneous abortion in female dental assistants. *Am J Epidemiol* **141**: 531–538.

Sharma R, Pervez S. (2005) Toxic metals status in human blood and breast milk samples in an integrated steel plant environment in Central India. *Environ Geochem Health* **27**: 39–45.

Skov T, Maarup B, Olsen J, *et al.* (1992) Leukaemia and reproductive outcome among nurses handling antineoplastic drugs. *Br J Ind Med* **49**: 855–861.

Stillerman KP, Mattison DR, Giudice LC, Woodruff TJ. (2008) Environmental exposures and adverse pregnancy outcomes: A review of the science. *Reproductive Sciences* **15**: 631–650.

Su SB, Lu CW, Kao YY, Guo HR. (2008) Effects of 12-hour rotating shifts on menstrual cycles of photoelectronic workers in Taiwan. *Chronobiol Int* **25**: 237–248.

Tang N, Zhu ZQ. (2003) Adverse reproductive effects in female workers of lead battery plants. *Int J Occup Med Environ Health* **16**: 359–361.

Taskinen H, Lindbohm ML, Hemminki K. (1986) Spontaneous abortions among women working in the pharmaceutical industry. *Br J Ind Med* **43**: 199–205.

Taskinen HK, Kyyrönen P, Liesivuori J, Sallmén M. (1995) Greenhouse work, pesticides and pregnancy outcome. An abstract. *Epidemiology* **6**: 109.

Torres-Sánchez LE, Berkowitz G, López-Carrillo L, *et al.* (1999) Intrauterine lead exposure and preterm birth. *Environ Res* **81**: 297–301.

Vahter M, Berglund M, Akesson A, Lidén C. (2002) Metals and women's health. *Environ Res* **88**: 145–155.

Wennborg H, Magnusson LL, Bonde JP, Olsen J. (2005) Congenital malformations related to maternal exposure to specific agents in biomedical research laboratories. *J Occup Environ Med* **47**: 11–19.

Windham GC, Lee D, Mitchell P, *et al.* (2005) Exposure to organochlorine compounds and effects on ovarian function. *Epidemiology* **16**: 182–190.

Chapter 16

Male Reproductive Disorders

Jens Peter Bonde* and Sin-Eng Chia[†,‡]

Introduction

Infertility is a common disorder among young people, while reduced libido and impotence rapidly increase in those over 50 years of age. These conditions have well-established causes related to the occupational environment, but are seldom reported to or recognized by work injury compensation authorities. This is possibly because capability for work is not affected by these disorders. The impact of male reproductive disorders extends beyond a reduction in quality of life and suffering in subfertile couples. It also possibly affects fertility rates at the population level.

The functioning of the male reproductive system is dependent on ongoing and highly specialized cell division, maturation and differentiation, which is highly vulnerable to environmental insult (Cooper and Kavlock, 1997; Lahdetie, 1995; Oliva, Spira and Multigner, 2001; Tas, Lauwerys and Lison, 1996).

Therefore, malfunction of the male reproduction system may serve as an early warning of environmental hazards. This was demonstrated

---

*The University of Copenhagen, Bispebjerg Hospital, Copenhagen, Denmark.
†Department of Epidemiology and Public Health, Yong Loo Lin School of Medicine, National University of Singapore.
‡Corresponding author. E-mail: ephcse@nus.edu.sg

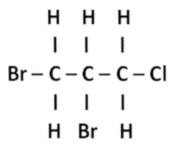

Fig. 1. The molecular structure of dibromochloropropane (DBCP).

in 1977 in California and in 1978 in Israel, when it was discovered that the nematocide dibromochloropropane (DBCP) (Fig. 1) caused severe testicular toxicity in exposed chemical plant (Whorton *et al.*, 1977) and agricultural workers (Potashnik *et al.*, 1978).

In some workers this compound caused azoospermia or severe oligospermia following exposure of a few months at low levels, without other signs of toxicity. Although the potency of this compound to disrupt spermatogenesis is unusually high, the DBCP tragedy points to the need to take seriously the potential risk of male reproductive toxicity.

In addition to infertility and impotence, male reproductive disorders of interest from an occupational point of view include cryptorchidism, hypospadias and testicular cancer, which may result from exposure of the developing fetal gonad in early pregnancy (Skakkebaek, Rajpert-De Meyts and Main, 2001). It is still uncertain whether exposure of the adult male may result in pregnancy failure or disorders in the offspring independent of maternal exposures and conditions (Anderson, 2003). Among some scientists the prevailing view is that exposure of the adult male to chemicals and ionizing radiation in general is unrelated to the occurrence of miscarriage, birth defects, growth retardation and cancer. There is, however, strong animal experimental evidence of male-mediated embryonal loss at dose levels not affecting fertility or sperm count (Trasler, 2003; Cordier, 2008; Robaire and Hales, 2003). We still do not know if the lack of unequivocal examples of male-mediated developmental toxicity in humans is due to methodological problems or the non-existence of this phenomenon.

Anatomy, Physiology and Mechanisms

The production of the male gamete, the spermatozoa, takes place in the seminiferous tubules in close association with the Sertoli cells (spermatogenesis) (Fig. 2). The main androgen, testosterone, is produced in the Leydig cells located in the interstitial base between the seminiferous tubules in the testis (steroidogenesis) (Lamb and Foster,

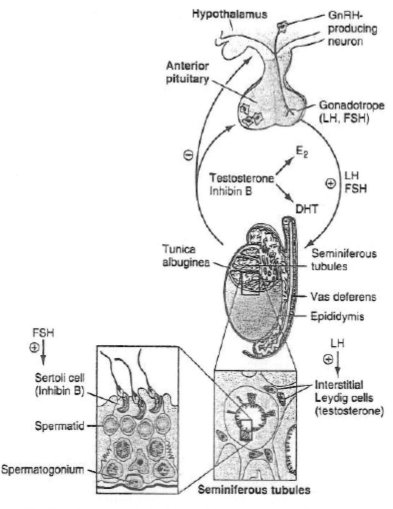

Fig. 2. Anatomy and physiology of the male reproductive system.

1988). Spermatogenesis as well as steroidogenesis is under strict hormonal regulation by coordinated hypothalamic-pituitary-gonadal interaction. Pulsatile secretion of gonadotropin-releasing hormone (GnRH) by the hypothalamus stimulates the secretion of luteinizing hormone (LH) and follicle-stimulating hormone (FSH) by the pituitary gland. These gonadotropins reach the testis where LH stimulates secretion of testosterone and estradiol from the Leydig cells and FSH binds to Sertoli cells and stimulates secretion of substances that support spermatogenesis. Testosterone exerts negative feedback inhibition on GnRH and LH secretion. Inhibin B secreted by the Sertoli cells exerts negative feedback inhibition on FSH by the pituitary.

Normal spermatogenesis requires a very high concentration of testosterone in the seminiferous tubule. The epididymis is essential for maturation of testicular immotile spermatozoa. During epididymal passage the spermatozoa gains motility and is stored in the distal part of the epididymis until ejaculation. Another accessory sex gland, the vesicula seminalis, provides nutrients for spermatozoa in the ejaculate and the prostate secretes a slightly acidic fluid rich in zinc and a number of enzymes facilitating semen liquefaction.

Spermatogenesis is a 72-day process that includes proliferation of spermatogonia, meiotic and mitotic cell division, differentiation, maturation and finally release of spermatozoa into the lumen of the seminiferous tubule (Lamb and Foster, 1988). Effects of reproductive toxicants (Fig. 3) depend on the stage of the spermatogenic cycle that is susceptible to damage (Scialli and Clegg, 1992). Toxicity to spermatogonia and Sertoli cells causes delayed effects that are permanent, if the damage is severe. Toxic substances that act on a later stage of spermatogenesis may have reversible effects on semen quality after a short delay.

Epidemiology

Infertility is defined as the inability of a couple to achieve pregnancy within one year of unprotected sexual relationship (Schill, Comhaire and Hargreave, 2006). According to this definition some 15% of couples in affluent countries are infertile (Luut, Kannaus and Olsen,

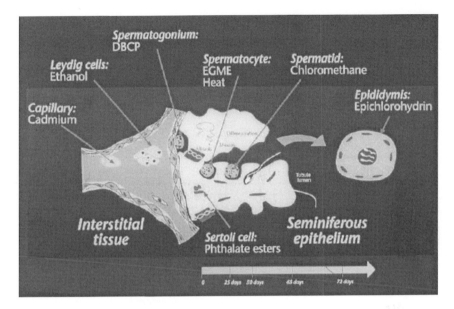

Fig. 3. Effects of reproductive toxicants on semen quality according to site of action.

1999). Male factors, most often in terms of poor semen quality, are the main cause of infertility in 35–40% of the cases (Schill, Comhaire and Hargreave, 2006). Fecundability is defined as the probability of fertilization during one menstrual cycle (Fig. 4). The fecundability in healthy couples is 20–30%, which means that about 3% of healthy couples will be categorized as infertile due to "bad luck" (Lamb and Foster, 1988). In populations where pregnancy planning is widespread, the time taken to conceive from discontinuance of contraception until fertilization is a sensitive functional measure of infertility that has been increasingly used in reproductive epidemiology to identify risk factors for infertility (Bonde *et al.*, 2006).

There are no good data to indicate whether population fecundity has changed in the past decades (Sallmen *et al.*, 2005). In modern societies many couples postpone having their first child until the woman is past 30 years. This will inevitably increase the frequency of infertility, because female fecundity declines dramatically after 30 years of age. There are indications that sperm count has declined

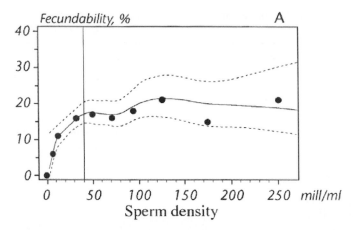

Fig. 4.   The probability of pregnancy according to sperm concentration in the ejaculate.
Source: Lancet (1998).

in some populations during some time periods (Giwercman and Bonde, 1998), but most often the evidence is circumstantial, because valid comparisons across time are difficult to derive. There is little doubt, however, that a large fraction of young men in some populations have sperm counts in the subfertile range below 40 million/ml (Andersen *et al.*, 2000).

The prevalence of male sexual dysfunction in terms of reduced libido, erectile dysfunction and ejaculation disorders is about 5% in the general male population. All types of male sexual dysfunctions increase with age. With respect to occurrence of pregnancy failures, the reader is referred to the chapter on female reproductive disorders.

Occupations at Risk, Common Occupational Causes

An overview of reported male reproductive hazards relating to human occupational exposure is provided in Table 1. More evidence is available from experimental studies in rodents than from human studies and therefore it is important to consult databases on reproductive toxicity that also include animal studies when investigating occupational risk to male infertility.

Table 1. Examples of Known and Suspected Occupational Hazards to Male Reproduction

Occupational Exposure	Male Reproductive Effect
Anesthetic gas	Malformations in offspring?
Dinitrotoluene and toluene diamine	Reduced semen quality?
Metals	
Welding	Infertility, reduced birth rate, reduced semen quality, spontaneous abortion in spouse?
Chromium compounds	Testis toxicity?
Cadmium	Testis capillary bed
Lead	Reduced semen quality
Manganese	Reduced birth rate?
Mercury vapor (metallic)	Infertility?
Oral contraceptives and sexual hormones	Gynecomastia, reduced libido, impotence, reduced testicular function?
Organic solvents	
Carbon disulfide	Reduced libido and impotence
Chlorinated hydrocarbons	Reduced semen quality?
Ethylene glycol ethers	Reduced semen quality
Halogenated hydrocarbons	Reduced semen quality?
Ethoxyethanol	Reduced semen quality
Persistent organochlorine compounds	
Polychlorinated biphenyls (PCB)	Reduced motility, damaged sperm chromatin
p, p'-DDE (a DDT metabolite)	Reduced sperm count
Dioxin	Reduced sperm count
Pesticides	
Carbaryl	Abnormal sperm morphology?
Chloroprene	Reduced semen quality?
Dibromochloropropane	Sterility, infertility, oligospermia
Ethylene dibromide	Reduced semen quality
Para-tertiary butyl acid	Reduced semen quality?
Chloroprene	Infertility?
Ionizing radiation, radium	Sterility, azoospermia oligospermia
Radar and microwaves	Reduced semen quality?
Radiant heat	Reduced sperm count

Box 1.   Websites on Reproductive Toxicity of Chemicals

REPROTOX provides comprehensive summaries, reviews and key original references to human and experimental data on selected chemicals and drugs. All aspects of human reproduction including male and female fertility and lactation are considered.

http://www.reprotox.org/

The **Center for the Evaluation of Risks to Human Reproduction (CERHR)** provides scientific reviews of the reproductive effects of chemicals.

http://cerhr.niehs.nih.gov/

The **National Toxicology Program (NTP)** provides data on comprehensive reproductive toxicology studies.

http://ntp.niehs.nih.gov/

The **Developmental and Reproductive Toxicology and Environmental Teratology Information Center (DART/ETIC)** provides references to book chapters, reviews, reports and original papers on the reproductive and developmental effects of chemicals.

http://toxnet.nlm.nih.gov/cgi-bin/sis/htmlgen? DARTETIC

A list of websites providing data on the reproductive toxicity of chemicals is provided in Box 1. Moreover, only a limited number of the listed agents and exposures are well-established risk factors for infertility in humans. These include ionizing radiation, inorganic lead and some pesticides.

Metals

Inorganic lead

The male reproductive toxicity of lead in terms of reduced semen quality, disruption of sex hormonal regulation and reduced fertility has been known for a long time. Suggested mechanisms include direct effects on the seminiferous tubule, disruption of the endocrine regulation of spermatogenesis or both. Very high exposure levels above 80 μg/dl blood are associated with impotence and decreased libido, which probably is of cerebral origin. Many occupational semen studies have demonstrated reduced sperm count and other signs of reduced semen quality at exposure levels of 30–60 μg/dl blood and this evidence is supported by compelling evidence in mice, rabbits and some rat strains (Apostoli *et al.*, 1998). An international European study points to a threshold around 45 μg/dl, below which effects on sperm count seem unlikely (Bonde *et al.*, 2002). These findings are consistent with some studies, but not others, of time to pregnancy in occupationally exposed populations (Joffe *et al.*, 2003). In any case, it should be borne in mind that the lowest effect level of 45 μg/dl of lead in blood is an average group threshold, which does not necessarily apply to all individuals.

Some men are expected to be more vulnerable than others. The individual susceptibility could be influenced by genetic polymorphisms that modify the toxicokinetics of lead. Male infertility because of exposure to inorganic lead probably occurs much more often than recognized by occupational health authorities.

Mercury

In mice the early stages of spermatogenesis are susceptible to toxic effects of mercury at dose levels not producing systemic toxicity. In humans there are case data linking occupational exposure to mercury with testicular toxicity (Ernst, 1993), but systematic evidence is limited.

Manganese

Histopathological changes in testicular tissue have been shown to occur in different animal species following doses that were not otherwise toxic. An earlier epidemiological study revealed a decline in birth rate in workers exposed to high levels of manganese dust (Gennart *et al.*, 1992), but this finding has not been corroborated by other studies. Several epidemiological studies have indicated reduced semen quality and increased frequency of subfertility in welders who were exposed to manganese, among other metals and agents (Bonde, 1993). However, whether the effects observed in welders are due to manganese is not known.

Cadmium

In rodents, cadmium produces severe testicular damage at low doses, which seems to be due to damage of the testicular capillaries.

Boron

The most sensitive adverse health endpoint of boron, including boric acid and borax, in animal toxicological studies is the reproductive system where testicular effects are consistent across several species (Chapin and Ku, 1994). The reproductive effects in rats start with reversible inhibition of spermiation (the release of mature spermatozoa from the Sertoli cells into the seminiferous tubule). This effect is seen after dose levels in the range of 20–25 mg boron per kg. Higher dose levels and longer treatment periods lead progressively to reduced sperm counts and degeneration of the seminiferous tubules and finally testicular atrophy with loss of sperm cells (Ku *et al.*, 1993). So far, effects on sperm count have not been documented in humans, but the evidence is limited (Scialli *et al.*, 2010).

Organic Solvents

Few human studies indicate that exposure to high levels of carbon disulfide in the workplace is related to increased occurrence of reduced libido and impotence as well as reduced semen quality (Vanhoorne, Comhaire and De Bacquer, 1994). Animal as well as human data on male reproductive effects of other widely used solvents such as styrene, toluene, xylene, benzene and mineral spirits are limited. Ethylene glycol ethyl ether is a highly specific male reproductive toxicant in several animal species and several large occupational studies with adequate exposure documentation have corroborated male reproductive toxicity in humans (Tielemans *et al.*, 1999).

Pesticides

Following the discovery of the severe reproductive effects of dibromochloropropane (DBCP), evidence has accumulated that some other compounds such as ethylene dibromide (which is structurally related to DBCP), 2,4-dichlorophenoxyacetic acid and DDT are male reproductive toxicants in humans (Ratcliffe *et al.*, 1987; Aneck-Habn *et al.*, 2007). For the occupational physician the evidence in humans of the effects of various pesticides is of limited value in view of the vast and ever-increasing number of compounds. In the individual case, emphasis must be on work history, exposure to specific chemicals and animal experimental evidence.

Radiation

Ionizing radiation in the workplace is an established risk factor for testicular damage. The testis is one of the most radiosensitive tissues of the body and spermatogonia are the most radiosensitive cells of spermatogenesis. A temporary reduction in sperm count occurs after a radiation dose of 0.15 Gy, while a single exposure above 2 Gy may cause permanent azoospermia (Rowley *et al.*, 1974). Non-ionizing high-frequency electromagnetic radiation among military radar equipment operators and telecommunication workers has been associated with reduced semen quality (Weyandt *et al.*, 1996; Hjollund, Bonde and Skotte, 1997), but there is no evidence that this type of radiation has biological effects at exposure levels not causing increased temperature of affected tissues. There is no evidence that electromagnetic radiation of extremely low frequency has an impact on male reproductive function (Hjollund *et al.*, 1999).

Radiant Heat and Sedentary Body Posture

The testes are located outside the body to keep their temperature below the core temperature. It is well established that elevation of the testis temperature impairs and even inhibits spermatogenesis. External heating of the testis for a short period of time results in a dramatic but temporary decrease in sperm count. This occurs after a delay of 6–8 weeks. Men working in hot occupational environments such as welders, foundry workers, ceramic workers and bakers may have reduced sperm counts because of radiant heat exposure of the testes (Bonde, 1992; Figà-Talamanca *et al.*, 1992). Disruption of testicular heat regulation may also be the cause of delayed conception in taxi drivers (Figà-Talamanca *et al.*, 1996). Sedentary office work is related to increased scrotal temperature, but there is no clear evidence that it is related to reduced sperm counts (Hjollund *et al.* 2002; Stay *et al.*, 2004). In fact, several large occupational studies do not indicate poor semen quality in white collar workers.

Clinical Approach to Commonly Presenting Disorders

Work-related male infertility is suspected when a hazardous workplace exposure is present in a worker with reduced semen quality that is not explained by a specific andrological disease (infection of the accessory sex glands, varicocele, congenital disorders) or specific medical disorder (endocrine disease, kidney failure, liver cirrhosis, respiratory tract disease).

In general, there are four criteria that must be fulfilled to establish that a case of infertility most likely is caused by a specific occupational exposure:

1. The adverse reproductive effect in terms of reduced libido or reduced quantity or quality of semen, for example, must fit with what is known about the adverse effects of the suspected hazardous exposure.
2. The exposure must be sufficient to cause the adverse effect. Occupational history is the main tool for obtaining information on the type, intensity and duration of an exposure. The mere presence of a toxic compound is not sufficient to cause damage. It is necessary to estimate the extent of exposure. Measurements of concentration in ambient air and biological monitoring data may greatly increase the validity of the exposure assessment. When considering hygienic standards it should be kept in mind that the criteria for standard-setting seldom account for subclinical adverse effects on the male reproductive tract.

3. It is important to consider the timing of exposure relative to the adverse effect. Irreversible effects of earlier exposures are difficult to document. If, however, discontinuation of an ongoing exposure is associated with an increased semen quality, e.g. in terms of increase in sperm count during subsequent weeks or months, it speaks in favor of causal associations. Chemical agents operating in the final stages of spermatogenesis (e.g. some pesticides) may have effects on sperm motility that may disappear in the weeks after cessation of exposure. On the contrary, chemical agents operating in the early stages of spermatogenesis may have effects lasting for several months after cessation of exposure, because the duration of human spermatogenesis is three months.

4. Other causes must be excluded. The occupational physician should consider alternative disorders that could explain the infertility. Sometimes, it may be necessary to consult an andrologist or urologist to ascertain other possible work-related factors that could have been contributory, for example, stress or lifestyle factors.

Management and Prevention

Occupational effects on male fertility depend critically on the timing of exposure. Men can often recover from testicular damage caused by temporary exposure in the workplace. It is therefore crucially important to keep in mind that a worker presenting with infertility may be exposed to reproductive hazards in the workplace. Infertility is not a prescribed occupational disorder in any country, and male infertility is not explicitly compensated by occupational health law acts. Nevertheless, identification of occupational reproductive disorders, including male infertility, is important for the individual worker who may be able to recover if the exposure is eliminated.

In cases of couples being investigated for infertility, it would be necessary for the attending physician to take an occupational history and consider if work factors could be contributory factors. If indicated, it would be useful to refer the male or female to an occupational physician for further evaluation and management.

Recognition of individual cases of work-related infertility may also promote general preventive measures in the workplace, including identification of potential hazards and appropriate regulation spanning the entire range of possible interventions from the complete ban of a chemical to restricted use, encapsulation/enclosure of the workplaces, exhaust ventilation, use of personal protective equipment and provision of information to exposed workers.

Case Study 1: Infertility

An unskilled 38-year-old man (BMI 27 kg/m^2) had been unsuccessful for more than a year in trying to achieve pregnancy with his wife (a 35-year-old nurse aide with a BMI of 31 kg/m^2). Both were in good health and were current smokers (10 cigarettes a day). The couple had a healthy child, aged seven years. Their previous preferred method of contraception was the pill.

Following primary school the man worked in agriculture for some years, then became a truck driver in various companies. Three years earlier, he started his current unskilled but well-paid full-time job in a car battery manufacturing company. His task in the clearing department entailed exposure to radiant heat and dust-containing inorganic lead. His blood lead increased, according to the mandatory lead monitoring program, from less than 5 μg/dl blood to 45 μg/dl blood within the first half a year of employment. It then declined to slightly lower levels around 35–40 μg/dl.

Lead is a possible main or contributing cause of the secondary infertility of this couple. Other established risk factors include the woman's age, male and female obesity and cigarette smoking, particularly in the woman. The infertility work-up did not reveal urogenital anomalies such as tubal occlusion or polycystic ovaries in the woman, while semen examination revealed low sperm counts (8 and 12 million/ml in two samples taken two weeks apart following four days of sexual abstinence). The FSH level was slightly elevated, pointing to a peripheral cause of hypogonadism. Serum testosterone and LH were in the normal range. The man was transferred to the battery store department, and subsequently his blood lead level declined to less than 10 μg/dl and his sperm count increased to 65 million/ml after one year. A little later, his wife became pregnant.

Case Study 2: Counseling — Male-mediated Developmental Toxicity

A male greenhouse worker became worried that his unborn child could have malformations because of paternal exposures in the ornamental flower greenhouse, where he had been employed for the past 12 years without interruption. His main work task was related to the growth of roses, namely spacing of cultures (10% of the time), picking and potting (25% of the time), nipping and cutting (25% of the time) and application of pesticides with a spraying device (20% of the time). The cultures were treated with various pesticides year-round but most intensely during the summer and autumn. Pesticides used included insecticides (imidacloprid, pirimicarb), fungicides (procloraz, fenarimol, vinclozolin) and growth inhibitors (paclobutrazol). When spraying he used gloves and a fresh-air helmet.

Several of the chemicals (pirimicarb and vinclozolin) have shown reproductive toxicity in experimental studies, but there is no available data indicating effects in pups following paternal exposure. During counseling, the patient should be reassured. There is no consistent evidence to indicate increased risk of malformation following paternal exposures in this particular occupational environment.

References

Andersen AG, Jensen TK, Carlsen E, *et al.* (2000) High frequency of suboptimal semen quality in an unselected population of young men. *Hum Reprod* **15**: 366–372.

Anderson D. (2003) Overview of male-mediated developmental toxicity. *Adv Exp Med Biol* **518**: 11–24.

Aneck-Habn NH, Schulenburg GW, Bornman MS, *et al.* (2007) Impaired semen quality associated with environmental DDT exposure in young men living in a malaria area in the Limpopo Province, South Africa. *J Androl* **28**: 423–434.

Apostoli P, Kiss P, Porru S, *et al.* (1998) Male reproductive toxicity of lead in animals and humans. ASCLEPIOS Study Group. *Occup Environ Med* **55**: 364–374.

Bonde JP. (1992) Semen quality in welders exposed to radiant heat. *Br J lnd Med* **49**: 5–10.

Bonde JP. (1993) The risk of male subfecundity attributable to welding of metals. Studies of semen quality, infertility, fertility, adverse pregnancy outcome and childhood malignancy. *Int J Androl* **16**: 1–29.

Bonde JP, Ernst E, Jensen TK, Hjollund NH. (1998) The relation between semen quality and fertility: A population based study of 430 first pregnancy planners. *Lancet* 1172–1177.

Bonde JP, Joffe M, Apostoli P, *et al.* (2002) Sperm count and chromatin structure in men exposed to inorganic lead: Lowest adverse effect levels. *Occup Environ Med* **59**: 234–242.

Bonde JP, Joffe M, Sallmen M, *et al.* (2006) Validity issues relating to time-to-pregnancy studies of fertility. *Epidemiology* **7**: 347–349.

Chapin RE, Ku WW. (1994) The reproductive toxicity of boric acid. *Environ Health Perspect* **102**: 87–91.

Cooper RL, Kavlock RJ. (1997) Endocrine disruptors and reproductive development: A weight-of-evidence overview. *J Endocrinol* **152**: 159–166.

Cordier S. (2008) Evidence for a role of paternal exposures in developmental toxicity. *Basic Clin Pharmacol Toxicol* **102**: 176–181.

Ernst E. (1993) Autometallographic detection of mercury in testicular tissue. *Reprod Toxicol* **7**: 469–475.

Figà-Talamanca I, Cini C, Varricchio GC, *et al.* (1996) Effects of prolonged autovehicle driving on male reproduction function: A study among taxi drivers. *Am J lnd Med* **30**: 750–758.

Figà-Talamanca I, Dell'Orco V, Pupi A, *et al.* (1992) Fertility and semen quality of workers exposed to high temperatures in the ceramics industry. *Reprod Toxicol* **6**: 517–523.

Gennart JP, Buchet JP, Roels H, *et al.* (1992) Fertility of male workers exposed to cadmium, lead, or manganese. *Am J Epidemiol* **135**: 1208–1219.

Giwercman A, Bonde JP. (1998) Declining male fertility and environmental factors. *Endocrinol J Metab Clin North Am* **27**: 807–830.

Hjollund NH, Bonde JP, Skotte JH. (1997) Semen analysis of personnel operating military radar equipment. *Reprod Toxicol* **1**: 897.

Hjollund NH, Skotte JH, Kolstad HA, Bonde JP. (1999) Extremely low frequency magnetic fields and fertility: A follow up study of couples planning first pregnancies. The Danish First Pregnancy Planner Study Team. *Occup Environ Med* **56**: 253–255.

Hjollund NH, Storgaard L, Ernst E, *et al.* (2002) The relation between daily activities and scrotal temperature. *Reprod Toxicol* **16**: 209–214.

Joffe M, Bisanti L, Apostoli P, *et al.* (2003) Time to pregnancy and occupational lead exposure. *Occup Environ Med* **60**: 752–758.

Ku WW, Chapin RE, Wine RN, Gladen BC. (1993) Testicular toxicity of boric acid (BA): Relationship of dose to lesion development and recovery in the F344 rat. *Reprod Toxicol* **7**: 305–319.

Lahdetie J. (1995) Occupation and exposure-related studies on human sperm. *J Occup Environ Med* **37**: 922–930.

Lamb JC, Foster P. (1988) *Physiology and Toxicology of Male Reproduction*. London: Academic Press.

Luut S, Kannaus W, Olsen J. (1999) Regional differences in waiting time to pregnancy: Pregnancy-based surveys from Denmark, France, Germany, Italy and Sweden. The European Infertility and Subfecundity Study Group. *Hum Reprod* **14**: 1250–1254.

Oliva A, Spira A, Multigner L. (2001) Contribution of environmental factors to the risk of male infertility. *Hum Repro* **16**: 1768–1776.

Potashnik G, Ben-Aderet N, Israeli R, *et al.* (1978) Suppressive effect of 1,2.dibromo-3-chloropropane on human spermatogenesis. *Fertil Steril* **30**: 444–447.

Ratcliffe J, Schrader SM, Steenland K, *et al.* (1987) Semen quality in papaya workers with long term exposure to ethylene dibromide. *Br J Ind Med* **44**: 317–326.

Robaire B, Hales BF. (2003) Mechanisms of action of cyclophosphamide as a male-mediated developmental toxicant. *Adv Exp Med Biol* **518**: 169–180.

Rowley MJ, Leach DR, Warner GA, Heller CG. (1974) Effect of graded doses of ionizing radiation on the human testis. *Radiat Res* **59**: 665–678.

Sallmen M, Weinberg CR, Baird DD, *et al.* (2005) Has human fertility declined over time? Why we may never know. *Epidemiology* **16**: 494–499.

Scialli AR, Bonde JP, Bruske-Hohlfeld I, *et al.* (2010) An overview of male reproductive studies of boron with emphasis on studies of highly exposed Chinese workers. *Reprod Toxicol* **29**: 10–24.

Scialli AR, Clegg E. (1992) *Reversibility in Testicular Toxicity Testing.* Boca Raton, Florida: CRC Press.

Schill WB, Comhaire FH, Hargreave TB. (2006) *Andrology for the Clinician.* Berlin; New York: Springer.

Skakkebaek NE, Rajpert-De Meyts E, Main KM. (2001) Testicular dysgenesis syndrome: An increasingly common developmental disorder with environmental aspects. *Hum Reprod* **16**: 972–978.

Stay J, Hjollund NH, Mortensen JT, *et al.* (2004) Semen quality and sedentary work position. *Int J Androl* **27**: 5–11.

Tas S, Lauwerys R, Lison D. (1996) Occupational hazards for the male reproductive system. *Crit Rev Toxicol* **26**: 261–307.

Tielemans E, Burdorf A, te Velde ERT, *et al.* (1999) Occupationally related exposures and reduced semen quality: A case-control study. *Fertil Steril* **71**: 690–696.

Trasler JM. (2003) Translational research in male mediated developmental toxicity. *Adv Exp Med Biol* **518**: 279–284.

Vanhoorne M, Comhaire F, De Bacquer D. (1994) Epidemiological study of the effects of carbon disulfide on male sexuality and reproduction. *Arch Environ Health* **49**: 273–278.

Weyandt TB, Schrader SM, Turner TW, Simon SD. (1996) Semen analysis of military personnel associated with military duty assignments. *Reprod Toxicol* **10**: 521–528.

Whorton MD, Krauss RM, Marshall S, Milby TH. (1977) Infertility in male pesticide workers. *Lancet* **2**: 1259–1261.

Section 2

Special Issues in Occupational Medicine

Chapter 17

Ethics in Occupational Medicine

David Koh and See-Muah Lee[†,‡]*

Introduction

The occupational physician functions at the interface between the employer (management) and the employee (non-management or trade union). It is important to recognize that the physician's primary duty is to protect the worker from ill health as a consequence of work.

A further area of concern is that of confidentiality of information. This has become a major issue in recent times because of the increasing use of biomarkers as well as the increasing computerization of health data.

The ethical principles of a doctor in medicine — autonomy, non-maleficence (doing no harm), beneficence (doing good) and justice — first championed by Childress and Beauchamp in 1965 are just as relevant in the doctor–worker relationship in occupational health as the doctor in the traditional therapeutic relationship.

*Department of Epidemiology and Public Health, Yong Loo Lin School of Medicine, National University of Singapore.

†Department of Epidemiology and Public Health, Yong Loo Lin School of Medicine, National University of Singapore, Diabetes Clinic, Khoo Teck Puat Hospital, Singapore.

‡Corresponding author. E-mail: see_muah_lee@nuhs.edu.sg

To perform his role effectively, the occupational physician will have to engage the works supervisors and the employers to understand the health and safety risks associated with the job. Besides the employers and management, other parties such as the state regulatory authorities, work representatives and insurers all have a vested interest in being informed and given notice in the event of any suspected or confirmed work-related illness. In some ways, it may not be possible to operate strictly within the confidential domain of a doctor–patient relationship if the interests of the patient and his co-workers are to be protected and promoted.

The occupational physician must not take sides with either the management or the trade union in the discharge of his duties. This may appear obvious but conflict of interest may arise, as the physician is often paid by management. His role as an impartial expert can be particularly sorely tested in an atmosphere of tense industrial relations. In this context it is always important to fully apprise both management and trade unions of the ethical responsibilities of a physician.

Case Study 1: Autonomy

A worker consulted his doctor several times for an eczematous rash. After several treatments, the doctor suspected that the rash could be due to some unidentified workplace allergen. The doctor sought the patient's consent for this clinical information to be released to his employer. The worker refused, fearing economic reprisals.

Ethical points for consideration

What is the purpose of disclosure?

A causal relationship, if confirmed, will assist the doctor in the management of his patient. It could also be argued that the disclosure is to alert the management to the possible harmful nature of the products to enable remedial measures to be taken. This could be an especially compelling argument in the case where large numbers of employees are exposed, compared to a small workplace where the number of employees is small.

What is the extent of harm?

If it is a minor skin condition, the need to disclose may be less as opposed to another condition with potentially fatal consequences, such as occupational asthma. Disclosure under such circumstances, even where the worker has accepted the risk of self-endangerment and refused consent for disclosure, could qualify on the grounds of "public interest" and therefore be ethically justified. If it is a condition which on analysis poses a threat to the safety of others, again the "public interest" argument may prevail to override the consent of the worker. Examples include a poorly controlled epileptic patient operating in a safety-sensitive environment.

Case Study 2: Health Risk Assessment

An environmental exposure measurement for a certain hazard mandated by legislation has been carried out. The majority of the measurements were within normal limits and the management has used these results, sanctioned by the occupational physician, to repel allegations of unsafe working conditions by the workers. In any case, the management has advised the occupational physician that the workers, though admittedly working under hazardous conditions, have been compensated more favorably compared to workers in the other departments.

Ethical points for consideration

How accurately do the environmental exposure readings
represent a safe working condition?

Exposure measurements are part of the total information matrix in a health risk assessment. They cannot be considered in isolation to prove (management interest) or to disprove (worker interest) a safe work environment in a dispute, which in some cases may have overtones of an industrial conflict. The evidence has to be objectively evaluated against other factors, such as the tasks of the workers, the duration of the exposures and the environmental control measures. An exposure measurement, even if properly undertaken by accredited experts, does not replace the need for primary prevention efforts in the workplace to reduce exposure as much as reasonably practicable.

Is it ethically acceptable to pay workers more to compensate for higher-risk jobs?

Workers are free to choose and negotiate their terms of employment with their employers, including the voluntary assumption of work-related risks. To some it may appear paternalistic and unacceptable to interfere with this, so long as the laws of the land are not violated.

However, the more ethically tenable view is that whilst payment may be increased for higher-risk jobs, the financial incentive should not replace the need for measures to minimize such risks as much as reasonably practicable. A globalized workforce with transient migrant labor across the world has made such issues all the more pressing.

Case Study 3: Commercial Secrecy

A factory manufacturing electronic components recently introduced a new cocktail mix of solvents in one of its processes. This improves the quality of the product and shortens the processing time. However, workers using this solvent cocktail reported minor skin itch. Some felt giddy after working with the new solvent mix. This occurred in spite of the use of respirators, gloves and other protective clothing while handling the solvent mix.

The occupational physician requested information on the chemical composition of the new solvent cocktail but the technical management was not keen to release the information, stating that it was a "commercial secret" which gave the company an edge over its rivals. Besides, the health complaints were felt to be relatively minor in nature, and the technical management stated that the workers were already provided with gloves and respirators to protect themselves adequately.

Ethical points for consideration

What is the duty of the occupational physician with respect to such "trade" information?

The doctor who obtains information about a business during the course of his work has an ethical duty to maintain the confidentiality of such information. This duty also extends to all staff as well as subsequent parties (e.g. medical laboratory workers whose expertise may be required) who may also have access to such information.

In a similar vein, should the doctor wish to publish the findings in medical journals, it would be best if the employers are given notice and a chance to discuss the findings. In the most extreme case, which is very unlikely, if a pressing "public interest" need arises for the disclosure of information that has been intentionally suppressed because of a grave endangerment to health, then legal advice has to be sought.

Is there a way to obtain the required information with minimal risk to the business interests of the employer?

This should be properly explored before a foreclosure of the possibilities of a medical investigation.

References

Beauchamp TL, Childress JF. (2001) *Principles of Biomedical Ethics*, 5th edn. Oxford: Oxford University Press.

Faculty of Occupational Medicine. (2006) *Guidance on Ethics for Occupational Physicians*, 6th edn. London: FOMRCP.

International Commission on Occupational Health. (2002) *International Code of Ethics for Occupational Health Professionals*. Rome: ICOH (http://www.icohweb.org/site_new/ico_core_documents.asp).

Chapter 18

Health Screening and Periodic Medical Examinations

*See-Muah Lee**, *Michael Wong*[†] *and John-Wah Lim*[‡,§]

Introduction

Screening is the presumptive identification of unrecognized disease or defect by the application of tests, examinations or other procedures, which can be applied rapidly. Screening tests sort out apparently well persons who apparently have a disease from those who probably do not (US Commission on Chronic Illness, 1957).

The United Kingdom National Screening Committee has defined screening as a public health service in which members of a defined population, who do not necessarily perceive they are at risk of or are already affected by a disease or its complications, are asked a question or offered a test, to identify those individuals who are more likely to be helped than harmed by further tests or treatment to reduce the risk of a disease or its complications (UK NSC, 2000). This introduces the risk-benefit concept, thus "acknowledging that screening can harm as

*Department of Epidemiology and Public Health, Yong Loo Lin School of Medicine, National University of Singapore. Diabetes Clinic, Khoo Teck Puat Hospital, Singapore.
[†]Health for Life, Khoo Teck Puat Hospital, Singapore.
[‡]Department of Epidemiology and Public Health, Yong Loo Lin School of Medicine, National University of Singapore.
[§]Corresponding author. E-mail: john_wah_lim@nuhs.edu.sg

well as help — a response perhaps to the increasing public climate of complaint and litigation" (Holland, Stewart and Masseria, 2006).

The appeal of health screening lies in the assumption that examinations can detect risk factors and/or disease early so that timely intervention can increase the prospect of cure and reduce the cost of care.

Very often, screening is targeted at, and offered to, asymptomatic and apparently healthy individuals in the selected population, e.g. women, adolescents and others. In occupational health, workers are often screened as part of fitness to work examinations, or because of special exposures at work.

In this respect, screening is different from tests that are applied to patients seeking consultation for an existing health problem with a doctor in a traditional therapeutic relationship.

Methods, Principles and Criteria

Methods adopted in screening range from self-assessment questionnaires at the very basic to very comprehensive consultations with all manner of sophisticated laboratory investigations, including genetic screening and whole body imaging.

In 1968, Wilson and Jungner (1968) established the principles and criteria on which screening should be based. The following should be taken into account when considering whether a condition or a particular set of risk factors ought to be screened:

1. Is the condition important?
2. Is the condition treatable?
3. Does the condition have a recognizable latent or asymptomatic stage?
4. Is the condition prevalent?
5. Is the screening test acceptable, safe, sensitive, specific, easily done and affordable?

Sensitivity, Specificity and Predictive Value

The sensitivity of a test is its ability to detect those with the condition being tested for. A test with 100% sensitivity will produce a positive test result for everyone affected by the condition with no false negatives. Every negative test result is a true negative. It is possible for the test result to be a false positive, i.e. giving a positive test result for individuals who do not have the condition — this depends on the specificity.

The specificity of a test is its ability not to detect those who do not have the condition being tested for. A test with 100% specificity will produce a negative test result for everyone not affected by the condition with no false positives. Every positive result is a true positive. However, it is possible for the test result to be a false negative, i.e. giving a false negative result for individuals who have the condition — this depends on the sensitivity.

It is extremely rare to have a screening test that is 100% sensitive and 100% specific — that would be the gold standard reference.

The likelihood of anyone with a positive test result actually having the disease, or the positive predictive value, depends on the prevalence of the condition in the tested population. If the prevalence is low, there will be a greater likelihood of false positive results, compared to a targeted screenee population where the prevalence is higher and the detection of true positives is higher. While the sensitivity and specificity are constant characteristics of any screening test — assuming that there is a gold standard reference to which the screening tests can be compared — the predictive values vary with the prevalence of the condition. Selection of the test populations therefore is critical to the success of the screening exercise. It helps to sharpen prediction rates and improve efficiency.

The definitions are represented algebraically in Table 1.

Case Study 1: Health Screening

Consider a hypothetical program using fecal occult blood (OB) to screen for colorectal cancer in an adult population of 300 participants, with eight cases of colorectal cancer (Table 2).

Using the same screening method, if the prevalence of colorectal cancer were to increase from 8 (2.6%) to 20 (6.6%), e.g. if the screening population of 300 participants is now in an older age group, the

Table 1.   Sensitivity, Specificity and Predictive Value

	Disease or Condition		
Test Result	Present	Absent	
Positive	a	b	Positive predictive value $[a/(a+b)] \times 100\%$
Negative	c	d	Negative predictive value $[d/(c+d)] \times 100\%$
	Sensitivity $[a/(a+c)] \times 100\%$	Specificity $[d/(b+d)] \times 100\%$	

Table 2.   Fecal Occult Blood Screening for Colorectal Cancer in a Population of 300

		Colorectal Cancer		
		Present	Absent	
Fecal occult Blood screening	Positive	True positive 6	False positive 17	Positive predictive value 26%
	Negative	False negative 2	True negative 275	Negative predictive value 99%
		Sensitivity 75%	Specificity 94%	

number of true positives will increase to 15 and the false positives will remain at 17, resulting in an increased positive predictive rate of 47% (Table 3).

Number Needed to Screen

The number needed to screen is defined as the number of people that need to be screened for a given duration to prevent a death or adverse event (Rembold, 1998). This can be used for planning and prioritizing screening strategies for various conditions. It can be directly calculated

Table 3.   Fecal Occult Blood Screening for Colorectal Cancer in a Population of 300

		Colorectal Cancer		
		Present	Absent	
Fecal occult Blood screening	Positive	True positive 15	False positive 17	Positive predictive value 47%
	Negative	False negative 5	True negative 263	Negative predictive value 98%
		Sensitivity 75%	Specificity 94%	

from clinical trials of disease screening, or it can be estimated from clinical trials of treatment and the prevalence of the so far unrecognized or untreated disease. To allow for comparisons, it is necessary for the number to be normalized to a duration standard. Thus, Rembold in his study determined that mammography significantly reduced deaths from breast cancer with a number needed to screen of 2451 for five years for women aged 50–59. The estimated number needed to screen for hypertension to prevent all-cause death was 274 to 1307 for five years if detection was followed by treatment with thiazide diuretics.

Types of Screening and Periodic Health Examinations

Pre-employment Examinations and Fitness to Work

Candidates for jobs often have to undergo a medical examination before they are employed. The purpose of the examination is to screen for medical conditions that might affect their fitness to do the job. A risk assessment of the job should be ideally matched with the pre-employment medical examination.

Thus it can be seen that for many jobs, e.g. those of a sedentary nature, the work demands do not necessarily pose a health risk. In most cases, there is no medical reason why most candidates, including those with chronic medical conditions, should not be able to meet the work demands. More often than not, the pre-employment examination serves as a general screening for blood pressure, blood glucose and other basic clinical parameters. In fact some companies may opt for a health questionnaire instead for such cases.

In selected occupations, a more detailed assessment may be required. Health can affect work. An example would be the job of pilots. Traditionally they are required to have a high degree of physical fitness. Pilot error is a significant safety factor in aviation. Selection and review of their health status is therefore a continuing and stringent process.

Another example is the case of a health worker being screened for human immunodeficiency virus (HIV). Ostensibly, one of the aims is to minimize and protect patients from onward transmission of the virus from infected healthcare workers. Should all health workers be screened or should this screening be done only for healthcare workers performing exposure-prone procedures?

Work can also affect health. An example would be work in environments with asthmogenic exposure, such as to isocyanates. In such cases, the pre-employment medical examination would include a duty to forewarn workers about such risks. Periodic assessments of lung function may be required to enable early detection and management of occupational asthma in such cases (Lee and Koh, 2008a).

Biomarkers indicating exposure to hazardous substances in the workplace can sometimes be reliably detected. However, its effects, clinical significance and proposed response of action have to be clarified before they can be adopted for screening.

Apart from the medical aspects, pre-employment medical examinations are sometimes made use of by employers to protect their economic interests (Lee and Koh, 2008b). They may view candidates with risk factors and chronic illnesses, notwithstanding the fact that they can do the job, as being less desirable because of perceived costs. These are business decisions. Candidates should be put on notice about such economic criteria for employment. The implementation of these business decisions may require medical input from the doctors.

Subject to laws governing discrimination (sex, race, disability, sexual orientation), "it is still the law that an employer is free to choose who he wishes to employ, and may have quixotic reasons for rejecting apparently worthy candidates" Kennedy LJ (*Kapfunde v Abbey*, 1998).

Job Transfer Examinations

Before transferring to another job, it is sometimes necessary for a worker to undergo a medical examination. A job change may mean a change in risk. There could be exposure to physical, chemical, biological or psychosocial hazards not encountered previously. Sometimes the change in risk could be logistic or administrative, as would be the case for an employee with his family being relocated to a remote condition with limited access to healthcare. Consideration has to be given to complications that may require repatriation at a high cost, not to mention the disruption to business.

Return to Work Examinations

A period of prolonged illness with prolonged absence may have implications on fitness to work. Modern medicine has enabled the successful rehabilitation of patients. In some cases, however, the health status could be altered and a review may need to be carried out. An example would be the case of a fireman recovering from a coronary event. He must undergo an assessment before normal fire-fighting duties can be resumed.

Case Study 2: Return to Work

A 45-year-old boilerman consults his physician upon returning to work after a four-week absence following an appendicectomy. In all likelihood, acclimatization to work in a hot environment would have been lost. The physician in this case should inform the supervisor to reschedule his work periods in the hot environment, ensuring that the exposure is slowly increased over a period of two weeks or so to reduce the possibility of heat disorders.

Genetic Screening in the Workplace

Genetic screening can help identify asymptomatic workers with a genetic predisposition to occupational diseases. Examples include bladder cancer and certain forms of occupational asthma (Christiani, Mehta and Yu, 2008). Employees can then decide for themselves whether to assume this risk. Employers can also use the information to relocate susceptible workers to alternative work environments.

In reality, however, the practical utility is limited. The test sensitivity and specificity may not be optimal, prevalence of such occupational diseases may be low, and the positive predictive value of a positive genetic test, correspondingly, will be low. In addition to all these uncertain variables, one must still take into account the long latency, sometimes decades-long, for many of such occupational diseases to develop. Decisions based on such results may thus needlessly disadvantage the "genetically marked" worker. Resources otherwise devoted to environmental control efforts might also be sacrificed.

Case Study 3: Chronic Beryllium Disease (CBD)

The genetic marker for susceptibility to chronic beryllium disease was identified as early as 1995 (Saltini, 1995). The genetic marker consisting of the glutamic acid substitution for lysine or arginine at position 69 of the HLA-DPB1-0201 allele of the major histocompatibility complex ("Glu69") was found to be associated with an elevated risk of CBD. CBD provides a human model of pulmonary granulomatous disease produced by occupational exposure, occurring more frequently in those with a genetic predisposition (Cooper and Harrison, 2009).

The manager of a beryllium fabrication plant, in which beryllium exposure has been identified, is keen to implement genetic marker screening to identify workers who may be at a higher risk of the immune-mediated organ destruction as a result. He has sought your views.

Various studies have quoted the prevalence of CBD among exposed workers as somewhere between 2% and 16% (Fontenot and

Maier, 2005) and the longitudinal positive predictive value to CBD over time at 12% (Silver and Sharp, 2006). Although not ideal at the present for screening on a large scale, given our zeal for genetic science, it is conceivable that further refinements and improvements in the predictive positive value as a result of better genetic tests will be made in the future. When a positive test result indicates more likely than not (above 50%) that a person truly has the susceptibility, the arguments favoring privacy may have to be deferred to that of health protection. Indeed, the Dow Chemical Company was found in the invidious position of defending itself against legal action taken by the widow of a deceased employee for failure to include the employee in its cytogenetic testing program, which might have detected early biological indications of his development of leukemia from his workplace exposure to benzene (Olafson, 2000; *Shrusch v Dow Chem Co*, 2001).

There is no doubt, however, that genetic tests have been inappropriately used in the past. A case in point would be the genetic testing program for susceptibility to carpal tunnel syndrome conducted by Burlington Northern Railway Company (United States District Court, 2001; Schulte and Lomax, 2003).

Genetic information is highly sensitive and personal, with potential implications for insurance coverage. If linked to ethnic and racial groups, actions based on such genetic characteristics may be interpreted as being indirectly discriminatory on the grounds of race or ethnicity. Groups may inadvertently become stigmatized. Designing a workplace genetic testing program requires accurate and compelling scientific evidence, an understanding of the other mechanisms contributing to the disease, forward planning, sensitivity and skill in communication and, last but not least, expertise in the scientific aspects of genetic counseling that can be made comprehensible to the examinee. Workers should be fairly and honestly treated.

Executive Health Screening

These are comprehensive screening packages offered to participants. It gives a sense of the process being thorough and also costly. Some employers will sponsor this as a perk for their staff. It is essentially one form of periodic health examination, albeit more thorough (Hensrud and Rhodes, 2009).

Packages may be individually tailored in a way that is not commensurate with personal or occupational health risks but with seniority. At the high end of the spectrum, the executive health screening — also known as Master Health Checkups in India (Rank, 2009) — takes on an indulgent and elitist aura more redolent of services in an opulent hotel than a healthcare facility, catering to business titans, the rich and the powerful (Rank, 2008).

As a commercially driven and supply-sensitive activity (Rank, 2008), it is therefore a potentially lucrative revenue source for providers. Some view the provision of "an expensive and unproven niche" service (Rank, 2009) for a few, while the great majority is still medically underserved, as ethically untenable. It may be argued that an unproven service does not necessarily translate into harm or lack of benefit. Indeed, if privately funded, the argument of equity may perforce also be demoted in deference to the commercial rules of demand and supply. Argued from this angle, health screening at the high end becomes no different and no less or more ethical than the more well-off having better access to a more exclusive lifestyle and the luxuries of life.

Nevertheless, there will be clear instances of harm. An example would be the use of CT scan of the heart to determine calcium scoring. In its 2004 summary of recommendations, the US Preventive Services Task Force (USPSTF) concluded that the potential harms of routine screening for coronary heart disease in low-risk adults exceed the potential benefits (USPTSF, 2004). To offer such screening therefore may be unethical.

The USPSTF regularly reviews the evidence for the effectiveness of, and updates the recommendations for, clinical preventive services including screening. Screening for hypertension, diabetes and lipid profiles in adult populations are definitely worthwhile. Cervical cancer screening and mammography may also be considered for women.

There should be transparency in the design of such screening programs. The goals, limitations, evidence and rationale should be explained to the participants.

Properly designed, company-sponsored screening services need not be unethical or expensive and wasteful. Decisions should be guided by the Wilson and Jungner criteria. Evidence for benefits in terms of morbidity and mortality reduction should be sought.

Such screening services can also provide an opportunity for workers to express any health concerns they may have. Ethically thought out, they might even be the place where participants can be warned and educated about the numerous dubious screening services with questionable benefits on direct offer (Kue and Ashar, 2009). For employers concerned about employee health, it would be wise to devote resources not only to screening, but also to basic issues in primary prevention like engineering controls and personal protective equipment.

Employers also need to be guarded against unrealistic expectations of the financial returns from screening seen as a prevention program. Indeed it is very possible for healthcare costs to increase as a direct result of screening programs, in part due to abnormalities being pursued and interventions being introduced.

Case Study 4: False Negatives and False Positives

A department store decided to sponsor well-woman screening for its predominantly female workforce. Brenda and Christina attended the screening, which included a mammogram and a Pap smear. Brenda was declared fit, but was diagnosed as having breast cancer six months later. Brenda is wondering whether her cancer was negligently missed during the screening. Christina initially screened positive, but after undergoing further investigations, was told that her result was a false positive. Christina had a history of hysterectomy for benign disease three years ago.

People who accept the offer of screening must be instilled with the realistic limitations and expectations of such tests (Wilson, 2000). For a one-year screening interval, the sensitivity of first mammography ranges from 71% to 96% (USPSTF, 2003a). There will always be an irreducible minimum of false negative screens as in Brenda's case.

Similarly, a false positive screen as seen in Christina's case is also possible. The USPSTF recommends against routine Pap smear screening in women who have had a total hysterectomy for benign disease (USPSTF, 2003b). The harms of false positives have been documented (Mitchell and Giles, 1996; Sigurdsson, 1999).

On the other hand, it must be questioned if the screening program has been organized to keep these rates down to a minimum. This may involve double reading, rigorous program auditing and quality assurance.

The potential harms, which must be included in evaluations of the cost-effectiveness of screening programs, would, in the case of a false negative result, be false assurance and delays in seeking treatment when a problem develops. False positive results would also cause harm from the discomfort of further investigations, not to mention the distress and worry (Durojaiye, 2009).

Bias and Confounding When Evaluating Screening Programs

When evaluating the effectiveness of screening programs, lead-time bias and length bias must be taken into account.

The apparent long survival of a patient whose cancer has been detected by screening, followed by early intervention, may be partly due to lead-time bias. The screening brings forward the time of diagnosis, thus lengthening the time of knowledge of disease rather than actually prolonging survival.

Another factor that might confound evaluation is length bias. There could be a tendency for screening to favor the detection of less aggressive and less serious conditions. More rapidly advancing illnesses, by their very nature, will only be present asymptomatically for a short time, and are more likely to present as cases for diagnosis. Since more slowly progressing illnesses than aggressive conditions are found on screening, this also gives the erroneous impression that detecting these conditions early has improved survival.

Conclusion

Health screening has a long history. From its humble beginnings in the 1940s when it was adopted for the early detection of pulmonary tuberculosis via mass miniature radiography, it has since evolved into a health industry keeping pace with medical developments.

However, our ability to prevent illnesses through screening is limited by the accuracy of screening tests. Not all detected risk factors and conditions upon confirmation will be amenable to cure. There are also ethical considerations of not causing harm to participants. From the public health point of view, the economic costs of screening everyone in order to identify those at risk also need to be balanced against other priorities.

Health screening programs as a means of improving health must therefore be properly planned and justified. The intuitive logic that prevention is better than cure has a strong emotional appeal, but when applied to screening, is only valid for selected cases.

In occupational health, health screening is also done to yield information for job selection and occupational risk exposures. Notwithstanding this, the validity of such screening and the impact of such information on the participant and the employer must also be considered.

References

Christiani DC, Mehta AJ, Yu CL. (2008) Genetic susceptibility to occupational exposures. *Occup Environ Med* **65**: 430–436.

Cooper RG, Harrison AP. (2009) The uses and adverse effects of beryllium on health. *Indian J Occup Environ Med* **13**: 65–76.

Durojaiye OC. (2009) Health screening: Is it always worth doing? *Int J Epidemiol* **7**: 1.

Fontenot AP, Maier LA. (2005) Genetic susceptibility and immune mediated destruction in beryllium-induced disease. *Trends Immunol* **26**(10): 543–549.

Hensrud DD, Rhodes DJ. (2009) Executive physicals, correspondence. *New Engl J Med* **360**: 421.

Holland WW, Stewart S, Masseria C. (2006) *Policy Brief: Screening in Europe World Health Organization*, on behalf of the European Observatory on Health Systems and Policies.

Kapfunde v Abbey National PLC and Daniel. (1998) 46 BMLR 176 CA.

Kue P, Ashar B. (2009). Executive physicals, correspondence. *New Engl J Med* **360**: 422.

Lee SM, Koh D. (2008a) Lessons from an isocyanate tragedy. *Singapore Med J* **49**: 372–375.

Lee SM, Koh D. (2008b) Fitness to work: Legal pitfalls. *Ann Acad Med Singapore* **37**: 236–240.

Mitchell HS, Giles GG. (1996) Cancer diagnosis after a report of negative cervical cytology. *Med J Aust* **164**(5): 270–273.

Olafson S. (2000) Suit claims Dow shirked duty on cancer-testing of workers. *Houston Chronicle*, 12 August, p. A1.

Rank B. (2008) Executive physicals: Bad medicine on three counts. *New Engl J Med* **359**: 1424–1425.

Rank B. (2009) Executive physicals, correspondence. *New Engl J Med* **360**: 422–423.

Rembold CM. (1998) Number needed to screen: Development of a statistic for disease screening. *Br Med J* **317**: 307–312.

Saltini C. (1995) A genetic marker for chronic beryllium disease. In: Mendelsohn ML, Peeters JP, Normandy MJ (eds). *Biomarkers and Occupational Health: Progress and Perspectives*, pp. 293–303. Washington, D.C.: Joseph Henry Press.

Sbrusch v Dow Chem Co. (2001) 124 F. Supp. 2d 1090, 1091 (S.D. Tex. 2000).

Schulte PA, Lomax G. (2003) Assessment of the scientific basis for genetic testing of railroad workers with carpal tunnel syndrome. *J Occup Environ Med* **45**: 592–600.

Sigurdsson K. (1999) Trends in cervical intra-epithelial neoplasia in Iceland through 1995: Evaluation of targeted age groups and screening intervals. *Acta Obstet Gynecol Scand* **78**(6): 486–492.

Silver K, Sharp RR. (2006) Ethical considerations in testing workers for the -Glu69 marker of genetic susceptibility to chronic beryllium disease. *J Occup Environ Med* **48**(4): 434–443.

US Commission on Chronic Illness. (1957) Chronic Illness in the US, Vol. I. *Prevention of Chronic Illness.* Cambridge, Massachusetts: Harvard University Press.

United Kingdom National Screening Committee (UK NSC), Health Departments of the United Kingdom. (2000) *Second Report of the National Screening Committee*, October.

United States District Court, Northern District of Iowa. (2001) *US EEOC v Burlington Northern Santa Fe Railway Company*. Civ. No. C01–4013 MWB, EEOC's Memorandum in support of petition for a preliminary injunction. 8 February 2001.

United States Preventive Services Task Force (USPSTF). (2003a) *Breast Cancer Screening Summary of the Evidence*. http://www.ahrq.gov/clinic/uspstf/gradespre.htm (accessed 10 September 2009).

United States Preventive Services Task Force (USPSTF). (2003b) *Screening for Cervical Cancer Recommendations and Rationale*. http://www.ahrq.gov/clinic/uspstf/gradespre.htm (accessed 10 September 2009).

United States Preventive Services Task Force (USPSTF). (2004) *Screening for Coronary Heart Disease Recommendation Statement*. http://www.ahrq.gov/clinic/uspstf/gradespre.htm (accessed 10 September 2009).

Wilson JMG, Jungner G. (1968) *Principles and Practice of Screening for Disease*. Geneva: World Health Organization.

Wilson RM. (2000) Screening for breast and cervical cancer as a common cause for litigation. *Br Med J* **320**: 1352–1353.

Chapter 19

Assessment of Disability for Compensation

Kenneth Choy*,‡ *and Hock-Siang Lee*†

Introduction

All occupational injuries and diseases should be prevented by ensuring a safe and healthy work environment. However, where an occupational injury or disease has occurred, an employee may be eligible for certain benefits under a workers' compensation system. Almost all countries provide some form of entitlement to employees who sustain an occupational injury or illness.

Doctors may be called upon by insurance companies, employers and the court to give an assessment of the disability suffered by the employee as a result of the injury or disease.

Workers' Compensation Schemes

Many countries provide some form of entitlement or compensation benefit to employees if they develop an occupational illness or

*Occupational Safety and Health Specialist Department, Ministry of Manpower, Singapore.
†Occupational Safety and Health Specialist Department, Ministry of Manpower, Singapore.
Department of Epidemiology and Public Health, Yong Loo Lin School of Medicine,
National University of Singapore.
‡Corresponding author. E-mail: kenneth_choy@mom.gov.sg

injury. This may also extend to the survivors of the injured employee. Legislations requiring employers to compensate employees or their survivors are based on the principle of employers' liability that

> "an employer who carries out economic activities through labor and machines, creates an organization the operation of which, by its very nature, is likely to cause injuries to his employees. Thus he is liable for payment of compensation whether their occurrence is attributable to his negligence or even where there has been no fault at all" (Higuchi, 1986).

Before the introduction of workers' compensation legislation, injured workers had to sue their employers under common law, and they had to prove negligence on the part of their employers which was often difficult to prove. The workers' compensation system was designed to minimize and avoid a lengthy litigation process and facilitate payment of compensation to injured employees. It is based on a "no fault" principle: "If in any employment personal injury by accident arising out of and in the course of the employment is caused to an employee, his employer shall be liable to pay compensation..." (Work Injury Compensation Act, Singapore, 2008). The employee is entitled to compensation for injury even if he had been contributory to the accident, provided it had not been deliberate. Legislation on employment injury benefits is often called the "Workers' Compensation Act". Employers may be required to take out insurance against their liability under the Act.

Some countries, instead of requiring companies to take out their own insurance for workers' compensation purposes, have adopted a social insurance scheme to provide injured employees with benefits. One of the important features of social insurance is the principle of sharing risks and pooling resources. A social insurance scheme establishes a public channel through a government agency or a supervised agency, which is responsible for procedures for handling claims and the award and payment of benefits (Higuchi, 1986). In Sweden, the employees' injury insurance is financed totally by employers' contributions based on a percentage of their wage bill.

In some countries, special funds have been set up for payment of compensation to employees for certain diseases, e.g. in Hong Kong, a special fund was set up for payment of compensation to employees with pneumoconiosis and occupational deafness. These are chronic diseases which may have been contributed to by multiple employers over a period of time. The fund is administered by a government body and employers whose workplaces are deemed to expose employees to the hazard have to pay a levy. The fund may also be used for rehabilitation of affected employees. The advantage of such a funding scheme is that the employee can get compensation without the administrative difficulties of establishing and proportioning liability to individual employers. He also does not have to deal with the issue of time-limited liability. The disadvantage is that there is no incentive for the individual employer to improve health and safety for their employees to minimize such claims.

Almost all employment injury compensation schemes were initially applied only to manual workers. Non-manual workers were either excluded or were subject to a wage ceiling to qualify. In some countries, certain categories of employees may also be excluded. Employees who are not covered by the legislation would have to take their employers to court to pursue their claims for compensation. In Singapore, the former Workmen's Compensation Act (covering workmen, i.e. manual workers and non-manual workers with monthly earnings not exceeding $1600) was amended in April 2008 to cover all employees in general and was renamed the Work Injury Compensation Act (WICA) (WICA, 2008; MOM, WSH Council, 2008).

There are also various employee assistance schemes to assist employees who fail to get compensation for various reasons such as employers who are no longer around or where the employee is no longer eligible because he has exceeded the eligibility time bar for claims. This is particularly so for certain occupational diseases with long latent periods (e.g. silicosis and mesothelioma). An example of such a scheme is the Workers' Fund in Singapore (WIC [Workers' Fund] Regulation, 2008).

Benefits Payable

Benefits payable under the workers' injury compensation schemes usually comprise three areas:

(a) temporary incapacity benefits,
(b) permanent incapacity benefits,
(c) survivors' benefits.

a) *Temporary incapacity benefits* are payable for injuries or diseases from which complete recovery occurs, and where there are no lasting effects. Examples of such injuries include minor lacerations and fractures with no complications or, in the case of occupational diseases, an episode of irritant contact dermatitis. Benefits payable often include medical and hospitalization fees, although a ceiling may be set. The other benefits are essentially payment for lost wages for the period of "incapacity" when the employee was not able to work. Such payment is usually proportionate to the wage which the injured employee was receiving averaged over a fixed period preceding the accident. The injured employee may be entitled to full wages up to a certain period of incapacity, e.g. six months, after which he gets a reduced rate that could be for up to one year. This arrangement is to encourage the injured employee to return to work as soon as his injury has healed.

b) *Permanent incapacity benefits* are payable for injuries or diseases from which complete recovery is not possible, and where there are lasting residual effects. Such injuries include amputations of limbs and paralysis of part of the body. Examples of occupational diseases resulting in permanent incapacity are noise-induced deafness and silicosis. There is no treatment for such diseases; the pathological process is irreversible and the damage is permanent. Payment may be in the form of a lump sum or a periodical payment (a pension).

The amount payable is proportionate to the severity of the injury or disease. This is usually based on the reduction of earning capacity of the employee or to the loss of faculty. The amount payable also typically takes into account the average earnings of the employee during the period preceding the injury and his age; generally a younger employee would be entitled to higher compensation than an older one for the same type of injury. The degree of incapacity for a particular injury is then used to compute the actual quantum of compensation, taking into consideration other factors like maximum and minimum compensation limits.

c) *Survivors' benefits* are payable to families of workers who died. The quantum payable may be subject to maximum and minimum amounts prescribed for payment of incapacity benefits.

Assessment of disability

When a doctor is asked to assess disability, this usually refers to that of permanent disability or incapacity. Permanent incapacity means that there is some anatomic or functional abnormality or loss which remains after maximal medical, surgical or other forms of treatment have been given. There is nothing further that can be done to improve the incapacity and the assessing doctor considers the residual incapacity to be stable and not likely to progress or improve further at the time of the medical evaluation.

Where permanent incapacity exists, an assessment has to be made by the doctor who is aided in most instances by a guide or a schedule in the legislation. Guides are available which provide for assessments of the musculoskeletal, respiratory, renal, hearing, visual and other systems of the body. However, it is not possible to provide guidelines for every type of injury or situation and the doctor may have to make judgment calls by studying the available guides, the examples given and compare similar injuries to give a fair assessment of the particular case. Objections may arise from the employer, employee or the insurer as to the assessment made. In Singapore, such objections are referred to a panel of specialists (Senior Consultants) appointed by the Work Injury Compensation Medical Board whose decision is final by law.

Compensation for Occupational Injuries

Legislation on workers' compensation often uses the term "percentage of loss of earning capacity" and most countries have established schedules or lists of degrees of incapacity relating to different injuries. In some instances, the percentages set might have some degree of arbitrariness. There are variations among countries as to the details and impairment ratings for different injuries.

The schedules usually specify what equates to "permanent total incapacity" for which 100% loss of earning capacity is awarded. For example, the schedules in Singapore prescribe 100% loss of earning capacity for:

a) loss of two limbs,
b) loss of both hands or of all fingers and both thumbs,
c) loss of both feet,
d) total loss of sight,
e) total paralysis,
f) injuries resulting in being permanently bedridden.

Other injuries listed are given varying percentages below 100%, e.g. loss of thumb is awarded 30%, and loss of foot 55%.

The system devised by the American Medical Association (AMA, 2008) assesses impairment and relates it to the "whole man" by referring to appropriate tables. For example, anatomic loss or total functional loss of a thumb at the metacarpophalangeal joint is rated as 40% impairment of the whole hand. This is equated to 36% impairment of the upper extremity, which in turn is equated to 22% impairment of the "whole man". Where two or more impairments are involved, the value of each impairment is ascertained and transposed to the common denominator of the "whole man". Then, these values are combined rather than added to relate it to the "whole man".

Case Study 1

A 33-year-old female suffered a crush injury of her right hand when it was caught in a roller of a machine. As a result, she lost her right index, middle, ring and little fingers and had serious lacerations on her palm and wrist. A few months later, when her condition had stabilized following treatment, she was assessed for permanent incapacity by a doctor. She was found to have:

1. *loss of four fingers on her right hand at their metacarpophalangeal joints,*
2. *restriction of movement at her right wrist.*

The injuries were assessed as follows based on the guidelines used in Singapore Workmen's Compensation Medical Board, MOM (2006)

1. *loss of four fingers = 60%,*
2. *restriction of movements at wrist (subtotal = 6% [active dorsi-flexion to 40 degrees = 3%, active palmar-flexion to 50 degrees = 3%]).*

Since there are two types of injuries, the final total is obtained by referring to the combined values chart. This gives 62%.

Compensation for Occupational Diseases

Some occupational diseases may result in permanent incapacity and examples of such diseases are noise-induced deafness, occupational lung diseases, repetitive strain injuries and occupational poisonings. A list of compensable occupational diseases may be provided in the legislation on workers' compensation and the nature of the occupation in relation to each disease may also be prescribed. Countries with such a prescribed list system include France, the UK, India, the Philippines and Malaysia. Some countries do not have a prescribed list but claims would be accepted if it can be shown that the disease is due to work (e.g. Finland, the USA). Others adopt a mixed system, e.g. Singapore, Germany and Italy (Munich Re, 2002; ILO, 2002).

The principles of assessment for permanent incapacity follow that for occupational injuries. To illustrate this, some examples are given below.

Noise-induced Deafness

Noise is a common hazard in industry and noise-induced hearing loss is one of the most common occupational diseases in many countries, including Singapore. Many workers' compensation systems provide for compensation for noise-induced deafness. As noise-induced deafness is irreversible, compensation payable is for "permanent incapacity".

In the diagnosis of noise-induced deafness, other causes of deafness should be considered and excluded. In addition, there should be a confirmed history of adequate occupational exposure to noise. The doctor has to assess the severity of the hearing loss and determine the percentage incapacity based on the guide or prescribed schedule. In Singapore, the minimum impairment qualifying for worker's compensation is 50 dB average hearing loss (AHL) over the 1, 2 and 3 kHz range in the better ear, based on air conduction.

Audiometry should be conducted in a proper booth and by a trained technician. As audiograms for the same person may vary over different times, for compensation purposes, it is important to check for consistency by comparing at least two audiogram readings.

Case Study 2

A 54-year-old shipyard worker has been exposed to high noise levels as a steelworker in various shipyards for the past 25 years. His audiogram showed a bilateral sensorineural hearing loss more pronounced in the high frequencies. His hearing thresholds ranged from 65 to 90 dB in all the frequencies tested. A repeat audiogram showed similar results. His AHL over 1, 2 and 3 kHz was 75 dB in the left ear and 60 dB in the right ear. Clinical examination and medical history did not reveal any other causes of hearing loss.

A diagnosis of noise-induced deafness was made. The AHL of the better ear was 60 dB. Based on the guidelines used in Singapore (see Table 1), the percentage incapacity was 15%. The guidelines provide for adjustment for presbycusis by discounting half a percent for each year that the age exceeded 50 years. The final incapacity award was 13% (15% minus 2%).

Table 1. Assessment of Hearing Loss

Hearing Threshold (dBA) (AHL: 1, 2 and 3 kHz)	Injuries or Accidents (Affected Ear) % Incapacity	Noise-induced Deafness (Better Ear) % Incapacity
50	3	5
55	5	10
60	8	15
65	10	20
70	13	25
75	15	30
80	20	40
85	25	50
90	30	60

Note: For sudden hearing loss resulting from accidents or injuries, assess each affected ear and add the percentage incapacities to get the total percentage incapacity.

Occupational Lung Diseases

Cases of occupational lung diseases, e.g. silicosis, asbestosis and occupational asthma, are assessed according to their lung function. A forced expiratory volume in the first second (FEV_1) and forced vital capacity (FVC) of 80% or more of the predicted values is considered "normal" and would normally mean that there is no disability (Table 2).

Silicosis and asbestosis are chronic diseases which may develop after the worker has stopped further exposure to silica or asbestos and has left his employment. These chronic diseases may progress with subsequent deterioration in lung function. Hence, a minimum degree of incapacity of 10% for radiologically definite silicosis and asbestosis cases may be awarded even if they are asymptomatic and the lung function tests are apparently normal at the time of assessment.

As asthma is a variable condition, assessing lung function on a particular day and after bronchodilator treatment may not be a fair assessment of the disability. Occupational asthma cases who require daily maintenance medication to control their symptoms, despite having been transferred from further exposure to the causative agent

Table 2.   Classification of Respiratory Incapacities Based on Lung Function Testing

Test of Pulmonary Function	0% No Impairment	10–25% Mild Impairment	30–45% Moderate Impairment	50–100% Severe Impairment
FVC	≥80% of predicted *and*	≥60 to <80% of predicted *or*	≥51 to <60% of predicted *or*	≤50% of predicted *or*
FEV$_1$	≥80% of predicted *and*	≥60 to <80% of predicted *or*	≥41 to <60% of predicted *or*	≤40% of predicted *or*
DLCO	≥80% of predicted *and*	≥60 to <80% of predicted *or*	≥41 to <60% of predicted *or*	≤40% of predicted *or*
VO$_2$ max ml/ (kg/min)	≥25	≥20 to <25	≥15 to <20	<15

for one year or more and who in the opinion of the assessing physician is unlikely to improve further, may be considered mildly impaired even though their FEV$_1$ is normal. These cases can be awarded incapacity of 5–20% depending on the minimum maintenance medication required to maintain control.

In Singapore, occupational asthma cases are first assessed based on spirometry results as for pneumoconiosis. However, if the spirometry is normal (i.e. FEV$_1$ > 80% predicted), cases of occupational asthma could be considered mildly impaired and awarded incapacity of 5–20% depending on the minimum daily maintenance medication required to maintain control (see Case Study 3). This is provided the patient has been transferred from further exposure to the asthma-causing agent for one year or more and who in the opinion of the assessing physician is unlikely to improve further.

Case Study 3

A 30-year-old female worker developed adult-onset asthma after six months of working in a furniture factory. Monitoring of her serial peak *expiratory flow rate showed improvement when she was away from work and deterioration during periods at work. Workplace inspection showed that she was exposed to wood dust and cyanoacrylate glue. A diagnosis of occupational asthma was confirmed based on a documented late asthmatic reaction during a specific bronchial provocation test to cyanoacrylate glue. She improved after she left the factory and was no longer exposed to the glue. She was assessed by a chest physician one year after she had stopped further exposure. Her FEV_1 and FVC were within normal limits. However, she continued to require daily inhaled low-dose steroids to control her asthma. On this regime of medication, she did not require any emergency treatment for her asthma.*

Based on the guidelines used in Singapore for asthma (see Table 3) (Workmen's Compensation Medical Board, MOM (2006)), she was awarded 10% permanent disability.

Table 3.   Assessment of Disability for Asthma Based on Medication Required

Minimum Medication Required	Percentage Incapacity
Bronchodilators only	5%
Low dose inhaled steroids	10%
High dose (> 800 μg/day) inhaled steroids or inhaled combination therapy (e.g. inhaled long acting beta2agonist plus inhaled steroids)	15%
Oral steroids	20%

Repetitive Strain Disorders of the Upper Limb

For repetitive strain disorders of the upper limb such as carpal tunnel syndrome and constrictive tenosynovitis, the work-relatedness of the condition must be established and the treatment optimized to ensure that the condition is stable. Assessments can be made according to the severity (e.g. mild, moderate or severe) of the specific condition or according to the restriction of range of motion. In the case of chronic persistent back or neck pain following documented injury, a 5% disability award can be made (Workmen's Compensation Medical Board, Singapore, 2006).

Occupational Poisonings

Occupational poisonings may result in kidney (e.g. cadmium or mercury poisoning) or liver damage (e.g. toxic hepatitis from certain chemicals, such as vinyl chloride monomer). These cases can be assessed according to the residual kidney or liver function.

Assessment of Other Systems

In diseases or injuries of the central nervous system, several areas of function may be impaired. Impaired functioning can occur in consciousness and level of awareness, mental status and integrative functioning, use and understanding of language, and in behavior and mood. The most severe of these categories is used to give a cerebral impairment rating and then the motor and sensory systems, gait and coordination are evaluated (Workmen's Compensation Medical Board, Singapore, 2006).

Future Challenges

Diagnosing a condition as work-related may be subjective and to objectively state the amount of incapacity may be even more complex. Also, with occupational risk factors shifting from the known to the unknown, tangible to intangible, physical to psychological, it is becoming more and more difficult to make an objective assessment of the degree of disability or impairment. There is a need to revise the traditional way in which assessment has been performed so as to be capable of dealing with psychological and "intangible" conditions, whilst providing fair systems for users and ensuring sustainability and financial viability (Munich Re, 2004).

Global climate change can have an impact on occupational diseases by increasing the risk of occupational diseases such as heat-related disorders, respiratory diseases due to pollens and cancers caused by ultraviolet radiation. The higher life expectancies and aging population in most countries suggest that tomorrow's workforce will have a larger share of older employees. The graying future workforce may have health risks associated with aging, resulting in more complex and costly medical treatment and prolonged care. Long-latency illnesses can also become more frequent with advancing age. As obesity rates in many countries continue to increase, more accidents could be expected as significantly overweight employees have been shown to suffer more on-the-job accidents. All these factors may put a strain on the viability of existing compensation schemes (Munich Re, 2009).

References

American Medical Association (AMA). (2008) *Guides to the Evaluation of Permanent Impairment*, 6th edn. Chicago: American Medical Association Press.

Higuchi T. (1986) Systems of employment injury protection: An international review. In: *Report on the Symposium on Employment Injury Protection for Developing Countries in Asia and the Pacific*, pp. 1–11. Bangkok: ILO Regional Office for Asia and the Pacific.

ILO. (2002) *R194 List of Occupational Diseases Recommendation.* http://www.ilo.org/ilolex/cgi-lex/convde.pl?R194 (accessed 23 June 2010).

Ministry of Manpower, WSH Council. (2008) *Work Injury Compensation Act: A Guide to the Work Injury Compensation Benefits and Claim Process.*

Munich Re. (2002) *Occupational Diseases: How Are They Covered Under Workers' Compensation Systems?* Munich: Munich Re Group.

Munich Re. (2004) *Assessing Disability: An International Comparison of Workers' Compensation System.* Munich: Munich Re Group.

Munich Re. (2009) *Future Challenges in Workers' Compensation.* A discussion paper by the Munich Re Centre of Competence for Workers' Compensation. Munich: Munich Re Group.

Workmen's Compensation Medical Board, Ministry of Manpower, Singapore. (2006) *A Guide to the Assessment of Traumatic Injuries and Occupational Diseases for Workmen's Compensation*, 5th edn. Singapore: Ministry of Manpower.

Work Injury Compensation Act (Chapter 354). (2008) In: *The Statutes of the Republic of Singapore.*

Work Injury Compensation (Workers' Fund) Regulation. (2008) In: *The Statutes of the Republic of Singapore.*

Chapter 20

Occupational Medicine Practice and the Law

See-Muah Lee[*,‡] *and David Koh*[†]

Introduction

The State has an interest in the regulation of medical practice, as it must, in all important spheres of public activity. The regulatory framework for this includes professional bodies, such as the national medical councils, which are vested with powers to investigate complaints and to sanction errant behavior, the law of tort, through which claimants who are harmed because of negligence can seek redress, and legislations. The law of contract would also be operable for agreed occupational health work by providers performed for employers.

Occupational health stands out as one specialty that is very much legislatively influenced, because of its essential interphase between the worker and his work environment. The protection of the health and safety of workers has long been acknowledged as a social right in all modern states. Not surprisingly, in all countries, there would be

*Department of Epidemiology and Public Health, Yong Loo Lin School of Medicine, National University of Singapore, Diabetes Clinic Khoo Teck Puat Hospital, Singapore.
†Department of Epidemiology and Public Health, Yong Loo Lin School of Medicine, National University of Singapore.
‡Corresponding author. E-mail: see_muah_lee@nuhs.edu.sg

legislation pertaining to health and safety at work. This would have an impact on the conduct of all parties responsible and accountable for the protection of the health of the worker, among them occupational physicians.

Ethics and the Law

An important hallmark of the profession is self-regulation. This takes effect through national bodies like the Singapore Medical Council in Singapore and the General Medical Council in the United Kingdom. The State grants such governing bodies the powers and, with them, the responsibilities for regulation of professional conduct.

The governing medical bodies would normally comprise senior and experienced members of the profession. Furthermore, perhaps mindful of the popular belief that "all professions are a conspiracy against the laity" (George Bernard Shaw), most such bodies would include some lay representation as well.

This right to determination of standards for its members would not be complete without the power to impose censures and penalties when members fall short of such standards, regardless of whether a harmed victim can be identified or not. The traditional principles in biomedical ethics — autonomy, beneficence and justice (Beauchamp and Childress, 2001) — are applicable to all physicians, including occupational physicians.

Many jurisdictions would allow for appeals against the decisions of the medical councils in a higher court of law. Reliance on medical ethics for the court decisions will play an important role (*R v General Medical Council & Simon Shorvon*, 2006), as would points of law. This has been extensively tested in the cases of the traditional therapeutic relationship of doctor and patient (*Foo Fio Na v Dr. Soo Fook Mun & Anor Federal Court*, 2006; *Chester v Afshar*, 2004) and biomedical research (Tay, 2007). There is no reason to believe that such reliance would not happen in occupational health.

One distinctive feature of occupational health is the interests of many stakeholders, such as employers, workers, government officials (such as factory inspectors), worker representatives and other technical experts; set against the backdrop of the work environment, instead of the traditional hospital or clinic setting. Specialty-specific guidances such as those provided in the International Code of Ethics for Occupational Health Professionals by the International Commission of Occupational Health and the *Guidance on Ethics for Occupational Physicians* by the Faculty of Occupational Medicine, United Kingdom, are helpful resources.

The status of workers, in any given situation, as patients construed in the traditional sense, has been perhaps a little over debated. How would biomedical guidelines apply? Indeed, what is the status of a worker at screening but not seeking care, or a pre-employment candidate at a medical examination? Each will have to be determined on its own merits, including an understanding of the purpose of such a determination.

Our guiding principle ought to be that of a universal respect for the dignity of all individuals. This will not change, regardless of the individual being one among a group affected by a management health decision, or a patient with a clinical problem for consultation.

Disclosure of Information: Ethics and the Law

Case Study 1: Sickness Absence

A company is trying to control its healthcare expenditure, which is increasing year by year. The human resource (HR) department has identified 20 workers with the highest medical expenditure and another 20 workers with the highest sickness absence. The HR department now wishes to know about their health conditions so that they can understand the reasons and help the workers maintain better health and productivity.

The doctor has a duty to maintain confidentiality of medical information that has been disclosed to him. Breach of confidentiality, that is, the disclosure of such information without consent, would be unethical (and, in certain countries, unlawful), for the purpose described.

Businesses have a legitimate interest in controlling costs. This applies to employee benefits and welfare. The containment of health-care costs is best achieved by the design of these benefits.

Doctors can assist in this through health protection and health promotion. But the disclosure of medical information without informed consent would be a step too far in the assistance of this business objective. When requesting consent, the doctors should also explain to the workers the purpose for which consent is sought.

The doctor who fails to offer and tries to limit access to reasonable healthcare violates medical ethics. When harm results, the doctor then faces the risk of litigation.

In the United Kingdom, the Data Protection Act 1998 goes a step further in prescribing the statutory right of access of the patient/worker to his own health and medical information.

As suggested in the Guidance on Ethics for Occupational Physicians (FOM, 2009), it is recommended that occupational physicians apprise the contracting parties of the fundamental ethical obligations of doctors. This can help pre-empt problems in contract terms and its interpretation that might run contrary to these obligations. The Guidance has also advised the need for occupational physicians, when preparing medical reports, to offer to show these reports to the workers or patients concerned before onward transmission to third parties, including employers.

The duty to maintain confidentiality of medical information is not absolute. The law may require disclosure, as in the notification of occupational illnesses, to the relevant authorities. In the event that the physician is the notifying person, then a delicate situation may also arise as to whether the employer should be informed as well. In most cases, it would be good practice to seek the agreement of the worker in letting the employer know. This would allow the employer to investigate and manage the risks accordingly and cooperate fully with the authorities.

Public interest, such as averting real harm to others, has also been cited as grounds for justifiably breaching the duty to maintain confidentiality of information. Such was the reasoning in *W v Edgell* (*W v Edgell*, 1990; UK Clinical Ethics Network, 2010).

Fitness to Work; Medicolegal Challenges

Case Study 2: Physical Harm

Coffee v McDonnell-Douglas Corporation (1972), 503 P2d 1366 Cal 1972

Mr. Coffee applied for a position as a pilot with an aircraft manufacturer. He was required to undergo a physical examination at the corporation's clinic. It included, among other investigations, blood tests for hemoglobin count and erythrocyte sedimentation rate, which were found to be abnormal. The blood test results were filed and time stamped by the clinic secretary without review by the doctors. Mr. Coffee was hired; several months later, he nearly collapsed and was discovered to have multiple myeloma.

Although the physicians, who were employees of the corporation, were exonerated, the corporation was nevertheless held to be negligent in failing to exercise due care in handling blood test reports taken in a physical examination they required Mr. Coffee to undergo.

Case Study 3: Economic Harm

Kapfunde v Abbey National PLC and Daniel (1998), 46 BMLR 176 CA

In the case of Kapfunde, the claimant revealed her sickle cell anemia and past history of chest infection in a health questionnaire as part of a pre-employment medical examination, directed by the prospective employer. Dr. Daniel, as an occupational health advisor, had to advise Abbey National whether a higher sickness absence could result. Dr. Daniel concluded that this was the case and the applicant was therefore assessed as unsuitable. She failed to obtain employment and sued the prospective employer and the physician Dr. Daniel, claiming a breach of duty of care owed to her directly by the bank, and that the doctor was a servant of the bank, pursuant to a contract of service as opposed to a contract for service.

Kapfunde's claim was dismissed on the basis that the doctor was neither an employee of the bank, nor was there any duty of care owed to her by the doctor. Furthermore, the doctor's professional recommendation, which resulted in the loss of an employment opportunity, was deemed to be within the range of reasonable responses and held not to be negligent.

These two cases clarify the extent and nature of the physician's legal duty when evaluating pre-employment fitness, when tort challenges occur (Lee and Koh, 2008). A tort is an injury resulting from a civil or private wrong. In order to succeed, tort claimants (in these cases, the workers) in negligence must establish a duty of care owed by the alleged wrongdoers (in these cases, the physicians and the employers), breach of that duty and harm resulting from the breach. All elements must be successfully proven.

In *Coffee*, the claim involved physical harm. The court rightly expects a non-negligent medical assessment, one which requires the exercise of reasonable skill and care. There is no duty to explore and discover all manner of illnesses at such examinations. Whether the standard of care was breached has to be judged in "the light of all the circumstances" (*Coffee*, 1972). Thus, the failure to pay regard to the abnormal results of tests that were ordered, whatever the reasons may be, was judged to be inexcusable. Furthermore, the senior physician of the team had given evidence that had he been aware of the abnormalities, it would have prompted further inquiry and disqualification for the job. In this particular case, the employer did have a procedural system directed to their physicians, which was unfortunately flawed and resulted in the oversight. The employers were therefore found liable.

It is highly probable that the physicians would have been liable had they not been employees but independent contractors. The legal doctrine of *"respondeat superior"*, which briefly translated from its Latin origin means "let the superior answer", is widely applied in employer–employee relationships. Thus not only would employers be themselves liable for their own negligent actions, they would also be generally held liable for the negligent actions of their employees at work.

Coffee should also serve as a deterrent to physicians against making careless and shoddy assessments. Implications of this can be far-reaching as illustrated by the example in Case Study 1 (fitness for overseas work in remote locations) in the chapter on cardiovascular disorders.

Furthermore, when it comes to the standard of care concerning the duty of disclosure, the courts have shown they can be quite vigorous in defending the examinee's interests. It would appear that the Bolam principle, espoused in *Bolam v Friern Hospital Management Committee* (1957), whenever the standard of clinical care is in dispute, has little application in such cases. Such a position has been taken in the landmark ruling of *Rogers v Whitaker* (1995) and followed again in the Malaysian case of *Foo Fio Na v Dr. Soo Fook Mun* (2006).

In *Kapfunde*, the claim involved economic interests. The claimant did not suffer physical harm from the actions of the physician. While her disqualification from the job as a result of the doctor's recommendation meant an economic loss, the court declined to recognize a duty of care to protect her economic interests.

Where a defendant advises a claimant, and knows that the advice will be relied on by the claimant, and economic loss ensues, then under the Hedley principle (*Hedley Byrne & Co v Heller and Partners*, 1964), the loss was foreseeable and a duty of care arises.

It could certainly be argued that it is Abbey National PLC who is trying to minimize the financial risk and who relies on this advice, rather than the job applicant. In this case, a duty to the job applicant should not arise. Moreover, it is not up to the claimant to decide whether or not at this point to reject or accept the doctor's professional opinion as a condition for accepting the job. Therefore the Hedley principle cannot apply in this instance.

Case Study 4: A Legal Duty to Non-Patients

Kaiser v Suburban Transportation System (1965), 398 P.2d 14 (Wash, 1965)

In Kaiser, the defendant physician prescribed a sedating antihistamine to his patient, whom the physician knew to be a bus driver. After taking the first dose of the medication the following morning, the driver went to work and was involved in an accident after falling asleep while driving the bus. The driver had apparently felt groggy before the accident but continued to drive nonetheless. A passenger on the bus was injured in the accident and sued the doctor and the bus company.

The Washington Supreme Court noted that the evidence suggested that the doctor may not have informed his bus driver-patient of "the dangerous side effects of drowsiness or lassitude" from the drug and that expert evidence suggested that it was negligent not to do so.

In remanding the case, the court held that "the jury should be directed that (a) in the event it finds no warning was given to the bus driver as to the side effects of the drug, it shall bring in a verdict against the doctor; (b) in the event the jury finds the bus driver failed to exercise the highest degree of care, even though he was given no warning as to the side effects of the drug, the jury shall also bring in a verdict against the bus company and the driver; and (c) in the event the jury finds that a warning of the side effects of the drug was given to the bus driver, then the verdict shall be against the bus company and the driver only."

Thus, the basis of the doctor's duty to the non-patient bus passenger stemmed solely from the need to warn his patient, the bus driver, of the potential side effect of drowsiness.

This case has also lent strong support to the later decision of McKenzie v Hawaii Permanente Medical Group (2002).

Kaiser is particularly instructive for occupational physicians. An occupational physician who has certified fitness in a worker who subsequently injures a co-worker because of a medical condition that has not been properly evaluated, or which the worker has not been cautioned about, may in turn be sued by the co-worker. The necessity to warn and to advise cannot be overemphasized. An example would be a diabetic worker on insulin who, if considered stable and fit for employment, must be warned and be engaged in a discussion about hypoglycemia. This is especially important if there are safety implications in the job (Lee, Sum and Koh, 2009).

Coffee, Kapfunde and *Kaiser* also illustrate the complexity and tension that exist in occupational health work. *Coffee* and *Kapfunde* primarily involve challenges between the worker, or prospective worker, and the physician. *Kaiser* gives notice about liabilities involving injured third parties.

We should also be mindful that work in occupational health is often conducted within a contractual framework with employers. A legal duty thus exists to enforce competent performance of contractual obligations by the occupational health providers for the employers, a breach of which can also potentially result in a claim by the employer.

Occupational Health and Safety Legislation

The laws of most countries would mandate the duties of employers in the protection of workers in the workplace. In the developed countries, such legislations often have a long history. For example, in the United Kingdom, these date back to the Act for the Better Regulation of Chimney Sweepers and their Apprentices of 1788. In 1802, the Health and Morals of Apprentices Act was enacted, and the Factory Act followed in 1819. The legislations have been continuously reviewed and updated, and subsequently led to the passing of the Health and Safety at Work etc Act 1974.

These laws compel employers to think and reflect on their occupational health and safety responsibilities in the various areas of work. Duties, responsibilities and competency issues will need to be addressed. The duties spelt out under the law in the United Kingdom are qualified by the principle of "so far as is reasonably practicable". Modern health and safety laws at work are generally based on risk assessment, risk management by competent persons, training and the setting up of emergency response procedures and the sharing of information with workers.

One continual challenge of occupational health law must be the necessity of responding to developments in work practices, such as the introduction of new substances, and new methods or new information about old substances and old methods used in the workplace.

The administration and enforcement of the legislation is usually provided for by the establishment of agencies with responsibilities for occupational safety and health, such as the US Occupational Safety and Health Agency (OSHA).

Case Study 5: Stop Work Order

In 2002, eight workers from Chem-Solv Technologies in Singapore were admitted to the hospital for accidental poisoning by inhalation of toxic vapor, suspected to be nickel carbonyl (Joint Press Release MOM and NEA, 2002). The employer was involved in the reclamation and treatment of industrial waste products and servicing of chemical containers. Its operations include the collection of waste chemicals in drums and containers from various companies, as well as the incineration, processing and recycling of the waste products.

The Ministry of Manpower issued a stop work order to the company to stop all work on its premises, pending investigations and remedial measures. The ministry, in consultation with the National Environment Agency, imposed additional requirements for the safe processing and treatment of waste chemicals. This includes engineering measures such as local exhaust ventilation systems as well as the use of air-supplied respirators to protect workers.

The responsible agencies have the power to issue remedial orders and stop work orders, and impose fines and penalties such as imprisonment. While health and safety laws would contain provisions for prosecution and criminal sanctions, it also gives significant powers to issue notices such as improvement and prohibition notices. Giving advice and guidance on compliance, either directly to the business or indirectly through publications and planned events, has long been a cherished tradition.

Features of Occupational Health and Safety Legislation

Common features found in such legislation would cover areas such as requirements for the following.

Risk assessment

Employers should assess the risks to employees and others who may be affected by the work. Such assessments should include identification of significant hazards and the control measures. There should be arrangements in place for the effective planning, organization, control, monitoring and review of the preventive and protective measures, including the provision of personal protective equipment.

First aid and emergency measures

Adequate facilities must be provided. There should also be trained personnel, such as first aiders and rescuers, who must be readily available to respond to emergency situations.

Appointment of trained and competent persons

This is to ensure that employers have trained competent persons appointed to monitor and effectively control health and health problems.

Training in occupational health and safety and hazard communication

All employees should understand their role and responsibilities in preventing accidents and diseases and promoting health at work. They should be made aware of the preventive measures required and be given specific training on safe work procedures. Persons exposed to hazardous substances or processes have a right to know about the risks and the preventive measures. Information provided can be in the form of Safety Data Sheets (SDS), warning signs and labeling.

Statutory medical examinations

Persons employed in certain occupations, or who are exposed to prescribed hazards in the workplace may require medical examinations to ensure they are fit for such work, as well as to monitor their health and detect any early evidence of work-related ill health.

There may be requirements for such examinations to be performed by medical practitioners who have training in occupational medicine.

Reporting of occupational accidents and diseases

It is important that accidents and diseases caused by work are reported as soon as possible so that investigations can be conducted and measures implemented promptly to prevent recurrence of such cases.

Health and safety committees

Health and safety committees should comprise management as well as worker representatives. This partnership, in theory at least, would enable collective wisdom to be brought to bear on the interpretation and compliance to health and safety laws, bearing in mind the particular circumstances of the business. Their functions are to review safety and occupational health performance regularly, as well as to promote occupational health and safety. In some countries, the occupational health physician is a designated member of the committee.

Case Study 6: Breach of Statutory Duty in Civil Claims

Groves v Lord Wimborne (1892), 2 QB 402

In Groves, the claimant was a boy employed in the service of the defendant, working at a steam winch with revolving cog wheels. These cog wheels were dangerous to a person working the winch unless fenced. This failure to safeguard dangerous machinery was in contravention of the law. The plaintiff's right arm was caught by the cog wheels and injured. The employer was penalized £100 for breach of statutory duty. However, "not one penny of the fine imposed under the sections of the Act need ever

*go into the pocket of the person injured" (AL Smith LJ). The court saw
no reason to deny the claimant a cause of action under tort in respect to
the breach of the Factory Act.*

*For another case where breach of statutory duty was alleged, see
Novartis Grimsby Ltd v John Cookson (2007).*

Claims can arise in tort for breach of health and safety duties created by statute. Employees who are injured because of the employers'
breach of these duties would find the courts in general to be quite
sympathetic in respect to such breaches being applied as a cause
of action. Such claimants belong to the class for whose benefit the
legislation was enacted.

Self-Regulation

State resources are often not available for intensive inspection and
scrutiny of all workplaces. Moreover, legislation can never be completely comprehensive in addressing issues given the varied nature of
workplaces and work processes. The statutes will need to be interpreted
in the context of each workplace.

A responsible state would not condone risky and poorly managed
activities voluntarily undertaken by workers, induced perhaps by the
prospect of more pay. Thus, regulations are issued for specific activities deemed too hazardous or dangerous to be left to discretionary
management by the business. These regulations include those for
chemical handling (COSHH), work in confined spaces (Confined
Spaces Regulations, 1997), noise exposure (Control of Noise at Work
Regulations, 2005) and asbestos (Control of Asbestos Regulations,
2006), among many others.

Standards and Codes of Practice

Occupational health and safety legislation is often supplemented by
standards developed to provide more detailed guidelines and performance measurements for the purposes of compliance and/or
adoption of best practices.

Two examples of these standards are exposure standards that set limits on exposures to harmful substances (such as noise, radiation, chemicals) and Occupational Health and Safety Management Systems (OHSMS). Key components of OHSMS include policy setting, hazard and risk analysis, implementation of measures to manage risk, training and hazard communication and measures for continuous review and improvement. Audits of these management systems must be conducted at regular intervals to ensure that they remain relevant and are effectively implemented.

Codes of practice provide practical examples of good practice. Adherence to codes of practice, analogous to clinical practice guidelines, would have evidentiary value in court proceedings. These codes of practice would usually have been approved by the relevant regulatory bodies. Examples include those for respirator use and ear defenders (CP74, 2006; CP76, 2006). The regulatory bodies can exercise their powers in enforcing compliance, providing advice and, in the gravest of cases, prosecution.

Qualifying Disclosures

In many countries, there are laws to protect whistleblowers against reprisals by employers if they make disclosures which are in the "public interest". Such reprisals may range from detrimental treatment at work to outright dismissal. Disclosures about threats to health and safety are included as matters of public interest. They should logically be followed up with the employer or management.

However, if the worker is not comfortable with disclosures to the employers, he may do so to the authorities. In the United Kingdom, under the Public Disclosure Act 1998, these are prescribed bodies, which in the case of occupational health and safety issues would be the "Health and Safety Executive". To be protected by the law, the worker must make the disclosure in good faith and believe the disclosure to be substantially true.

Occupational Health Legislations and the Occupational Physician

The involvement of occupational health physicians as specialist service providers is often needed when health risk assessments are undertaken. This can be varied, from statutory medical examinations for workers, e.g. those exposed to prescribed hazards such as noise, to workplace assessment, e.g. noise level measurements. Reliance on such advice by employers which turn out to be inept or negligent could be potentially litigable (Lee, Sng and Koh, 2009). The case of the occupational health providers being invited to court to defend such decisions, though seldom heard of, is a distinct possibility.

Notification of occupational illnesses is also another statutory duty in most countries. This would follow a prescribed list in the regulations, which in the United Kingdom is the Reporting of Injuries, Diseases and Dangerous Occurrences Regulations (RIDDOR, 2005).

Compensation for Injuries Suffered at Work and Occupational Diseases

Medical assessment for purposes of compensation for injuries suffered at work can be part of the work of occupational health physicians. This activity is often performed together with specialists from the other allied medical specialties. For compensable occupational diseases, the list of diseases would usually be prescribed under legislation.

To succeed in such claims, the worker needs to prove his eligibility as a workman; that the injury or the occupational illness arose from the course of employment; and that there was incapacity. Death arising from work, of course, is compensable to the estate of the deceased.

Legislations such as the Workmen's Compensation Act will help expedite and simplify such claims, and avert the need for expensive tort litigation. Establishing legal fault and blameworthiness is normally not required for claims made under the Workmen's Compensation Act.

However, the compensation in monetary terms is usually formula fixed, and often much less than what could be obtained by pursuing the claim in civil courts (see Case Study 7). Compensation through the civil courts allow for additional damages to be awarded for pain, suffering and costs of continuing medical care. Statutory awards under the Workmen's Compensation Act are based mainly on loss of future income and medical expenses which are capped.

Tort litigation would involve establishing legal fault and blameworthiness in a highly charged courtroom atmosphere. The extent to which the injury was due to the carelessness of the injured can be subject to vigorous contention. Although fairly straightforward in most cases, the determination of whether an injury or illness arises out of employment can be, on occasions, open to dispute. Stress-related illness is one example (Shortt, 1995), as are musculoskeletal disorders.

Case Study 7: Workmen's Compensation

In 2008, Mr. Hafizul, a foreign worker from Bangladesh working at a construction site in Singapore, was injured (Vijayan, 2010). A 50 kg bag of cement fell on his back, fractured his spine and left him paralyzed from the waist down. He rejected the workmen's compensation of S$182,000 authorized by the Commissioner for Labour and decided to pursue the claim in the civil court. In June 2010, the High Court found in his favor and ordered the employers to compensate Mr. Hafizul S$910,000.

Conclusion

Many stakeholders are involved in occupational health. The agenda of these stakeholders may not be necessarily congruent. Profits and the bottom line would be pressing concerns for all commercial enterprises. Employment issues for workers would revolve round career progression, perks and pay. Safety, with its immediate consequences and impact, may tend to overshadow occupational health concerns, some of which have long latency before harms are obvious. Adherence to sound occupational health practice requires commitment, training, greater awareness and the resources of a multidisciplinary team. The state has an important role in balancing the interests of all these stakeholders, through the application of laws and regulations and the use of the "carrot and stick" approach.

Note and Acknowledgments

This chapter was written substantively in the context of the common law system, adopted from the legal system in England and practised in many English-speaking countries.

The authors acknowledge with thanks the late Dr. Denis D'Auria for his communication of his thoughts on the subject.

Appendix

Standard of Care

Bolam v Friern Hospital Management Committee (1957), 2 ALL ER 118

Bolam involved a claimant patient who underwent electroconvulsive therapy and suffered fractures as a result. Were the doctors liable for failing to administer muscle relaxants, a practice not uniformly adopted by all responsible doctors? "A doctor is not guilty of negligence if he has acted in accordance with a practice accepted as proper by a responsible body of medical men skilled in that particular art". The claim therefore failed.

Duty to Warn

Foo Fio Na v Dr. Soo Fook Mun & Anor Federal Court, Putrajaya Civil Appeal No: 02-20-2001(W), 29 December 2006 Judgment

Ms. Foo, described by the court as a bright young lady, sustained a neck injury in a road traffic accident. Subsequent treatment, which included two surgeries, was unsuccessful. She became paralyzed. The case was disputed from the trial court to the Court of Appeal and finally to the Federal Court. The Federal Court held that the Bolam test has no relevance to the duty and standard of care of a medical practitioner in providing advice to a patient on the inherent and material risks of the proposed treatment.

Rogers v Whitaker (1992), 175 CLR 479

In the Australian case of Rogers, the surgeon operated on Mr. Whitaker's right eye, which was blind to start with. The operation was not successful. He further developed the rather rare complication of sympathetic ophthalmia in the otherwise normal left eye, and as a result was left with no useful vision. Failure to warn was considered negligent. The court declined to follow the Bolam defence, which was that it was accepted practice among eye surgeons not to warn patients about the rare complication. Particularly in the field of non-disclosure of risk and the provision of advice and information, "it is for the courts to adjudicate on what is the appropriate standard of care after giving weight to the paramount consideration that a person is entitled to make his own decisions about his life".

Economic Loss

Hedley Byrne & Co v Heller and Partners (1964), AC 465

This is a case of economic loss resulting from wrongful financial advice from a bank about a client's creditworthiness — notoriously difficult to win in England — being given to the claimants. For such cases to succeed, there must be a special relationship arising where "it is plain that the party seeking information or advice was trusting the other to exercise such a degree of care as the circumstances required ... ought to have known that the enquirer was relying on him" (Lord Reid).

Duty to Non-Patients

McKenzie v Hawaii Permanente Medical Group, Civ. No. 98-00726 DAE Hawaii Supreme Court, 10 June 2002

Kathryn McKenzie was a minor who suffered serious injuries after being hit by a car driven by Mr. Wilson. The McKenzies and Wilson claim the accident occurred because Wilson fainted while driving due to the side effect of prazosin, of which he was not properly warned and of which he was not expected to know unless specifically addressed. In such cases the law can and does recognize a duty of care owed by the physician to such third parties (McKenzie). In doing so, the courts are not interfering with prescribing decisions, but imposing a legal duty to warn about foreseeable risks and side effects of the prescription choice.

Breach of Statutory Duty

Novartis Grimsby Ltd v John Cookson (2007), EWCA Civ 1261

Mr. Cookson had worked for Novartis in the production of dyestuffs from 1964. In 2001, he developed bladder cancer and alleged that this was caused by negligent exposure to beta-naphthylamine, among some other substances of varying carcinogenicity found in the dye manufacturing process. Throughout this period, the regulations regarding beta-naphthylamine use have been updated in tandem with new knowledge about its properties and health effects.

The process of making dyestuff consisted of mixing and heating various chemicals in liquid form in reaction vessels. The work environment to which the claimant was exposed was extremely dusty and the claimant alleged a breach of Section 63(1) of the Factories Act in force at that time. Furthermore it was alleged that the employer failed to warn the claimant of the risk of exposure and did not provide him with appropriate protective clothing. At one time, the claimant was given only a gauze mask and later a paper mask.

Having established that there was exposure and that the exposure was in breach of duty, the final issue of the claim turned on causation. An independent epidemiologist, invited to submit his views on the issue on causation, concluded that the risk of harm from smoking was probably greater compared to occupational exposure. However, Mr. Cookson's urologist did not agree and went on to prepare a full report refuting the findings of the epidemiologist. He referred also to the epidemiologist's own published work claiming that the risks due to smoking decreased with the passage of time after cessation. Mr. Cookson had by that time given up smoking for many years. The urologist also made references to the exposure levels to which Mr. Cookson was subjected.

The appeal by the employer, against the judgment of the lower court which found the employer liable, was subsequently dismissed.

Disclosure in the Public Interest

W v Edgell (1990), 1 ALL ER 835

The patient was a prisoner in a secure hospital following convictions for killing five people and wounding several others. He made an application to a mental health tribunal to be transferred to a regional unit. An independent psychiatrist, Dr. Edgell, was asked by W's legal advisors to provide a confidential expert opinion that they hoped would show that W was no longer a danger to the public. However, Dr. Edgell was of the opinion that in fact W was still dangerous. W's application was withdrawn. Dr. Edgell, knowing that his opinion would not be included in the patient's notes, sent a copy to the medical director of the hospital and to the Home Office. The patient brought an action for breach of confidence. The Court of Appeal held that the breach was justified in the public interest, on grounds of protection of the public from dangerous criminal acts. However, the Court said the risk must be "real, immediate and serious".

References

Beauchamp TL, Childress JF. (2001) *Principles of Biomedical Ethics,* 5th edn. Oxford: Oxford University Press.

Bolam v Friern Hospital Management Committee. (1957) 2 ALL ER 118.

Chester v Afshar. [2004]. UKHL41.

Coffee v McDonnell-Douglas Corporation. (1972) 503 P2d 1366 Cal 1972.

Confined Spaces Regulations. (1997) http://www.opsi.gov.uk/si/si1997/19971713.htm (accessed 23 Jun 2010).

Control of Asbestos Regulations. (2006) http://www.hse.gov.uk/asbestos/regulations.htm (accessed 23 Jun 2010).

Control of Noise at Work Regulations. (2005) http://www.hse.gov.uk/noise/regulations.htm (accessed 23 Jun 2010).

Control of Substances Hazardous to Health (COSHH). http://www.hse.gov.uk/coshh/index.htm (accessed 23 Jun 2010).

CP74. (2006) Code of Practice 74. Code of Practice for selection, use and maintenance of respiratory protection devises, approved under Workplace Safety and Health Act Singapore.

CP76. (2006) Code of Practice 76. Code of Practice for selection, use and maintenance of hearing protectors, approved under Workplace Safety and Health Act Singapore.

FOM; SOM. (2009) *Joint Statement to FOM & SOM Members, New GMC Guidance on Confidentiality.* http://www.som.org.uk (accessed 23 Jun 2010).

Foo Fio Na v Dr Soo Fook Mun & Anor Federal Court, Putrajaya. (2006). Civil Appeal No: 02-20-2001(W) 29 December 2006.

Groves v Lord Wimborne. (1892) 2 QB 402.

Health and Safety Regulations — A Short Guide. http://www.hse.gov.uk/pubns/hsc13.pdf (accessed 23 Jun 2010).

Hedley Byrne & Co v Heller and Partners (1964) AC 465.

Joint Press Release by the Ministry of Manpower and National Environment Agency on the incident at Chem-Solv Technologies at 29 Pioneer Sector 2 (2002).

Kaiser v Suburban Transportation System. (1965) 398 P.2d 14 (Wash. 1965).

Kapfunde v Abbey National PLC and Daniel. (1998) 46 BMLR 176 CA.

Lee SM, Koh D. (2008) Fitness to work: Legal pitfalls. *Ann Acad Med Singapore* **37**: 236–240.

Lee SM, Sng J, Koh D. (2009) The doctor in claims for work injuries and ill health: Legal pitfalls. *Ann Acad Med Singapore* **38**: 727–732.

Lee SM, Sum CF, Koh D. (2009) Legal issues in the management of patients with diabetes mellitus. *Singapore Med J* **50**(12): 1200–1206.

McKenzie v Hawaii Permanente Medical Group. (2002). Civ. No. 98-00726 DAE Hawaii Supreme Court, 10 June 2002.

Novartis Grimsby Ltd v John Cookson. (2007) EWCA Civ 1261.

R (on the application of Singapore Medical Council) (Claimant) v General Medical Council (Defendant) & Simon Shorvon (Interested Party). (2006) EWHC 3277 (Admin) QBD (Admin) (Davis J) 21 December 2006.

Reporting of Injuries, Diseases and Dangerous Occurrences Regulations (RIDDOR). (1995) UK.

Rogers v Whitaker. (1995) 175 CLR 479.

Shortt EDS. (1995) The compensability of chronic stress. *Can Pub Pol.* **21**: 219–232.

Tay CSK. (2007) Recent developments of informed consent in eye research. *Ann Acad Med Singapore.* **36**(Suppl): 56–60.

UK Clinical Ethics Network. (2010) http://www.ethics-network.org.uk/ethical-issues/confidentiality/legal-considerations (accessed 23 June 2010).

Vijayan KC. (2010) $1M awarded to paralysed Bangladeshi, *The Straits Times*, 24 June.

W v Edgell. (1990) 1 ALL ER 835.

Chapter 21

Medical Disaster Planning and Response

*Meng-Kin Lim**

Introduction

Few scenarios pose as great a challenge to occupational physicians as an industrial disaster resulting in mass casualties. The poisonous gas leak from the Union Carbide insecticide plant in Bhopal, India, in 1984 (Case Study 1) and the disaster at the Chernobyl nuclear power plant in Russia in 1986 (Case Study 2) cost thousands of lives and rank as two of the world's worst industrial disasters ever. These colossal events underscore the need for both prevention and preparedness.

It is not only the very large industrial plants, however, that need to be prepared. Every industrial facility, big or small, must have its own disaster management blueprint; first, to avert disaster, and second, to mitigate the effects and ameliorate the impact when disaster does strike. This chapter deals with the medical aspects of disaster planning and outlines the medical organization and support needed to effectively handle a disaster situation involving mass casualties in the workplace.

*Department of Epidemiology and Public Health, Yong Loo Lin School of Medicine, National University of Singapore. E-mail: ephlmk@nus.edu.sg

Case Study 1

On 3 December 1984, over 30 tons of methyl isocyanate, a chemical intermediate in the production of carbaryl, a commonly used pesticide, were accidentally released from a Union Carbide plant in Bhopal, India (Fig. 1). The incident occurred in the middle of the night. The nearby residents had no knowledge of effective evacuation plans or procedures. Between 50,000 and 100,000 people were affected enough to seek medical care of some type. While no precise figures are available (as it is often unclear whether the gas cloud was the cause of death, and many victims have taken years to die from the effects of exposure), India's Supreme Court put the death toll at 3800 in 1991 when it awarded $480 million in damages against US-based Union Carbide Corp and its Indian subsidiary. By 1994, 10 years to the day after the disaster, official government records showed 6495 people had died from exposure to toxic methyl isocyanate.

Case Study 2

On 26 April 1986, the overheating of a water-cooled nuclear reactor in Chernobyl in Ukraine resulted in a major nuclear disaster. About

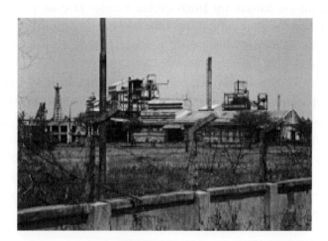

Fig. 1. The Union Carbide plant, Bhopal, India, the site of a chemical gas leak which killed and injured thousands.

30 people were killed immediately, and the nuclear discharge from Chernobyl spread across national boundaries. An estimated 150–200 million curies of radioactive material were released into the environment within the first 10 days. The highest concentrations of radionuclides fell over Ukraine, Belarus and Russia, and raised levels were found as far away as North America. By 1999, a dramatic rise in the incidence of childhood thyroid cancer had been documented in Ukraine in the years since the nuclear disaster. Experts estimate that several thousand more persons affected by the accident will die from cancer within the next several decades.

Definition of Industrial Disaster

The World Health Organization defines disaster as "a situation which implies unforeseen, serious and immediate threats to public health". This broad definition recognizes that disasters come in all forms, both natural (e.g. floods, earthquakes, volcanic eruptions) and man-made. There is no single universally accepted definition of an industrial disaster. Because of the lack of uniformity of definition, the true overall incidence of industrial disasters in the world is not known.

The Swiss Reinsurance Company has since 1970 maintained a limited access database for both global natural and man-made disasters, using a stringent criteria of at least one of the following for inclusion: 20 deaths or 50 injured or 2000 homeless or insured losses of >US$14 million (marine), >US$28 million (aviation), >US$35 million (all other losses), or total losses in excess of US$70 million. As of 2008, there are approximately 7000 entries in the database with 300 new entries per year. In contrast, the Spatial Hazard Event and Losses Database for the United States (SHELDUS), which was created and maintained by the University of South Carolina, and which uses much less stringent criteria, has recorded over 400,000 events in the United States alone, since 1960.

Table 1 shows selected examples of industrial disasters in various countries between 1970 and 2008.

From a practical point of view, we can take an industrial disaster to mean an event which causes casualties, the size and severity of

Table 1.   Selected Examples of Industrial Disasters in Various Countries (1970–2008)

Year	Place	Cause	Product	Deaths	Injured	Evacuated
1970	Osaka, Japan	Explosion	Gas	92	—	—
1974	Flixborough, UK	Explosion	Cyclohexane	23	104	3000
	Decatur, USA	Rail accident	Isobutane	7	152	—
1975	Beek, Holland	Explosion	Ethylene	14	1071	—
1976	Houston, USA	Silo explosion	Wheat	7	0	10,000
	Lapua, Finland	Explosion	Explosives	43	—	—
	Seveso, Italy	Leakage	Dioxin	0	193	730
1978	Los Alfaques, Spain	Road accident	Propylene	216	200	—
1979	Bremen, Germany	Mill explosion	Flour	14	27	—
1980	Mandir Asad, India	Industrial accident	Explosives	50	—	—
	Barking, USA	Industrial fire	Cyanide/Sodium	0	12	—
1981	Tocaoa, Venezuela	Explosion	Oil	145	1000	—
1984	Sao Paulo, Brazil	Pipeline explosion	Petrol	508	—	—
	Bhopal, India	Leakage	Methyl isocyanate	>2500	>10,000	>3,00,000
	San Juanico, Mexico	Boiling liquid expanding vapor explosion (BLEVE)	Liquid petroleum	600	7000	—
1986	Chernobyl, USSR	Nuclear accident	Nuclear power	direct: 31	500	112,000

(Continued)

(Continued)

Year	Place	Cause	Product	Deaths	Injured	Evacuated
1987	Harbin, PR of China	Explosion	Flax	49	—	—
	Dkajakarta, Indonesia	Fire	Textile	30	—	—
	Pampa, USA	Explosion	Chemicals	31	Severe damage	
1988	North Sea	Fire	Oil exploration platform	166	—	—
1989	Pasadena, USA	Explosion	Petrochemicals	23	—	—
2000	Enschede, Netherlands	Explosion	Fireworks	22	947	—
2003	Fengchen, Jiangxi, PR of China	Gas explosion	Coal	49	7	—
2003	Wangkou, Hebei, PR of China	Explosion and fire	Fireworks	35	91	—
2005	Texas City, USA	Explosion and fire	Oil	15	100	—
2008	Seoul, Korea	Explosion and fire	Flammable goods	40	10	—
2008	Deeg, Rajasthan, India	Explosion and fire	Fireworks	25	16	—

Sources: OECD statistics; Swiss Reinsurance Company.

which overwhelms the day-to-day medical resources available in the workplace. In other words, the two criteria that define an industrial disaster are: (a) an event has occurred in the workplace in which there are sick or injured victims needing simultaneous attention, and (b) there is a serious discrepancy between the number needing treatment and the treatment capacity immediately available, so that outside help and reinforcements are necessary.

Uncertainty in Planning

A major problem with medical disaster planning is the shroud of uncertainty surrounding the disaster being planned for. For instance, it is not possible to predict the number of casualties that will be involved, which in turn determines the resources that need to be kept in readiness. The casualty load remains an unknown factor until the disaster has occurred. The best one can do is to paint possible scenarios and plan according to certain assumptions.

Then, there is the need to know the types of casualties likely to be encountered, which will vary from industry to industry. For instance, burn injuries can be expected in disasters involving fire and explosion, e.g. an oil refinery fire (see Case Study 3). Smoke in confined spaces, as in ships and warehouses, can cause inhalational injuries and gas poisoning. Collapse of building structures tend to produce external bodily injuries such as crushed limbs. Moreover, civilians living nearby may need to be evacuated if the disaster is complicated by the environmental release of a wide variety of hazardous substances (see Case Studies 3 and 4).

Case Study 3

On 12 December 1999, at 11.13 am, a spark ignited a vapor leak from an oil container at the 40-year-old Thai oil refinery (Fig. 2) in Laem Chabang, about 50 miles southeast of Bangkok. Seven people were killed and at least 15 injured when a huge storage container exploded. There were about 35 people on duty when the explosion occurred. Firefighters battled the blaze throughout the night but the fire persisted, sending thick

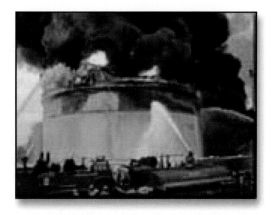

Fig. 2. Thai oil refinery fire in Laem Chabang, Thailand.

black smoke over the Gulf of Thailand. The fire spread from the first storage tank containing 1.5 million liters of fuel to three others containing 26 million liters of fuel. Four thousand residents living in the surrounding area had to be evacuated from their homes.

Case Study 4

On 12 February 1990, at approximately 1 am, a fire began in an outdoor storage area in Hagersville, Ontario, containing 14 million used tires. Arson was the suspected cause. The fire burned for 17 days, eventually consuming 12.6 million tires. This was the first tire fire of this magnitude in Canada and emergency response teams had to resort to trial and error in their efforts to combat it. Tire fires represent significant environmental problems due to the hazardous combustion products emitted into the air and ground, including benzene, toluene, xylene and oils. The environmental consequences of the Hagersville fire were severe, with considerable surface and groundwater contamination. Between 12,000 and 50,000 liters of oil were believed to have reached the water table. Soil contamination was limited to the burn area itself, but this still amounted to 11 acres, with an estimated 20,000 cubic meters of waste material. Due to the large amounts of air and water contamination during the fire, 1700 people were evacuated from a four-kilometer radius for 18 days.

Medical Planning for Industrial Disasters

Medical disaster planning cannot be done in isolation. Medical response plans are part of, and must therefore necessarily conform to, the overall disaster response plan for the particular industry, factory or workplace. Joint planning should be initiated at the senior management level. The planning team at the factory level is usually headed by someone senior and authoritative, who could be the plant's deputy general manager or the fire and safety manager. Members are drawn from the various departments involved in emergency rescue, firefighting, security, personnel, public relations, etc. The medical officer in charge of emergency medical response is invariably a member of this team.

While the exact timing, nature and extent of the disaster being prepared for cannot be known beforehand, disaster plans must nevertheless be clear and comprehensive enough, covering all anticipated actions that need to be taken upon activation, e.g. how to notify, mobilize and organize personnel resources, what command and control structure to adopt, and what communication channels would be used. Likewise, the medical plan must clearly state how key medical personnel are to be mobilized and recalled at short notice, spell out the respective roles of each member of the medical team, and detail how coordination is to be achieved with other teams and external agencies.

Plans should be tested, reviewed and updated on a regular basis. Regular meetings and frequent interactions between team members will ensure familiarity with each other's roles and requirements. In particular, command, control and coordination issues need to be ironed out beforehand. There should be flexibility to allow for the response to be stepped up in the event of escalating circumstances. Above all, the plan needs to be known and understood by everybody involved.

For completeness, the medical response plan should cover all stages of the disaster, i.e. before the event, during the event and after the event.

Pre-Disaster Activities

During this "quiet" phase, the responsibilities of various agencies and the lines of communication should be established and, once established, clearly made known to all. Specific steps should be taken to identify all available resources. Equipment and supplies need to be procured and pre-positioned at strategic sites.

Protective gear for medical rescue workers

There should be appropriate equipment at work sites to ensure the safety of rescue workers, including medical personnel. This should include safety helmets, safety boots, protective clothing against hazardous materials, and other items such as ear plugs, gloves and safety harnesses.

Medical equipment

Emergency medical equipment is best kept in clearly marked boxes that are both robust and portable. The contents should include splints, spinal supports, bandages and dressings and essential items such as airways, resuscitators and ventilators, and infusion sets. Stretchers and blankets should also be available.

Medical treatment area

Suitable sites should be pre-identified as possible medical treatment areas. These may be vacant lots, existing medical clinics or any areas that have good access to ambulance vehicles. The medical treatment area should be large enough for triage, i.e. sorting of patients according to clinical condition, and to accommodate treatment areas for severe, moderate and light casualties.

Communication equipment

Effective communication is a crucial aspect of any disaster response. Communication networks using equipment with compatible frequencies are essential, for coordination between medical teams and other rescue agencies. Walkie-talkies are very useful for medical personnel to communicate with each other. In addition, cellular phones and dedicated telephone lines can be used for direct communication between onsite medical teams and the hospitals.

Training of staff

All employees should be taught first aid and cardiopulmonary resuscitation. Medical staff should be trained in basic trauma life support skills. Ideally, all doctors should be trained to the level of advanced trauma life support (ATLS).

Troubleshooting

Always ask what can go wrong, where, and what the consequences of such problems are, especially in relation to specific hazards present in the workplace. Special consideration should be given to the danger of fire, explosion and toxic release, along with environmental damage. The possibility of floods, earthquakes and storms occurring concomitantly should not be ruled out. Moreover, each of the above may occur individually or in combination.

Disaster drills

Disaster drills are a must. Studies of many past disasters have found that in many instances, although disaster plans may have existed, they were not put into action, resulting in disorganization and even chaos when disaster struck. A recurring major theme was that key personnel did not fully understand the plan or their role in it.

Drills should be carried out at regular intervals, and in conjunction with other rescue agencies. They are extremely useful in showing up deficiencies either in the medical response plan or in the knowledge and skills of the staff. Often, only by going through the paces of a mock-up exercise can concepts not readily appreciated in the abstract — such as the effective management of limited space and time — be convincingly demonstrated.

The decisions made during the first few minutes of a disaster are crucial to the successful management and control of a disaster situation. It is therefore important that all personnel involved know when to activate a disaster response plan.

Activities During Disaster

Although the detailed circumstances may vary, the principles of medical management in a disaster, consisting of rescue, triage, stabilization and evacuation of casualties from the site, are generic and can be applied to all disaster situations.

Initial rescue

Upon activation, information about the nature of the disaster and a rough estimate of the number of casualties should be ascertained quickly. The medical team despatched to the site should report to an overall incident commander (usually a fire or safety officer). Care should be taken not to venture into any hazardous area unless cleared to do so. The freeing of injured persons from imminent danger should be left to personnel trained for such tasks. Although speed is important, care must be taken to ensure that aggravation of injuries does not occur during rescue.

The medical personnel on scene should make a quick assessment as to what additional help and resources are needed, and to communicate these requests as appropriate.

Activation of additional medical resources

Different countries have different systems of activating additional medical reinforcements. In Singapore, this is done either through the police (telephone 999) or the Singapore Civil Defence Force (995). In the event of a large-scale disaster, the medical resources of the armed forces are also activated.

Organization of disaster site

The disaster area is usually divided into three main zones. The police or security personnel should cordon off and establish an outer perimeter Safety Zone from which traffic is diverted. They should allow ambulances and authorized personnel to pass through designated entrances (and exits) into a second Inner Zone where rescue activities take place. This is where the medical First Aid Post should be, along with the command posts of the police, fire and other essential agencies. The First Aid Post should be located fairly close to, yet at a safe distance from, the exit of the third zone, which is the Danger Zone. The latter is a limited access zone because of the potential danger from fire, chemicals or smoke, and open only to specially equipped and trained personnel. Identification badges should be worn by rescue personnel to facilitate smooth access between zones.

The selection of the First Aid Post site is the medical officer's responsibility and should be done in consultation with the incident commander. The site should be clearly marked with signs. It should be large enough for subdivision into treatment sections for serious, moderate and light casualties. An ambulance assembly area should also be designated, distinct from the ambulance point for the loading of casualties.

Triage

Presented with multiple casualties requiring varying degrees of medical attention, it is important for the medical officer to be able to make a quick assessment and assign each casualty with an appropriate priority status for receiving treatment. This process, called "triage", is done not according to the severity of injuries but the immediacy of need for treatment, i.e. priority being given to those with life-threatening problems and who have the greatest chance of survival when given immediate treatment.

Singapore, along with many other countries, has adopted four triage categories as follows:

Priority I:
Serious casualties (tagged red) with life-threatening problems requiring immediate attention. Non-ambulant.

Priority II:
Moderate casualties (tagged yellow) requiring fairly urgent action. Non-ambulant.

Priority III:
Light casualties (tagged green). Minor injuries only. Ambulant.

Priority 0:
Dead casualties (tagged black).

Because casualties are passed from one person to another along the chain of care, the triage classification needs to be made known to others. Color-coded labels have been developed for this purpose. The color scheme in Table 2 has come about not by universally accepted convention but by common usage. In general, triage labels should be prominent and legible to medical personnel and stretcher bearers, easily secured to the casualty's body, and should allow for alterations to be made as the clinical condition changes.

Triage labels (see Fig. 3) designed by the American Civil Defense Association have gained popular usage in many countries. Because it has been endorsed by the International Civil Aviation Organization, these METTAG labels are used in many airports around the world. The labels are water-resistant and have a matching serial numbering system that allows for tracking of the casualty's movement and belongings throughout the various phases of evacuation and treatment.

Table 2.   Priority System of Triage

Color	Priority
Red	1
Yellow	2
Green	3
Black	0

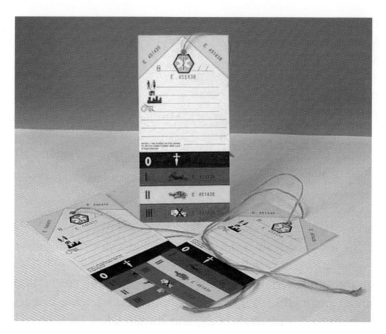

Fig. 3. METTAG triage labels designed and produced by the American Civil Defense Association.

Management of casualties

Given the urgency of the moment and the extremely stressful conditions typical of disasters, an instinctive knowledge of trauma life-support protocols, such as the "ABCs" advocated by the American College of Surgeons and the American College of Emergency Physicians, is indispensible. The priorities are:

A   Airway with cervical spine control
B   Breathing
C   Circulation
D   Disability assessment including neurological status
E   Exposure (undress the patient but prevent hypothermia)

It is outside the scope of this chapter to go into the techniques of emergency resuscitation and care of the trauma patient; but suffice to say, the more rapidly, efficiently and systematically the stabilization of casualties is carried out, the greater will be the chances of their survival.

Casualty evacuation

Two considerations should be maintained during casualty evacuation — the safety of the patient and the speed of transport.

Safety considerations require the continuous and uninterrupted care of the casualty during transportation. Trained nurses or paramedics in the ambulance should ensure that intravenous lines, catheters and tubes are all well anchored to the patient. There should be enough oxygen and intravenous fluids available for the duration of the trip.

Because the patient may deteriorate en route and require emergency resuscitation, there should ideally be no more than one Priority I casualty transported in an ambulance at any one time. Priority I casualties are most likely to run into complications en route to hospital. An ambulance officer cannot effectively deal with more than one resuscitation case in the cramped space of a vehicle.

The assistance of traffic policemen may be required to help clear the way. Do not underestimate the number of curious onlookers and motorists who may jam the exit roads. Police outriders may even be able to facilitate smooth passage past traffic lights.

In such circumstances, the availability of helicopters would of course be a boon; but smooth execution of "heli-casevac" requires both special skills and adherence to special procedures — thus emphasizing the need for prior planning, training and coordination with other agencies, such as the military.

Post-Disaster Activities

Forensic teams will have to carry out the arduous task of identification of remains.

Not to be forgotten is the psychological component of disasters. In the recent few decades, disaster managers have come to appreciate the widespread occurrence of psychological stress following disasters. Disaster victims, their relatives and rescue personnel are equally vulnerable.

Occupational physicians are in a good position to spot and manage post-traumatic stress disorder early, before they progress to chronic mental disability.

Follow-up should include psychological debriefing and counseling sessions. Some may require longer-term psychiatric follow-up. In addition to professional psychological support, the emotional support of family members, friends and social workers should also be encouraged.

A "business" debriefing session should also be conducted with all key personnel involved in the rescue operation soon after the event. The aim is to exhaustively review the actions taken during the disaster with a view to identifying procedural lapses and recommending improvements to the disaster response plan.

The occupational physician can help to identify the human factors and occupational safety lapses contributing to the disaster. Industrial disasters, unlike earthquakes and volcano eruptions, are not entirely "random" events that seemingly just happen; they are caused. Post-disaster investigations of the Bhopal disaster, for example, revealed that the workers had reported prodromal leaks, exposures and maintenance problems but these were not taken seriously. It goes to show that a weak emphasis on workplace health and safety, and a lack of disaster preparedness, together make a sure recipe for disaster to occur — or, for that matter, to recur!

Conclusion

Disasters are by their very nature unpredictable, it is nevertheless possible to plan for them. Although they are by definition characterized by chaos and confusion, the greater the degree of pre-disaster planning and organization, the higher will be the chances of bringing order to an otherwise uncontrollable situation. The aim is always to plan in such a way that when an emergency arises, a swift and effective response can be mounted to contain or minimize the effects of the incident, and to restore normality as soon as possible.

But ultimately, of course, every disaster will present with its own unique set of problems and therefore no single plan, or even multiple plans, can possibly provide all the answers to all possible situations. Hence, the occupational physician responding to an industrial disaster situation must exercise leadership, clear thinking and adapt under the most trying of circumstances. He can best do this if he is sufficiently prepared.

References

American College of Surgeons. (1997) *ATLS: Advanced Trauma Life Support for Doctors.*

Gunn SWA. (1990) *Multilingual Dictionary of Disaster and International Relief.* The Netherlands: Kluwer Academic Publishers.

Kelly RB. (1989) *Industrial Emergency Preparedness.* New York: Van Nostrand Reinhold.

Auf der Heide E. (1989) *Disaster Response: Principles of Preparation and Coordination.* St. Louis: CV Mosby Company.

Chapter 22

Aviation and Diving Medicine

Gregory Chan* and Wee-Tong Ng[†,‡]

Humans, in pursuance of expanding areas for activity, have entered foreign and hostile environments such as seas and aerospace. In doing so, they have come under various biological, physical and psychological stresses of unconventional nature, which need to be endured. The application of medical knowledge to study the interaction between such environments and humans and to further promote the diagnosis, treatment and prevention of disorders formulate the two themes discussed together in this chapter: aviation medicine and diving medicine.

Aviation medicine is also called flight medicine and aerospace medicine; diving medicine is also called undersea medicine. Both are considered subfields of the preventive specialty of occupational and environmental medicine but are sometimes associated with emergency medicine, as in the case of decompression sickness which is related to both themes. Indeed, both themes share wide commonalities in involving pressure excursions, operational changes in body attitude and position, controlled breathing sources, and critical dependence on supportive mechanisms and protective equipment.

---

*Division of Occupational Health, Senior Occupational Health Physician and Dive Control Officer, Office of Safety, Health and Environment, National University of Singapore.
†Department of Geriatric Medicine, Singapore Aeromedical Centre.
‡Corresponding author. E-mail: wtng@pacific.net.sg

Consequently, the two themes are often discussed together in textbooks and even combined in the names of professional organizations, e.g. "Danish Society of Aviation and Diving Medicine".

Aviation Medicine

Introduction

Man was not born to fly. The aviation environment is foreign to the evolution of normal human physiology and our sense mechanisms, especially those senses involved in proprioception and our orientation to the world around us. Hence, the basic aviation environment, though the natural habitat for birds, is by nature hazardous to the human body, as it never evolved to adapt to that environment.

Although aviation is only barely over a hundred years old, the pace of progress in the last century has resulted in high-technology aircraft that paradoxically increase the hazards to the pilot. This is especially true for military pilots, where current and next-generation combat aircraft continue to stress the limits of human physiology.

Aviation medicine is a specialized subset of occupational medicine that manages the issues associated with flight and the flight environment. The specialty encompasses all aspects of aviation, from private pilots, ballooning and gliders to commercial and military aviation. Within these various forms of aviation, the spectrum of care ranges from the management of occupational disease and aviation physiology training for aircrew to fitness to fly assessments.

The practice of aviation medicine requires an understanding of the aviation environment, the hazards associated with flight, human physiology at altitude and the different job and task requirements of the various forms of aviation. In this respect, the approach taken in aviation medicine is no different from the practice of mainstream occupational medicine, where the medical practitioner requires a working knowledge of the worker's job demands, environment and hazards, and then correlates this with the health of the worker.

Case Study 1

A 26-year-old pilot of a private jet plane was cruising at 28000 feet (8534 meters) when he realized he was feeling a little dizzy and breathing faster than usual. He rapidly scanned his instruments and discovered that the cabin pressure had risen to almost 18000 feet (5486 meters), from the normal 6000 feet (1829 meters). He quickly descended the aircraft to below 10000 feet (3048 meters) where he made further checks which indicated that the aircraft cabin pressurization system was faulty.

What the pilot was experiencing were the insidious effects of hypoxia. Had the pilot not been alert to the situation and recognized the imminent danger, he would have eventually lost consciousness and become comatose. Constant education and demonstrations of the effects of hypoxia to pilots are the mainstays in the prevention of hypoxic incidents, when aircraft oxygenation or pressurization systems fail.

Case Study 2

A 22-year old trainee fighter pilot was completing a training flight with an instructor. As he descended from 25000 feet (7620 meters), he felt an intense pain over his cheeks. The pain was so severe that he handed control of the aircraft to his instructor. As the aircraft descended further, the pain increased until he felt a sharp tearing sensation across his cheeks. The pain then subsided and he felt a warm sensation in his oxygen mask. Taking the mask off, he saw that there was blood pouring out from his nose and it had accumulated in his mask. The instructor landed the aircraft quickly and the trainee was sent to the medical center.

The pilot trainee had developed a cough and rhinitis two days prior to the flight. However, he self-medicated on the morning of the flight to stop the rhinitis. Although he had symptomatic relief, his upper respiratory tract infection (URTI) had caused swelling of the mucosa around the outlets of the maxillary sinus. During descent, the closed cavities of the maxillary sinuses could not equalize with the external environment, hence the resultant air volume contraction on descent caused a pressure gradient which resulted in the eventual rupture and tearing of the mucosal membrane of the maxillary sinuses. The pilot would be grounded for 3–6 months to allow the sinus membranes to heal.

Pilots and aircrew need to be educated on the dangers of flying with an URTI or other inter-current illnesses. They should seek medical attention upon feeling unwell and should not self-medicate if they intend to fly.

Hazards and Effects of the Aviation Environment

Low-pressure environment and the onset of hypoxia

Hypoxia, due to the effect of altitude, is the result of a reduction in oxygen tension (partial pressure of oxygen) at the point of inspiration. The pressure exerted at sea level by the weight of the atmosphere is 760 mmHg. This pressure decreases as the altitude increases. The concentration of oxygen in the environment is constant (20.9%) up to about 100,000 feet (30,480 meters) of altitude. Thus, at sea level, the partial pressure of oxygen at the point of inspiration, at the level of the trachea, is equal to 149 mmHg ($0.209 \times (760 - 47)$), where the 47 mmHg constant represents the contribution of water vapor. Therefore, hypoxia occurs at altitude due to a *decrease in atmospheric pressure* as altitude increases, since the concentration of oxygen and the contribution of water vapor do not change with increasing altitude up to 100,000 feet.

The effects of acute hypoxia can be insidious, manifesting mildly at lower altitudes (below 10,000 feet or 3048 meters) as impairment of night vision, narrowing of peripheral vision and mild psychomotor and memory impairment. At higher altitudes, the physical, psychomotor and cognitive effects are greater, resulting in personality changes, loss of judgment and decision-making capabilities, euphoria, sensory loss, muscular incoordination and cyanosis. There is also the natural physiological effect of concurrent hyperventilation due to the hypoxia, resulting in dizziness, neuromuscular irritability, paresthesia and carpopedal spasms. When the hypoxia becomes severe, loss of consciousness and death will result.

Hypoxia is prevented by either aircraft cabin pressurization or the provision of oxygen via a well-fitted mask, utilized singularly or in combination. Cabin pressurization creates a pressure gradient between the cabin and the external environment, thus the pilot, crew and passengers will experience a pressure as close to sea level as possible. Providing oxygen changes the inhaled oxygen concentration from 20.9% to any value up to 100%. However, although high oxygen values are used in certain circumstances, extended exposure to oxygen concentrations above 40% is not recommended due to the risk of oxygen toxicity and the resultant damage to the lungs.

Commercial airliners utilize cabin pressurization as the primary strategy against hypoxia, successfully designing cabins to be pressurized such that the occupants are exposed to only the equivalent at 5000–8000 feet (1524–2438 meters) in the cabin when the true altitude is over 30,000 feet (9144 meters). Oxygen is available and this is provided in the form of emergency oxygen systems that drop masks from the ceiling of the cabin, should the cabin pressurization be compromised.

Military fighter aircraft cannot be pressurized to this extent due to combat performance reasons and thus most fighter aircraft will have a cabin pressure equivalent to exposure at an altitude of 18,000–20,000 feet (5486–6096 meters) when the aircraft is over 30,000 feet (9144 meters). Therefore, military fighter pilots will wear an oxygen mask at all times to increase the oxygen concentration and hence the oxygen tension at the point of inspiration.

The vast majority of helicopters implement neither cabin pressurization nor the provision of oxygen. Therefore, helicopters often have an operational ceiling under 10,000 feet (3048 meters), to minimize the effects of hypoxia.

Pilots and aircrew are often trained, in a hypobaric chamber, to experience and recognize the onset of hypoxia. In this setting, the training session is often videotaped to demonstrate to the trainee the cognitive and coordination dysfunction when hypoxic.

Sub-atmospheric pressure changes and decompression sickness (DCS)

Although the clinical syndrome of decompression sickness in divers and compressed air workers (Caisson disease) was recognized in the 1850s, it was not until the advent of high-altitude flight in the 1930s that it was described in the aviation environment.

During ascent, as previously mentioned, the atmospheric pressure decreases. Thus the partial pressure exerted by the various component gases will also decrease in tandem. In the case of DCS, the gas of interest is nitrogen.

At ground level, the tissues and blood of the human body contain dissolved nitrogen. The partial pressure of this nitrogen in the human body is equal to that of the nitrogen in inspired air. During ascent, the fall in the partial pressure causes the body tissues to release the nitrogen into the blood, for excretion via the lungs. However, as the solubility of nitrogen in blood is low, the rate of fall of the absolute pressure in the tissues is greater than the rate of fall of the partial pressure of nitrogen in those tissues. Thus, the tissues become supersaturated with nitrogen. This supersaturation of the tissues will eventually give rise to the formation of nitrogen bubbles within the tissues. It is this formation of nitrogen bubbles in the tissues or the embolism of these bubbles to other tissues that result in the clinical syndrome of DCS.

DCS can manifest as joint pain ("bends"), skin disturbances (itching, tingling, "creeps"), respiratory disturbances (tightness of chest, difficulty taking breaths, "chokes"), neurological disturbances (paresthesia, convulsions, "staggers"), visual disturbances (blurring, scotomata, hemianopia) and ultimately cardiovascular collapse.

A decrease in the altitude will usually result in rapid recovery and amelioration of the symptoms. Severe cases may require hyperbaric compression treatment but this is uncommon as the severity of sub-atmospheric DCS is often less than that of compressed air DCS.

Sub-atmospheric DCS does not occur below an altitude of 18,000 feet (5486 meters). The incidence below 22,500 feet (6858 meters) is extremely low, with DCS becoming a significant threat only above 22,500 feet. The risk of DCS for passengers in commercial airliners is non-existent, as the cabin pressure is kept at 5000–8000 feet (1524–2438 meters), but for one important exception. A passenger who has exposed himself to pressures greater than 1 bar (diving or compressed air workers) in the preceding 24 hours can develop DCS symptoms on a commercial flight, even though the cabin altitude is only 5000–8000 feet. High-altitude ballooning and military aircraft at high altitudes are the other groups at risk of DCS.

Other personal factors that increase the risk of DCS include increasing age, obesity, recent joint injury, infection, inter-current illness and a previous episode of DCS.

DCS is prevented primarily through cabin pressurization. As long as cabin pressure can be maintained at less than 18,000 feet (5486 meters), then the risk of DCS is considerably diminished. However, if prolonged exposure to high altitudes is unavoidable, the principal method of prevention is through the inspiration of 100% oxygen. Pure oxygen is administered for an hour pre-flight to wash out the body's nitrogen. The protocols for the pre-administration of 100% oxygen are customized according to the differing needs of the various aircraft and flight profiles. The common users of this strategy are high-altitude parachutists, pilots of special military aircraft and astronauts.

Pressure change and barotrauma

Boyle's law explains that the relationship between pressure and volume is inverse. Hence, as pressure falls, the volume (of air) increases and vice versa. During aircraft ascent, as the altitude increases, the atmospheric pressure falls and therefore the air volume in the cavities of the human body will increase. The converse is also true; as the altitude decreases, during descent, the atmospheric pressure increases and the air volume in the cavities will decrease. In the human body, the impact of this air volume change is important in the closed or semi-closed cavities, namely the lungs, middle ear, paranasal sinuses and the gastrointestinal tract.

In the lung, the elasticity of lung tissue and the size of the tracheal lumen allow free exchange of air from the lungs. Therefore, when the air volume in the lung changes, during ascent or descent, it is rapidly equalized with the external environment. The exception occurs when a closed glottis (e.g. during breath-holding) is combined with sudden extreme volume changes. This can occur during rapid decompression of a pressurized cabin. If the cabin of a passenger airliner is compromised during high-altitude cruising flight, the cabin altitude of 5000–8000 feet (1524–2435 meters) will rapidly equalize with the real altitude of 30,000 feet (9144 meters); in effect, a rapid ascent of 22,000–25,000 feet (6709–7620 meters). If a passenger closes his glottis during this event, and the rapid lung expansion exceeds his normal total lung volume, this will result in barotrauma to the lung. Lung tissue and blood vessels will tear, resulting in surgical emphysema, hemothorax and generalized gas embolism as air enters the torn blood vessels.

The middle ear communicates with the external atmosphere by way of the Eustachian tube, which opens into the nasopharyngeal space. The Eustachian tube is a passive one-way valve, so during ascent, as volume increases, the air equalizes passively through the tube. However, during descent, as the air volume in the middle ear decreases, the Eustachian tube remains closed and does not passively allow air to flow back to the middle ear. Therefore, the Eustachian tube must be actively forced opened in this instance via swallowing, yawning or the deliberate act of a Valsalva or Frenzel manoeuvre. If the Eustachian tube is blocked, due to disease or illness, e.g. an upper respiratory tract infection, the tympanic membrane will become distorted and will eventually rupture either during ascent or descent.

The paranasal sinuses are small cavities, situated in the bones of the face and skull. They drain into the nose either via ducts or directly by a hole in the wall of the sinus. Barotrauma to the sinuses occurs more often during descent, usually due to mucosal inflammation secondary to illness or infection, which results in blockage of the duct or drainage hole. The resulting inability to equilibrate air volumes during descent leads to intense pain and eventual tearing and damage of the mucosal lining of the sinus wall, with resultant hemorrhage into the sinus cavity.

Barotrauma, resulting in visceral damage to the gastrointestinal tract, as a result of air volume expansion or contraction, has not been described in the literature. The commonest symptoms occur during ascent as air volume increases. If this air is not vented via the mouth or anus, a sensation of abdominal fullness and mild abdominal discomfort may occur. Severe pain is extremely rare. With experience, frequent flyers will avoid gas-forming foodstuffs (e.g. peas, beans, carbonated drinks) which can exacerbate the discomfort.

Severe pain in the teeth has been described during ascent (aerodontalgia). This is due to the expansion of air that is trapped between the tooth substance and a deep cavity filling. This was seen with the older generation of dental fillings and aerodontalgia is now rarely experienced with modern dental materials and methods.

Temperature and hypothermia

The ambient temperature varies according to the altitude. From sea level to approximately 58,000 feet over the equator, the fall in temperature during ascent is linear, from +15°C to −53°C at a lapse rate of 2°C every 1000 feet (304.8 meters). Thus, hypothermia can occur with unprotected exposure to altitude. Most aircraft implement cabin-conditioning systems to maintain the temperature in the cabin at homeostatic levels. Helicopters rarely traverse over 10,000 feet (3048 meters) for engineering reasons as well as reasons of hypoxia. Thus, the main groups at risk are high-altitude ballooning enthusiasts and parachutists. Appropriate clothing and warming attire is often worn by these groups to prevent hypothermia.

Ozone and pulmonary edema

Ozone exists in the Earth's atmosphere as a band, called the ozonosphere, which stretches from 40,000 feet (12,192 meters or 12.2 kilometers) to 140,000 feet (42,672 meters or 42.7 kilometers). Ozone is a strong oxidant and, when inhaled at a sufficient concentration, causes pulmonary edema. If the concentration is high enough, the resultant pulmonary edema can be fatal. As ozone is only present above 40,000 feet, the only passenger aircraft at risk was the Concorde, which routinely flew at supersonic speeds at altitudes of 50,000 to 60,000 feet (15.2 to 18.3 kilometers). Special filters were installed in the aircraft to break down ozone before it entered the cabin. The entire Concorde fleet was retired in 2003 after 27 years of service and at present there are no commercial aircraft that operate at those altitudes.

Cosmic radiation

At sea level, the effect of cosmic radiation is mitigated due to collision and degradation of protons, electrons and neutrons with atmospheric molecules. At higher altitudes, this degradation effect is lessened and the levels of cosmic radiation are higher. It is estimated that commercial aircrew receive a dose not exceeding 6 mSv per year, which is within the maximum allowable dose for radiation workers (20 mSv/year). These studies were conducted on the Concorde, which flew higher than other airliners. Thus, it is expected that the cosmic radiation doses experienced on normal commercial aircraft are even lower.

Other Important Hazards

High-performance aircraft, G-force and G-induced loss of consciousness (G-LOC)

High-performance aircraft, such as military fighter aircraft and hyper-agile stunt aircraft, function in a three-dimensional space. Therefore, the human body, during high-performance flights, will experience acceleration in all three axes. By convention, this acceleration is termed "G", which is a multiple of the acceleration due to the force of gravity ("g") which equals 9.8 ms^{-2}. Therefore, if a pilot is described to have experienced 3 G, it implies that his body had experienced acceleration of 29.4 ms^{-2}. This acceleration is experienced in three axes, which is conventionally denoted as G_x, G_y and G_z with a plus or minus sign in front to denote the direction of the acceleration.

In aviation, the accelerative force of concern is $+G_z$. The direction of this accelerative force is such that it causes blood to draw away from the brain and towards the feet. Therefore, when the $+G_z$ forces are high enough to overcome the blood pressure in the brain, the brain will experience no blood flow, which will result in a loss of consciousness. This phenomenon is termed G-induced loss of consciousness (G-LOC). This is clearly a hazard as sudden incapacitation of the pilot will lead to loss of control and probable eventual loss of aircraft and pilot.

There are three principal strategies for combating G-LOC. The first is via engineering efforts on the aircraft itself, to integrate a pilot seat with an optimal seat angle, to reduce the effect of $+G_z$ acceleration. The second is by wearing a G-suit, a special suit composed of numerous air bladders. The inflation mechanism is integrated into the aircraft, with automatic inflation of the bladders as $+G_z$ increases during certain air manoeuvres. These bladders compress against the legs, to prevent pooling of blood. The third method is by the execution of an anti-G straining manoeuvre (AGSM), a special modified Valsalva effort against a closed glottis. The AGSM increases the intrathoracic pressure which translates into an increase in the blood pressure to the brain. The AGSM is the most effective method to prevent G-LOC at high $+G_z$ exposures. However, it must be actively taught to the pilots and the technique checked periodically to ensure compliance and correct execution.

Spatial disorientation

The human system of orientation depends on three organs: the eyes, the vestibular system (saccule, utricle and the semi-circular canals) and the organs of proprioception. Of these three, the eyes are the most powerful, with the visual cues able to override conflicting vestibular and proprioceptive cues. However, the aviation environment is able to degrade, confuse and mislead these three organs of orientation. With night, fog or snow, visibility can be degraded to such an extent to obviate any visual cues. The human vestibular and proprioceptive systems are conditioned to function at normal gravity, i.e. 1 G. Under the influence of high G forces, these two systems may mislead the brain with regards to the body's true position in the air.

Through a combination of the many factors in aviation that can degrade the human system of orientation, there are hundreds of illusions and phenomenon that are described in which the perceived orientation is erroneous. Spatial disorientation is a major cause of aircraft incidents and accidents and thus its prevention is important to aviation safety.

Spatial disorientation is prevented primarily through education. Pilots are taught the mechanics of various common illusions and the principles behind the weaknesses of our orientation mechanisms in the aviation environment. The common illusions can also be demonstrated in a spatial disorientation trainer, a special simulator that can replicate certain illusions. Lastly, aircraft systems are designed to compensate for some of these illusions, warning the pilot when certain aircraft parameters, which may lead to unsafe flight conditions, are met.

Fitness to Fly

In the early days of aviation, the principal cause of air accidents was design defects or engineering lapses. However, as the aviation industry matured and tackled these issues, aircraft became much safer and the main cause of mishaps became human error. Incapacitation or mishap due to a medical condition is part of the causal chain attributed to human error.

Fitness to fly for pilots and aircrew is governed by two broad principles, that of flight safety and performance. Flight safety refers to the ability to conduct flight operations in a manner that does not put at risk the aircraft or its occupants. The ability to fly an aircraft and manage its on-board systems is degraded by illness, injury, physical and mental incapacitation. Performance refers to the ability to execute an assigned task with the aircraft to the highest capability of the pilot. Both flight safety and performance are usually closely intertwined in the basic assigned task. For example, the basic task in civil aviation is to fly an aircraft, carrying passengers or cargo, from one destination to another. The pilot is expected to complete this assigned task without accident or mishap. Performance may be determined or measured by punctuality of the flight, avoidance of turbulence to increase passenger comfort and a smooth landing. In the military, the pilot's task is complicated by the concept of aerial combat, where there is an adversary whose purpose is to destroy your aircraft. The performance of the military pilot is not just to maintain safe flight operations, but to conduct air combat with the aim of destroying enemy aircraft or targets, without loss of his own aircraft or life.

The workload of a pilot in a complex modern cockpit is high. This complexity is accentuated in the military cockpit where the aircraft is extremely agile and there are additional demands such as weapon management, electronic countermeasures and life support systems. Thus, even minor ailments and symptoms may cause a dramatic reduction in the capability of the pilot to function adequately. Seemingly minor complaints such as a mild abdominal discomfort or headache can have profound effects on flight performance and safety, as the cognition and workload capacity of an individual degrades markedly if distracted by pain or discomfiture.

Hence, all inter-current illness, injury and prescribed medication are assessed for flight fitness, with both safety and performance as the guiding parameters. If a condition or its attendant treatment results in physical or mental degradation, e.g. sedation, fatigue, blurring of vision, nausea, headache, etc, then the pilot or aircrew will be deemed unfit for flight operations and will be grounded for the appropriate duration. In certain circumstances, where the risk of incapacitation is low, the pilot may be allowed to fly under restriction, e.g. to fly as a co-pilot only, with another qualified pilot.

Diving Medicine

Introduction

Occupational divers work in a unique environment. Its "uniqueness" is twofold. First, the working environment is underwater; and second, the environment is hyperbaric. Man was not created to exist naturally in such environments. For this reason, occupational diving is considered highly hazardous work.

Types of Occupational Divers*

The various categories of occupational divers are listed below.

Construction divers

Construction diving is the most common form of occupational diving, and regarded as the most dangerous. It includes any work involving the inspection, construction, maintenance, repair, alteration, demolition and removal of any structure, wall or building. The work can be conducted in any water body such as a canal, harbor, drainage system, river, dam, pipeline or reservoir; work can be done on a ship, raft, wreck, buoy or any obstruction to in-water navigation.

Military, police and search and rescue divers

This group of divers is sometimes classified together with construction divers because of the highly hazardous nature of their diving work. Their work is specialized with specific in-water tasks such as explosive ordnance and military actions (Fig. 1). They may also conduct construction diving activities involving military or coastal police vessels.

Aquaculture divers

Fish, shellfish and aquatic plant farms will engage aquaculture divers. These divers are involved in the growth and harvesting activities. Fishermen divers used to exist in the past and were well-known to have suffered decompression sickness, but they have since been replaced by better diving technology. These aquaculture divers may also conduct underwater maintenance and repair work without the conduct of any construction diving activities.

---

* Adapted from "Guidelines for Occupational Diving 2004" published by the Departement of Labour, Wellington New Zealand.

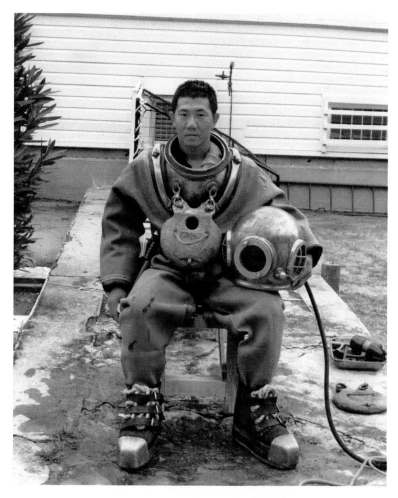

Fig. 1.   Naval mine clearance diver.

Research divers

Research or scientific diving is undertaken by researchers who conduct scientific activities pertaining to the underwater environment. The spectrum of research diving activities includes inspection, deployment of scientific equipment, collection of specimens or data, maintenance and retrieval of scientific equipment. These research divers are usually part of a research, educational or conservation facility. There is no conduct of any construction diving activities.

Recreational dive instructors

These divers instruct and supervise recreational divers as well as those who are learning the various skill sets for diving. They comprise instructors, divemasters and dive controllers.

Photographic divers

These divers conduct filming and photographic activities underwater.

Tourism divers

Tourism divers bring diver tourists on a guided tour underwater. This may be in the open sea or within the confines of an aquarium.

Risks Associated with Occupational Diving

The inherent risks associated with diving arise because man is not meant to exist underwater. The human physiology relies on a living environment where man breathes air (not just oxygen) at atmospheric pressure (sea level). Only a few medical conditions related to diving are described briefly in this section while the potential injuries arising from such work have been omitted.

Changes in the environmental pressure

When a diver is in the water, he is weightless. But there is the pressure of the water column acting upon him in addition to the 1 atmospheric pressure (or 1 bar) at sea level. The additional pressure is known as hydrostatic pressure and increases by approximately 1 bar for every depth of 10 meters of water.

Barotrauma

The air-filled organs within our bodies are affected by changes in pressure (in accordance with Boyle's law). As pressure increases (as in during descent into the water), the volume of the air decreases provided the temperature remains constant. Conversely, as pressure decreases (during ascent towards the surface), the volume of air increases. Simply put:

$$\text{Pressure } 1 \times \text{Volume } 1 = \text{Pressure } 2 \times \text{Volume } 2 = \text{Pressure } 3 \times \text{Volume } 3$$

The types of air-filled organs include the lungs, external and middle ear, sinuses, gut and dental caries. Injuries occurring as a consequence of pressure changes are known as barotraumas. They are described as barotraumas of descent or ascent, depending on when the injury occurs.

The symptoms of barotraumas also depend on the organ affected as well as the presence of complications. The most common barotrauma is that of the middle ear when the Eustachian tube becomes blocked for various reasons.

The most dangerous type of barotrauma is that of the lungs. Barotrauma of the lungs can have three complications: cerebral air-gas embolism, pneumothorax and subcutaneous/mediastinal emphysema. Lung barotrauma can result because of breath-holding during a rapid ascent. Its symptoms are rapid, occurring within minutes upon reaching the surface, and include sudden loss of consciousness, localized muscle weakness and sensory deficits. Definitive treatment is by recompression treatment and hyperbaric oxygen therapy.

Case Study 3

A young tourism diver presented with right-sided hemiplegia with right facial weakness almost immediately after breaking the surface. He had been showing some diver tourists the marine life at the diving resort when one of the tourists dropped her camera. The tourist went to retrieve her camera but got into a bit of a problem and panicked. He rushed to help the struggling tourist and had to manually haul her to the surface from a depth of approximately 8 meters. He lost consciousness at the surface and awoke with right-sided weakness. He was managed by the neurologist at the hospital on the presumptive diagnosis of a cerebrovascular accident with little improvement. The diver's employer requested a diving physician's assessment. He was treated in the recompression chamber urgently with marked improvement almost immediately. The diagnosis was that of pulmonary barotrauma with cerebral air-gas embolism.

Decompression sickness (DCS)

Another pressure-related disorder is known as decompression sickness (DCS). It is also known by other names such as the "bends" or Caisson disease.

Henry's law states that the amount of any given gas that will dissolve in a liquid at a given temperature is a function of the partial pressure of the gas that is in contact with the liquid and the solubility coefficient of the gas in the particular liquid. As a large percentage of the human body is water, more gas will dissolve in the blood and body tissues as depth increases, until the point of saturation is reached. Air, being made up of about 79% nitrogen and 21% oxygen, will continue to dissolve in the body as the diver descends until the point of saturation. The amount of nitrogen dissolved is referred to as the nitrogen load, and the nitrogen loading will depend on the depth and duration of the dive.

As the diver ascends, nitrogen will gradually return from its dissolved state to the gaseous state. When enough of these bubbles form, they can affect various organ systems within the body, causing a range of symptoms by mechanical disruption of the tissue functions or via secondary inflammatory pathways. Decompression sickness can be classically described as Type 1 (painful joints or "bends" and skin manifestations) or Type 2 (central and peripheral nerve disorders, cardio-respiratory system). There may also be a delayed presentation in the long bones known as dysbaric osteonecrosis that can present at least six months later.

The risk factors include that pertaining to the dive profile (repetitiveness, depth, duration, dive pattern), the type of gas used (enriched air has a theoretically reduced risk for the same dive) and the individual medical status (gross obesity, previous injuries, right-to-left shunts in the heart and previous decompression sickness have all been described to promote risk). The treatment of decompression sickness is by recompression and hyperbaric oxygen therapy (Figs. 2 and 3).

Case Study 4

A young researcher presented with fatigue, lapses in memory and inability to concentrate. She had just completed an intensive week of diving, collecting coral samples and recording data, as she rushed to meet her research project timelines. She did not consider the possibility of decompression sickness as her dives were shallow (less than 15

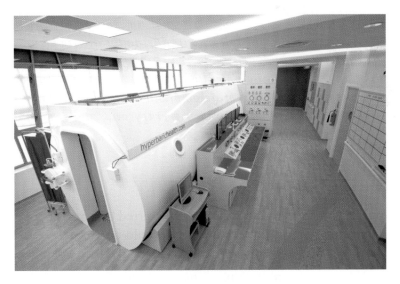

Fig. 2.   Recompression chamber facility.

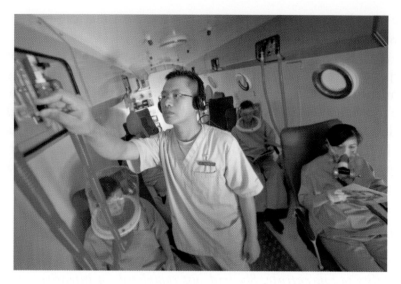

Fig. 3.   Hyperbaric nurse in the recompression chamber during hyperbaric oxygen therapy.

meters). Upon evaluation, the dive profile was consistently about 10–12 meters at the deepest and she would stay in excess of two hours at a go. She also made multiple ascents during the dive to bring samples or equipment, and she made repetitive dives, averaging three dives per day. She was also noted to be grossly overweight. In view of the risk factors, a diagnosis of decompression sickness was made. She was treated with hyperbaric oxygen therapy and made a complete recovery.

Changes in partial pressure of gas used

Dalton's law states that the total pressure exerted by a mixture of gases is equal to the sum of the pressures that would be exerted by each of the gases if it alone were present and occupied the total volume.

$$P_{Total} = Pp_1 + Pp_2 + \cdots + Pp_n$$

where *Pp* denotes the partial pressure of the particular gas component.

In a gas mixture, the portion of the total pressure contributed by a single gas is called the partial pressure of that gas. The two primary components of air are nitrogen and oxygen.

Nitrogen narcosis

A high concentration of nitrogen present in our bodies has a narcotic effect on our central nervous system. A number of diving fatalities have been attributed to nitrogen narcosis. This clinical syndrome occurs frequently at depths beyond 35 meters, but it is readily reversible. Some effects include impairment of reasoning, judgment, memory, concentration, attention, loss of coordination and hallucination. It has sometimes been described as the "rapture of the deep". Some individual factors increase the likelihood of nitrogen narcosis, including anxiety, inexperience, alcohol consumption, fatigue, cold water and carbon dioxide retention. One can develop tolerance with frequent exposure to a particular depth.

Oxygen toxicity

Some divers use enriched air (with higher partial pressures of oxygen) or even pure oxygen in the course of their work. Oxygen breathed at partial pressures of more than 1.6 atmospheric pressure places the diver at significant risk of oxygen toxicity affecting the central nervous system. The symptoms are wide-ranging and include dizziness, nausea, twitching, agitation, disorientation, hearing loss and convulsion. It has been said that the risk of oxygen toxicity increases with the oxygen partial pressure used, exposure time, exercise, cold and carbon dioxide retention.

Toxicities arising from other gases used, such as carbon dioxide and helium, can also occur.

Hazards of the water environment

The underwater environment comes with its own set of physical challenges. For instance, marine life can be pretty to look at but there are numerous dangerous marine animals that can cut, sting or poison the unsuspecting diver. The diver can also be subjected to aspiration and hypothermia.

Near drowning

Near drowning occurs when there is aspiration of water into the lungs. Hypoxemia can develop and may result in acute respiratory distress syndrome, hypoxic brain damage, cardiac arrhythmias, electrolyte disturbances and multi-organ failure. The early clinical presentation includes dyspnea, blood-stained frothy sputum, tachypnoea and cyanosis. Recovery is usually complete, and some cases have been known to survive even with 15–45 minutes of immersion. Thus, resuscitation for drowning cases must always be attempted.

Hypothermia

Hypothermia is a medical condition in which the body loses significant heat to disrupt normal bodily functions, and occurs when divers dive in waters colder than body temperature for an extended time period. The effects of hypothermia vary between divers and are influenced by individual factors (e.g. body fat, cold adaptability and type of insulation used) and the work environment (e.g. type of activity, water temperature and duration of exposure).

Hypothermia is broadly classified into three groups based on the core temperature of the body:

- Mild hypothermia (35–33°C): shivering, fatigue and loss of dexterity;
- Moderate hypothermia (33–30°C): less shivering, muscle weakness and confusion;
- Severe hypothermia (less than 30°C): no shivering, increased muscle stiffness, loss of consciousness and no apparent vital signs.

The lethal lower limit of core temperature in humans is 23–25°C. Prevention of hypothermia during diving is possible with appropriate insulation and adequate fluids to ensure good hydration.

Diving Techniques

Occupational divers can use a variety of diving techniques and breathing gases in the course of their work. The choice of breathing apparatus and the gases used depends on the nature of work, the need for mobility, the time period required to complete the work and the depth of the dive. It also depends on the diving support available such as access to medical care, recompression chambers and live-in chambers for deep saturation dives.

The divers may do breath-hold diving (or skin diving) whereby no specialized equipment is used. Historically, female Japanese ama divers used breath-hold diving to retrieve shellfish and some still do today. The self-contained underwater breathing apparatus (SCUBA) used in diving ranges from the common open-circuit types to semi-closed and closed rebreathing circuits used by technical divers. In other instances, the diver may use surface-supplied diving.

There are also different gases that can be used by the divers. They include compressed air, nitrogen-oxygen mixtures (sometimes referred to as oxygen-enriched air or NITROX), helium-oxygen mixtures (HELIOX) and even pure oxygen.

Prevention of Diving-related Disorders

The health risks in diving can be reduced significantly in various ways. Before each dive, a risk assessment is to be conducted such that a reasonable dive plan can be constructed. The dive plan will incorporate the control measures throughout the dive based on the environment (weather, type of dive vessel, depth of dive, etc), the nature of work (manual lifting, welding, filming, scientific experiments, etc) and the well-being of the diver. The dive plan also incorporates the type of compressed gas to be used, the breathing apparatus, as well as the choice of dive tables or dive computers.

Other essential safety control measures include being adequately trained and proficient in occupational diving and competent in doing the work required. There are various certifications available in different countries. In addition, the diver himself must also be medically fit to dive.

Medical Fitness to Dive

The conduct of medical examinations to assess fitness to dive in the occupational diver has the following objectives:

- To meet the legislative requirements;
- To meet the relevant commercial diving medical standards;
- To ensure that the candidate is able to conduct the diving activities safely without injury to self or others;
- To ensure that diving does not aggravate any underlying medical condition in the candidate.

The medical examination should be done by a physician trained in the field of diving medicine and familiar with the work environment of the particular diving candidate. The challenge to the physician is that he has to consider both the interests of the employer and the candidate without compromising professional and ethical standards. Such fitness to dive examinations should be done prior to engagement, periodically and following an extended period of non-diving due to a medical event (such as hospitalization or prolonged sick leave). This forms part of the medical surveillance program for occupational divers.

The scope of the diving medical examination usually comprises a health questionnaire with a declaration, a physical examination and a series of investigations. The routine investigations could comprise audiometry, spirometry and chest X-ray. Where indicated, further tests to evaluate the severity of the underlying medical condition (e.g. methacholine or hypertonic saline challenge tests, CT scan of the thorax, exercise stress test) as well as baseline investigations such as long bone X-rays may be required.

The outcome of the diving medical examination would fall into one of these groups:

- Fit to dive with no restriction;
- Fit to dive with restriction;
- Temporarily unfit to dive;
- Permanently unfit to dive.

There are absolute and relative medical contraindications to diving. A list is shown in Table 1.

Table 1.   Some Medical Contraindications to Diving

Risk of sudden death

- Asthma
- Coronary artery disease
- Intracranial aneurysm or atrioventricular malformation
- Other cerebrovascular disease
- Cardiac arrhythmia
- Severe hypertension
- Congestive heart failure

Impaired consciousness

- Drugs
- Epilepsy
- Diabetes mellitus
- Cardiac arrhythmia
- Transient ischemic attacks

Impaired judgment

- Drugs
- Psychosis
- Severe anxiety
- Severe depression
- Claustrophobia

Risk of disorientation

- Tympanic membrane perforation
- Inner ear disease
- Uncorrected poor visual acuity

Impaired mobility

- Spinal cord disease or injury
- Neuromuscular disease
- Obesity
- Poor physical fitness
- Pregnancy

Risk of barotrauma

- Asthma
- Spontaneous pneumothorax
- Pulmonary cysts, fibrosis, scars, bronchitis, chronic obstructive airway disease
- Blocked Eustachian tubes
- Acute or chronic respiratory infections

Risk of decompression sickness

- Obesity
- Acute physical injury
- Spinal cord disease or injury
- Intracardiac shunts
- Pregnancy

Source: Edmonds C *et al.* (2002) *Diving and Subaquatic Medicine*, 4th edn.

References

Aviation Medicine

Barratt MR, Pool S. (eds). (2008) *Principles of Clinical Medicine for Space Flight*. New York: Springer Science + Business Media, LLC.

Davis JR, Johnson R, Stepanek J, Fogarty JA. (eds). (2008) *Fundamentals of Aerospace Medicine*. Philadelphia: Lippincott Williams & Wilkins.

Rainford DJ, Gradwell DP. (eds). (2006) *Ernsting's Aviation Medicine*, 4th edn. London: Hodder Arnold.

Rayman RB. (2006) *Clinical Aviation Medicine*, 4th edn. New York: Professional Publishing Group.

Diving Medicine

Bove AA. (2003) *Bove and Davis' Diving Medicine*. Philadelphia: Saunders.

Brubak A, Neuman T. (2003) *Bennett and Elliott's Physiology and Medicine of Diving*, 5th edn. London: WB Saunders.

Edmonds C, Lowry C, Pennefather J, Walker R. (2002) *Diving and Subaquatic Medicine*, 4th edn. London: Arnold.

Guidelines for Occupational Diving (2004) New Zealand: Occupational Safety and Health Service, Department of Labour, Wellington.

SS511: Code of Practice for Diving at Work (2010) Singapore: Spring Singapore.

Technical Advisory for Inland/Inshore Commercial Diving Safety and Health (2009) Singapore: Workplace Safety and Health Council.

Chapter 23

Prevention of Occupational Diseases

David Koh and *Judy Sng**,†

Occupational diseases are by definition, restricted to the working population and are caused by excessive exposure to specific chemical, physical, biological or psychosocial agents in the workplace. As the causes of these diseases are known and environmental in origin, these diseases can be prevented.

The basic aim of preventive medicine is to stop the occurrence of disease in the individual or a specific population group. This is usually achieved by attempts to reduce the risk of contracting a disease. If this is not possible, then activities targeted at early detection of disease may be undertaken, before symptoms and signs manifest or the disease becomes irreversible.

Several levels of prevention are recognized (Table 1).

Primary prevention reduces the disease occurrence by eliminating the causal agent or preventing the agent from causing damage. For example, the prevention of noise-induced hearing loss could be achieved through elimination of the source of noise, or the use of ear protectors.

*Department of Epidemiology and Public Health, Yong Loo Lin School of Medicine, National University of Singapore.
†Corresponding author. E-mail: ephjsgk@nus.edu.sg

Table 1.   Prevention of Occupational Diseases

Primary Prevention	Secondary Prevention
Control of new hazards	Screening — early detection of effects
Control of known hazards	
Environmental monitoring	Periodic medical examinations
Biological monitoring	
Identification of vulnerable workers (pre-employment medical examinations)	
Substitution	
Engineering controls to minimize exposure	
Personal protective equipment	

Secondary prevention detects early effects of harmful exposure or disease before they manifest as clinical symptoms and signs. Examples are the regular monitoring of blood lead (BPb) levels among lead-exposed workers and conducting regular audiograms among workers working in noisy environments. If early effects are detected, corrective action is introduced to the work environment, and the worker temporarily removed from further exposure to prevent progression. In many instances, the early health effects are reversible.

Tertiary prevention aims to minimize the consequences in persons who already have disease. This activity is largely a curative and rehabilitative procedure. Primary and secondary prevention will be the focus of this chapter.

General Health Promotion and Prevention of Disease

In many situations, occupational health services provide total healthcare to the working population. In the past, occupational health services were only concerned with occupational disease. This compartmentalization may have been for the convenience of the physician rather than the worker. In recognition of the intimate two-way relationship between work and disease, it is widely accepted today that a more holistic approach to occupational health is appropriate. Such an approach allows for the use of the workplace as the focal point for general health promotion and disease prevention activities.

Health is not only the absence of disease; it is also the presence of optimal physical, mental and social well-being. Health promotion has been defined as the process of enabling people to increase control over their health and thereby improve it. Health promotion is thus a continuum of activities ranging from management of disease, prevention of disease and promotion of optimal health. Appropriate national policies such as smoking prevention can be instrumental in the achievement of health promotion objectives in the workplace. Health promotion activities for employees in their workplaces have the following advantages: convenient location, a readily available target group, peer pressure to conform to healthy lifestyle, workers accustomed to receiving and following health and safety advice from health workers, and facilities available for incorporation of healthy lifestyle practices, e.g. canteen.

In the newly industrializing countries (NICs), rapid economic growth invariably changes disease patterns from predominantly infectious diseases to lifestyle-dependent diseases such as cancer and atherosclerotic disease (Koh and Sng, 2009). A correlation between lifestyle and selected diseases is shown in Table 2.

The workplace is also increasingly recognized as an important focal point for the implementation of substance abuse prevention programs.

Table 2. Lifestyle Factors as Risk Factors for Selected Diseases

Disease	Unhealthy/ Unsafe Behavior	Lack of Exercise	Stress	Smoking
Cancer	*		*	*
Ischemic heart disease	*	*	*	*
Stroke	*	*	*	*
Diabetes mellitus	*	*	*	
Accidents	*		*	*

Besides an improvement in health, there are also several additional benefits of health promotion programs. Studies have shown that workplace health promotion programs can reduce healthcare costs, decrease sickness absenteeism, increase job performance, decrease work-related injuries and reduce employee turnover.

Prevention of Work-related Diseases

The World Health Organization has identified the following diseases as being work-related: behavioral and psychosomatic illness, hypertension, ischemic heart disease, chronic non-specific respiratory disease and musculoskeletal disorders.

Work-related diseases have multiple causes which may frequently include workplace factors. Such diseases are not exclusively seen among working populations. Furthermore, working conditions and exposures need not be risk factors in every case. These diseases may be work-related in a number of ways: they may be partially caused or exacerbated by adverse workplace exposures.

Case Study 1

Mr. L was a 52-year-old furniture factory manager who died of an acute asthmatic attack after being exposed to diisocyanate vapor. He had a history of asthma which was poorly controlled in the past few months, requiring emergency treatment at the family clinic. Many of his asthmatic attacks had been provoked by exposure to diisocynate fumes from spray-painting works at his factory.

Case Study 2

Mr. T is a 30-year-old man who worked as a technician in a semiconductor manufacturing company (Fig. 1). He suffered from worsening neck and shoulder pain which was only temporarily relieved by analgesics. On enquiring about the nature of his job, it was found that he had to clean the spin coater many times a day. The machine was placed on a low bench, requiring him to work with his neck flexed for prolonged periods.

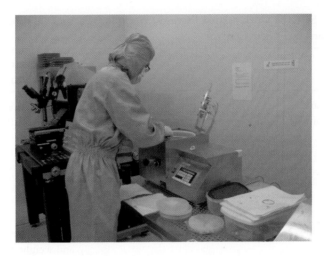

Fig. 1.   Mr. T at his workbench.

The workplace and non-occupational factors associated with each disease are shown in Table 3. In order to prevent work-related diseases, the associated workplace factors should be minimized to safe levels. In addition, it is not only necessary to reduce workplace factors contributing to disease; the known non-occupational risk factors for disease should also be identified and controlled.

For the business traveler or expatriate worker, travel-related illness such as infections and sleep disorders from jet lag are work-related. Thus, preventive activities would include immunizations, giving advice on how to avoid travel-related infections as well as general advice on management of jet lag and food hygiene.

Prevention of Occupational Diseases

Occupational diseases are caused by exposure to physical, chemical and biological agents in the workplace. Psychosocial factors causing ill health have been dealt with in the previous section and in the chapter on mental health.

Occupational diseases account for a relatively small percentage of overall morbidity. However, they offer great scope for prevention as their causal agents are known and exposure can often be controlled

Table 3.   Selected Work-related Diseases, Workplace Factors, Non-occupational Risk Factors and Their Control

Disease	Adverse Workplace Factors	Risk Factors and Control
Behavioral and psychosomatic illness	Stress caused by a) work overload b) work underload c) shift work d) career development e) migration/travel f) role conflict g) role ambiguity	Type A behavior; reduction of organizational stress
Hypertension	Stress	Stress relief, screening, diet and weight control
Ischemic heart disease	Stress Workplace exposures, e.g. CS_2, CO Lack of physical exercise	Stress relief, screening for risk factors and intervention
Chronic non-specific respiratory disease	Dusts and irritants	Smoking; control of dusts and irritants
Musculoskeletal disorders	Ergonomic factors: weight bearing, trauma, whole body vibration, poor work posture	Ergonomic design, healthy back program

and maintained at safe levels. The occurrence of occupational disease must be viewed as a failure of prevention.

Case Study 3

Two production lines in an electronics factory that assembled printed circuit boards (PrCBs) had to be shut down because all the workers complained of itch of the hands and fingers. They noted that the problem started when a new "dusty" PrCB was used.

Examination of the workers revealed only excoriation marks. Skin stripping with adhesive tape after the workers washed their hands showed fiberglass spicules in the epidermis (Fig. 2). Samples of the PrCBs from the production line and two other unaffected lines were examined. The sample from the problem line showed the most free fiberglass from the edge of the PrCB (Fig. 3). The diagnosis was fiberglass itch from PrCBs.

   The problem was resolved by requesting workers to apply powder, wear cotton gloves, and wash their hands during breaks. At the same time, other measures were taken. These included the use of sharper cutting tools to

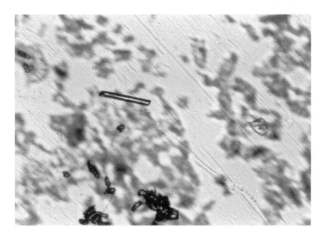

Fig. 2.   Skin stripping of worker, showing fiberglass.

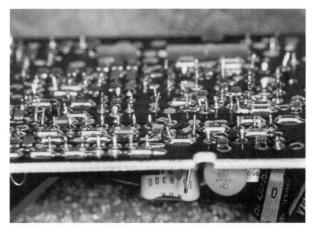

Fig. 3.   Fiberglass could be found at the free edge of the printed circuit board.

minimize free fiberglass at the edge of the PrCBs, and vacuuming of the free edges before the PrCBs were sent to the assembly lines. Plans were also made to inform the supplier to produce PrCBs with less freely dislodged fiberglass.

Case Study 4

A group of display artists working in a retail store complained of tiredness, loss of concentration, exhaustion and difficulty in sleeping. They worked with solvent-based paints to prepare the sales displays in a fairly confined space.

They were young, fit and had no previous health problems. Clinical examination by the company doctor did not reveal any remarkable findings. Liver function tests were performed and showed that liver transaminase enzymes were raised, indication of some form of subclinical liver injury (other causes of hepatic damage, e.g. viral hepatitis, alcohol ingestion, were excluded). Workers with more severe symptoms were sent for neurophysiological assessment, with inconclusive results. It was not possible to ascertain the exact chemical constituents of the solvent from the suppliers.

In spite of the lack of a definitive diagnosis, the management was advised of the risk of solvent exposure, and work in the confined area was stopped. The potential hazard was communicated to the staff concerned through several dialogue sessions. Staff were also briefed on the control measures to be taken while working with the solvents. Subsequently, a management decision was taken to reduce solvent usage in decorative work. All solvent spray work was relocated to another part of the workplace, which had proper ventilation and exhaust fans. Workers undertaking work using solvents wore masks, gloves and other personal protective equipment, and worked for shortened periods at these operations. Following these changes, all the workers recovered uneventfully.

Primary Prevention of Occupational Diseases

Primary prevention refers to efforts to reduce the occurrence of occupational disease by eliminating the cause or preventing harmful exposure to the agent.

Control of new hazards

Animal toxicity studies of chemicals to be used in industry are a reasonable predictor of potential health hazards to humans. On the basis of these studies the legislation in manufacturing nations would control the usage of certain chemicals in industrial processes. The limitation is that such controls apply only to the new chemicals which are to be introduced into the market. For instance, it is estimated that only 10% of pesticides in current usage have undergone such toxicological evaluation. In addition, animal toxicity studies often do not provide adequate information on long-term human health effects, such as cancer causation.

Control of known hazards

Several countries have legislation to ban the use of substances known to be harmful to human health. Since 1991 the United Nations has compiled and regularly updated a "Consolidated List of Products Whose Consumption and/or Sale Have Been Banned or Severely Restricted by Governments". This publication is a tool which helps governments to keep up-to-date with regulatory decisions taken by other governments and assists them in considering the scope for eventual regulatory action. In 1989, the United Nations Environment Program (UNEP) evolved a mechanism of Prior Informed Consent (PIC) procedure to inform governments of banned agents so that appropriate action could be taken for their control (Table 4). Chemicals which have been banned or severely restricted in at least five countries have further information made available through Decision Guidance Documents.

By means of such documents the UN system aims to prevent importing countries from unknowingly using substances already banned in other countries for health reasons. Chemicals banned for health reasons in the country of manufacture should not be manufactured solely for export.

Control of exposure

Successful prevention of occupational disease could be achieved by limiting exposure to harmful agents to what are considered as safe levels. There are two mechanisms to monitor exposure: environmental and biological monitoring (Table 5).

Table 4.   Chemicals Subject to the Prior Informed Consent Procedure

2,4,5-T and its salts and esters	Toxaphene
Aldrin	Dustable powder formulations containing
Binapacryl	a combination of benomyl at or
Captafol	above 7%, carbofuran at above 10%,
Chlordane	thiram at or above 15%
Chlordimeform	
Chlorobenzilate	Methamidophos (soluble liquid
DDT	formulations of the substance that
Dieldrin	exceed 600 g active ingredient/l)
Dinitro-ortho-cresol (DNOC)	Phosphamidon (soluble liquid
and its salts	formulations of the substance that
Dinoseb and its salts and esters	exceed 1000 g active ingredient/l)
1,2-dibromoethane (EDB)	
Ethylene dichloride	Methyl-parathion (emulsifiable
Ethylene oxide	concentrates [EC]) at or above
Fluoroacetamide	19.5% active ingredient and dusts
HCH (mixed isomers)	at or above 1.5% active
Heptachlor	ingredient)
Hexachlorobenzene	Asbestos (crocidolite, actinolite,
Lindane	anthophyllite, amosite, tremolite)
Mercury compounds including	Polybrominated biphenyls (PBB)
inorganic mercury compounds,	Polychlorinated biphenyls (PCB)
alkyl mercury compounds	Polychlorinated terphenyls (PCT)
and alkyloxyalkyl and aryl	Tetraethyl lead
mercury compounds	Tetramethyl lead
Monocrotophos	Tris (2,3-dibromopropyl) phosphate
Parathion	
Pentachlorophenol and its salts and esters	

Source: UNEP, http://www.pic.int/en/Table7.htm (accessed 20 June 2010).

Table 5.   Types of Monitoring and Screening in Prevention of Occupational Disease

Primary Prevention			Secondary Prevention
Ambient ← air	Environmental → monitoring	Permissible level (TLV)	Screening Early detection of disease
Internal ← dose	Biological → monitoring	Biological exposure index (BEI)	Periodic medical examination

Environmental monitoring

Environmental or ambient monitoring is undertaken to measure external exposure to harmful agents. This is to ensure that environmental levels are kept within permissible levels so as to prevent the agent from causing disease. The concept of permissible levels assumes that for each substance there is a level of exposure at or below which the exposed worker does not suffer any health impairment.

There are limitations when permissible levels of exposure are applied. Such levels are based on current understanding of health effects which may not be complete (especially for long-term effects such as carcinogenesis and reproductive system effects). Previously unsuspected health risks have arisen from substances assumed to be comparatively safe, e.g. glycol ethers in the electronics industry and spontaneous abortions. As such, every effort must be made to keep exposure levels as low as possible.

The determination of permissible levels are based on several considerations, such as the physical and chemical properties of the substance (including the nature and amount of impurities), toxicological studies (using animal models) and available human data.

In some countries, the permissible level is a set point above which exposure should not occur, and is used for enforcement of legislation. For example, threshold limit values (TLVs) are permissible levels for workplace exposure recommended by the American Conference of Governmental Industrial Hygienists (ACGIH). There are three categories of TLVs (Table 6):

(1) Threshold limit value – time-weighted average (TLV-TWA),
(2) Threshold limit value – short-term exposure limit (TLV-STEL),
(3) Threshold limit value – ceiling (TLV-C).

Biological monitoring

Biological monitoring is the examination of the worker for the presence of a toxic substance or its metabolite. The measurement value obtained by biological monitoring is evaluated as a health risk by comparing it with the corresponding biological exposure index (BEI)

Table 6.   Threshold Limit Values of Selected Agents (ACGIH, 2009)

Substance	TWA (ppm/mg/m^3)	STEL/C (ppm/mg/m^3)	Notations	TLV Basis — Critical Effects
Acetaldehyde	—	C 25 ppm	A3	Eye and URT irritation
Acrylamide	0.03 mg/m^3	—	Skin, A3	CNS, dermatitis
Asbestos (all forms)	0.1 f/cc	—	A1	Pneumoconiosis, lung cancer, mesothelioma
n-butyl acrylate	2 ppm	—	SEN, A4	Skin, eye and URT irritation
Chlorine	0.5 ppm	1 ppm	A4	Irritation
Chloroacetone	—	C 1 ppm	—	URT and eye irritation
Lead and inorganic compounds, as Pb	0.05 mg/m^3	—	A3, BEI	CNS and PNS impairment, hematologic effect
Lead chromate				
as Pb	0.05 mg/m^3	—	A2, BEI	Male repro damage
as Cr	0.012 mg/m^3	—	A2	teratogenic effect, vasoconstriction
Mercury				
Alkyl compounds	0.01 mg/m^3	0.03 mg/m^3	Skin	CNS and PNS impairment, kidney damage
Aryl compounds	0.1 mg/m^3	—	Skin	CNS impairment, kidney damage
Elemental and inorganic forms	0.025 mg/m^3	—	Skin, A4, BEI	CNS impairment, kidney damage
Wood dusts				
Western Red Cedar	0.05 mg/m^3	—	SEN, A4	Asthma
All other species	1 mg/m^3	—	—	Pulmonary function
Carcinogenicity				
Oak and beech		—	A1	
Birch, mahogany, teak, walnut		—	A2	
All other wood dusts		—	A4	

ppm = parts per million; URT = upper respiratory tract; CNS = central nervous system; PNS = peripheral nervous system; Pb = lead; Cr = chromate; BEI = biological exposure index; SEN = sensitizer.

or biological limit value (BLV). The BEI is based either on the relationship between the intensity of exposure and the biological levels of the toxicant (or its metabolite), or on the relationship between the biological level and health effects.

Biological exposure indices (BEI) as used by the ACGIH (2009) for some toxicants are shown in Table 7.

Identification of susceptible workers

Pre-placement/employment medical examination aims to achieve proper job placement according to the mental and physical capabilities

Table 7. Biological Exposure Indices (BEIs) of Some Chemical Toxicants (ACGIH, 2009)

Toxicant	BEI	Source	Sampling Time
Carbon monoxide			
Carboxyhemoglobin	3.5% of hemoglobin	Blood	End of shift
Carbon monoxide	20 ppm	End-exhaled air	End of shift
Cadmium and inorganic compounds	5 μg/g creatinine	Urine	Not critical
	5 μg/L	Blood	Not critical
***n*-hexane**			
2,5-hexanedione	0.4 mg/L	Urine	End of shift at end of work week
Lead	30 μg/100 ml	Blood	Not critical
Mercury (inorganic)	35 μg/g creatinine	Urine	Pre-shift
	15 μg/L	Blood	End of shift at end of work week
Phenol	250 mg/g creatinine	Urine	End of shift

of the worker. During such examinations and job placements, susceptible workers can be identified and their exposure limited to prevent
adverse health effects. Such tests are also undertaken with different
objectives, e.g. to protect other workers and the general public; for
insurance purposes; and to obtain baseline information on health and
fitness.

There are genetic disorders that may make a worker more vulnerable to certain workplace exposures. One example is a deficiency in
red cell glucose-6-phosphate dehydrogenase (G6PD), which increases
susceptibility to hemolytic anemia. As such, G6PD-deficient individuals should be protected from exposure to hemolytic agents. Another
example is alpha-1 antitrypsin (AAT) deficiency. Persons with AAT
deficiency are at high risk of developing chronic obstructive pulmonary disease and should not be allowed to work with substances
that can worsen respiratory function.

Similarly, lifestyle factors such as smoking, alcohol consumption
and pre-existing diseases such as chronic bronchitis, liver or kidney
disease may increase the susceptibility to certain toxicants.

Engineering controls

Engineering controls minimize or eliminate hazards at the source.
This is a preferred means of prevention. Unlike other measures, such
as the use of personal protective equipment, engineering controls do
not rely on workers' compliance for their effectiveness.

Engineering controls could include the following:

- Removal (or replacement with safer alternatives) of toxic hazards
  in the manufacturing process, e.g. using a cadmium-free brazing
  filler in Case Study 5, or using a benzene-free organic solvent.
- Automation, enclosure or segregation of a work process to minimize worker exposure.
  (In such situations, exposure could still occur among maintenance
  and repair staff.)
- Modifications to reduce the emission of hazards form the work
  process, e.g. dampeners or mufflers to reduce vibration or noise,

reducing the open surface area for the evaporation of volatile toxic agents.

- Application of exhaust ventilation to remove hazardous fumes, vapors or dust in the work process.

It is often more cost-effective to incorporate the engineering controls at the initial setting up of the work process. Such controls should also be considered when new processes or machinery are introduced to existing manufacturing operations. It is important that the effectiveness of the engineering controls be monitored periodically, and maintenance carried out when necessary.

Case Study 5

Brazing is a process where a filler metal (of lower melting point than the two metals to be joined) is melted and allowed to flow by capillary action into a close fitting joint of two metals. A common type of brazing filler metal is a copper-zinc-silver-cadmium alloy. This is used to join brass, cast iron, nickel or stainless steel.

Torch brazing was performed in a factory that manufactured compressors. A review of the safety data sheet of the filler revealed that it contained a significant amount of cadmium. Cadmium is a nephrotoxic agent that is used to reduce the melting point of the filler metal. While cadmium-free alloys are available, these cost more, as a higher silver content is needed to achieve an equivalent melting temperature.

Environmental monitoring showed that cadmium levels in the air were above the recommended threshold limit values in that country. Biological monitoring of exposed workers showed that a large proportion of exposed workers had blood cadmium values higher than 10 μg/L, the recommended biological exposure index in that country. (The BEI for cadmium in blood recommended by the ACGIH is 5 μg/L [ACGIH, 2009]).

The health risk was found to be unacceptable and, as a result, the brazing alloy used was replaced with a cadmium-free substitute.

Redesign of the workstation or process

Redesign of the workstation, to reduce unnecessary and repetitive bending or to prevent excessive stretching to the limit of the range of movement of the workers, can minimize ergonomic hazards (Fig. 4).

In the case of computer operators, the use of adjustable equipment, the positioning of the workstation to reduce glare, and appropriate work rest pauses can prevent the development of eyestrain and musculoskeletal complaints.

Administrative controls

Administrative controls may be a viable alternative or additional measure to reduce worker exposure to occupational hazards. These measures could take the form of job enlargement and job rotation, restriction of hours of work at a hazardous operation, or even temporary job re-assignment. Prevention of travel illness for frequent business travelers (such as immunization, advice on food safety and hygiene) could be considered as a form of administrative control of occupational hazards.

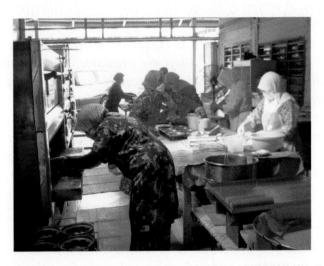

Fig. 4.   Ergonomic improvements in this workplace could reduce the risk of musculoskeletal disorders among the workers.

Training workers to recognize work hazards, how to work safely, and what to do in the event of an emergency or when occupational diseases occur is another important aspect of prevention.

Personal protective equipment

The use of personal protective equipment is often widely practised. It has its merits, a major one being its relative low cost, and it is especially useful for short-term or occasional exposure to occupational hazards.

However, protective equipment has to be properly selected to be effective against specific hazards, e.g. the choice of appropriate gloves for use with a particular solvent. Workers have to be trained to use the equipment correctly and to ensure that it is working effectively, e.g. the use of respirators and respirator fit testing. Worker compliance in the use of the equipment must be high; otherwise the protective effects may be less than desired, e.g. hearing protectors. Finally, personal protective equipment have to be regularly maintained and replaced when necessary.

The Occupational Safety and Health Administration (OSHA, 1995) stipulates that personal protective equipment should not be used as a substitute for engineering, work practice and/or administrative controls. Instead, personal protective equipment should be used in conjunction with these controls to provide for employee safety and health in the workplace.

Secondary Prevention of Occupational Disease

Secondary prevention is the detection of disease at an early stage before the worker would normally seek clinical care. For such an activity to be truly preventive, detection of the disease in the preclinical, asymptomatic or early symptomatic stage must be of benefit to the workers. This means that the pathological process must be reversible on discontinuation of exposure and prognosis better than if it were detected at later stages.

Screening for disease

The discussion on screening for disease in this chapter is confined to early detection of disease. It must be proven that such early detection of disease is of benefit to the worker. Otherwise, it is not considered a screening procedure.

Biological monitoring may sometimes be wrongly classified as a screening procedure. This is not accurate as the purpose of biological monitoring is to detect the presence of a toxicant or metabolite so as to keep exposure levels within safe limits. Thus biological monitoring precedes screening as it is not necessarily indicative of disease, whereas screening is to detect early disease (Table 8).

Recent advances in monitoring and screening

Technological advances in molecular biology over the last few decades have offered more sophisticated techniques that can be used to study the role of specific exogenous agents and host factors in causing ill health.

These advances have resulted in the development of newer molecular biomarkers of exposure, response and genetic susceptibility. These include measurements for structural gene damage, gene variation and gene products in cells and body fluids, e.g. oncogenes and tumor suppressor

Table 8.   Levels of Prevention in Occupational Disease

	Primary Prevention	Secondary Prevention	
Pre-employment medical examination			
Periodic medical examination	Measurement of toxicant or metabolite	Early detection of asymptomatic disease	Screening
Biological monitoring	Measurement of health effects	Measurement of health effects	
Molecular biomarkers	Not proven	Not proven	

genes, DNA adducts, gene products and genetic polymorphisms and metabolic phenotypes in environmentally exposed populations.

An understanding of biochemistry and genetics at the molecular level, and specific knowledge of metabolism, mechanisms of action and epidemiology have become increasingly important. This is necessary in order to address the major question of the validation and relevance of these molecular biomarkers.

For example, the availability of genetic tests to identify susceptible workers raises issues of ethics, individual privacy, right to work and the relevance of such tests. Several studies have presented data on the association between environmental measurements and various biomarkers for internal and biologically effective doses, genetic polymorphisms and early response markers (Table 9).

There are limitations to individual molecular biomarkers in assessing health risk, and environmental diseases are multifactorial in nature. It is likely that a combined approach which examines several of these biomarkers simultaneously will increase our understanding of the complex issue of disease mechanisms and further refine the process of risk assessment.

In the last few decades, OMICS technologies have emerged as new biomarker discovery tools that can potentially be applied to occupational and environmental health practice. The five most developed OMICS technologies are genotyping, transcriptomics, epigenomics, proteomics and metabolomics. At present, their use has largely been limited to research studies. Examples of utilization of OMICS technologies have been in the investigation of the effects of benzene and arsenic on human health (Vlaanderen *et al.*, 2010).

In this chapter, screening is defined as the detection of disease at an asymptomatic or subclinical stage. The following are certain criteria to be fulfilled prior to screening:

(i)   The screening test/procedure is validated as being able to detect the disease at an asymptomatic stage.

(ii) Early intervention in the management of the disease is of benefit to the individual screened and facilities are locally available for its management.

Table 9.   Examples of Molecular Biomarkers Measured in Occupational Health Studies

Molecular Biomarkers	Application	Study Population
Exposure marker		
8-hydroxy-2-deoxyguanosine (8-OHdG)	Oxidative stress and increased cancer risk from exposure to benzene, chromium, cobalt, fine particulate matter (PM2.5)	Petrol station attendants, electroplating workers, boilermakers
PAH-DNA adduct	Workplace and community exposures and exposure to cigarette smoke, and risk of lung cancer	Foundry workers, coke oven workers, general community in industrial areas
Early effect markers		
p53 tumor-suppressor gene or its protein product	Specific fingerprint mutation in certain gene codon and risk of liver, breast, lung, and esophageal cancer	Radon-exposed miners, vinyl chloride monomer workers, general population with environmental exposure to AFB1
H-*ras* and K-*ras* gene or its protein product	Increased risk of various cancers, e.g. lung, liver and bladder	Firefighters, hazardous waste workers, foundry workers, vinyl chloride monomer workers
Host susceptibility markers		
Functional polymorphisms in GST genes	Increased risk of lung cancer with exposure to indoor cooking fumes (wood smoke, cooking oil fumes)	Cooks, kitchen workers (especially Asian-style cooking)
CYP1A1 polymorphism	Increased risk of lung cancer with exposure to Benzo(a)pyrene	Foundry workers
NAT2 polymorphism	Increased risk of bladder cancer	Workers exposed to arylamine and hydrazine

Sources: Koh, Seow and Ong, 1999; Pilger and Rüdiger, 2006; Hosgood, Berndt and Qing, 2007.

(iii) The physician undertaking the screening procedure is not the one who will subsequently treat the disease. This is important as it eliminates the potential for observer bias, particularly in situations where there exists a financial benefit in over-diagnosing for treatment. Such a problem will not arise where the physician is a salaried employee — as opposed to a physician whose income is influenced by the number of interactions and consultations undertaken.

Often, the usual physician–patient relationship does not prevail in screening procedures as the person screened is asymptomatic and has not sought medical opinion for an ailment. Screening is undertaken on "well" persons who are invited for screening and a disease diagnosed as a consequence of this intervention.

Periodic medical examinations

Periodic medical examinations are undertaken on occupational groups in order to effect primary or, failing that, secondary prevention of disease.

In many countries, by convention most employees undergo pre-employment medical examinations. The main focus of such examinations is not necessarily as a pre-placement procedure but rather for assessing routine fitness for work as well as for medical insurance needs. In some countries, there are legal and administrative regulations mandating pre-employment and periodic medical examinations.

Statutory medical examinations

An example of statutory examinations can be found in Singapore, where since 1985, all workers exposed to a list of prescribed hazards have to undergo pre-employment and periodic medical examinations (Table 10). Such examinations are to be conducted by physicians trained in occupational health and registered with the Ministry of Manpower.

In addition, periodic examinations are required for other categories of workers such as migrant workers, food handlers, professional drivers and radiographers.

Table 10. Prescribed Hazards Requiring Medical Examinations under the Workplace Safety and Health (Medical Examinations) Regulations

1. Arsenic and its compounds
2. Asbestos
3. Benzene
4. Cadmium and its compounds
5. Raw cotton
6. Lead and its compounds
7. Manganese and its compounds
8. Mercury and its compounds
9. Excessive noise
10. Organophosphates
11. Perchloroethylene
12. Silica
13. Tar
14. Pitch
15. Bitumen
16. Creosote
17. Trichloroethylene
18. Vinyl chloride monomer
19. Any occupation or process carried out using compressed air

Source: Ministry of Manpower, Singapore (2010).

Notification of occupational diseases

Most countries require the statutory notification of occupational diseases to the government. Notification should be done upon the suspicion of occupational disease. The notified case is subsequently investigated and confirmed by the relevant government specialists. Either the employer or health practitioner who sees the worker can notify the government. In many countries, a list of notifiable occupational diseases is available.

Notification serves as an additional means of control of occupational diseases, undertaken by occupational health and safety professionals in the public sector. It initiates a chain of events, which often includes investigation and confirmation of the index case, and active case finding of other affected persons.

Recommendations for specific preventive measures in the workplace are then prescribed. The authorities would follow up by ensuring that the recommendations have been implemented. If necessary, further evaluation of the effectiveness of the preventive measures can be made. An example of a notification form is given in Fig. 5. In Singapore, such a form in hard copy is no longer available, as there is presently an online electronic notification process.

Figure 6 summarizes the continuum of various means of prevention in occupational health practice.

Tertiary Prevention

Tertiary prevention activities are largely curative and rehabilitative procedures. Workers should be removed from further exposure, and the appropriate medical treatment given if indicated. Examples of appropriate treatment include the rendering of first aid promptly after an injury, chelation for severe cases of heavy metal overexposure, and hyperbaric treatment for cases of compressed air illness.

Disaster planning

Occupational health personnel can also assist in planning for disasters in the workplace and community. Services such as the fire and emergency response services are essential in dealing with disasters in the workplace that may affect the community. As such, planning and practice drills should be done jointly with the relevant local community agencies. This topic is covered in an earlier chapter.

Post-illness or post-injury evaluation

An evaluation of the health status of an employee returning to work after a prolonged absence from work due to illness or injury is important. The aim is to ensure that the worker has sufficiently recovered from the illness or injury, and that he or she is fit to return to work.

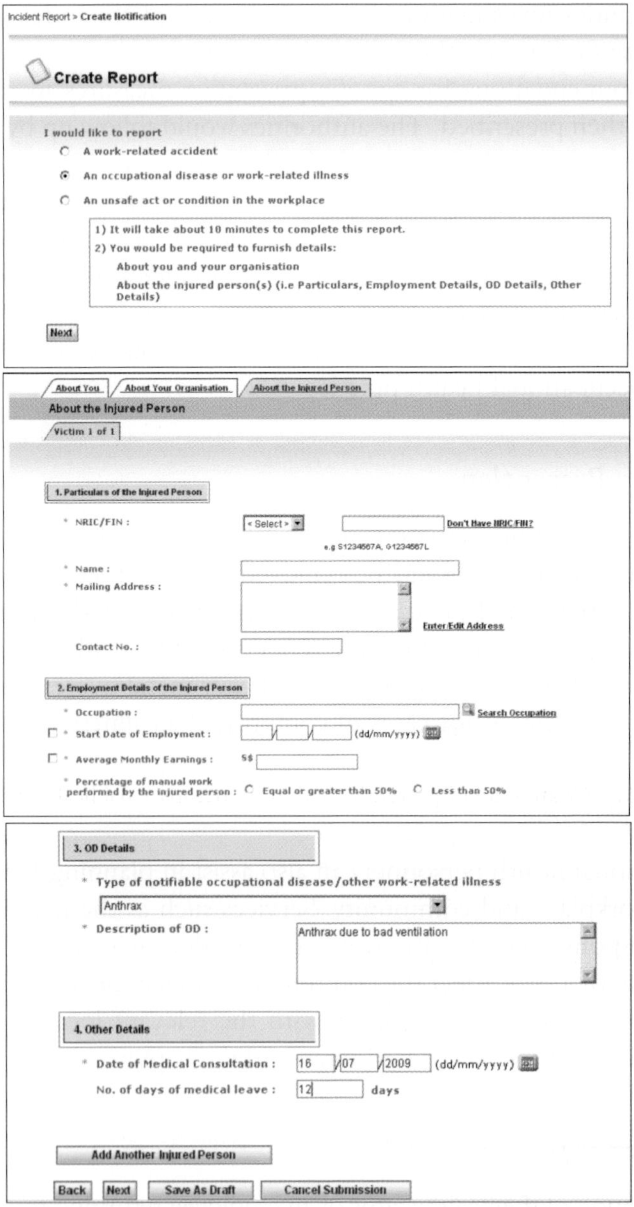

Fig. 5.   Online notification of occupational diseases in Singapore.

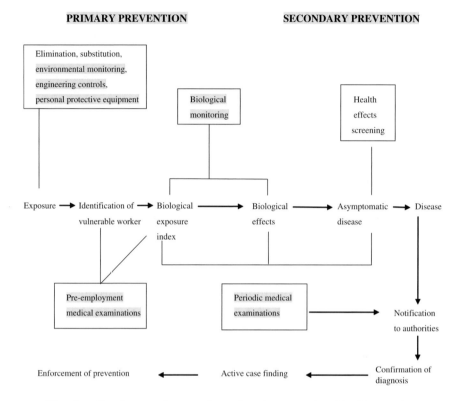

Fig. 6.   Continuum of preventive actions in occupational health practice.

Two issues to consider are:

— Can the worker perform his or her duty without adverse health and safety risks to himself/herself or fellow workers?
— Should he or she return to full-time unrestricted duty, or should some modified, restricted or alternative duty be given?

Rehabilitation

Rehabilitation of workers is another important aspect of occupational healthcare. Management, fellow workers, occupational health professionals and the injured worker have to work together to ensure that suitable alternative duties are provided, and that any work restrictions or physical limitations are understood.

There should be clear short-term and long-term goals in rehabilitation, and alternative duties should be meaningful and contribute to production (ACOM and ACRM, 1987). Sometimes, the use of external rehabilitation resources may be needed.

Workmen's Compensation

In many countries, workers who are injured at work, or fall ill from hazardous work exposures are eligible for compensation. Employers who carry out economic activities through labor and machines create an environment that may cause ill health in employees. Thus employers should be liable for payment of compensation to workers if they are injured or fall sick because of the work.

Legislation concerning employment injury benefits is often called a Workmen's Compensation Act. Employers may be required to insure against their liability under the Act. The workmen's compensation system is designed to minimize litigation and facilitate payment of compensation to injured workmen. It is based on a "no fault" principle. In different countries, certain categories of workers, e.g. domestic helpers, may be excluded.

Assessment of disability for compensation is covered in a previous chapter.

Evaluation of Prevention Programs

Evidence for the success of prevention programs has increasingly been documented. There have already been several Cochrane reviews produced on the effectiveness of various preventive strategies in occupational health practice. (Cochrane reviews are systematic reviews of primary research in human healthcare and health policy that investigate the effects of interventions for prevention, treatment and rehabilitation.)

These include reviews on interventions for musculoskeletal disorders, smoking, injuries and poisonings, infectious diseases and mental health, and cover primary, secondary and tertiary prevention strategies (Table 11).

Table 11. Selected Cochrane Reviews in Occupational Health

Musculoskeletal disorders

Back schools for non-specific low-back pain

Manual material handling advice and assistive devices for preventing and
treating back pain in workers

Multidisciplinary biopsychosocial rehabilitation for subacute low-back
pain among working age adults

Physical conditioning programs for improving work outcomes in workers
with back pain

Work conditioning, work hardening and functional restoration for workers
with back and neck pain

Multidisciplinary biopsychosocial rehabilitation for neck and shoulder
pain among working age adults

Biopsychosocial rehabilitation for upper limb repetitive strain injuries in
working age adults

Ergonomic and physiotherapeutic interventions for treating work-related
complaints of the arm, neck or shoulder in adults

Multidisciplinary rehabilitation for fibromyalgia and musculoskeletal pain
in working age adults

Smoking

Workplace interventions for smoking cessation

Injuries and poisoning

Alcohol and drug screening of occupational drivers to prevent injury

Alkalinization for organophosphorus pesticide poisoning

Interventions for preventing injuries in the agricultural industry

Interventions for preventing injuries in the construction industry

Oximes for acute organophosphate pesticide poisoning

Infectious diseases

Antibiotics for preventing leptospirosis

Antiretroviral post-exposure prophylaxis (PEP) for occupational HIV exposure

Influenza vaccination for healthcare workers who work with the elderly

Vaccines for preventing hepatitis B in healthcare workers

Mental health

Interventions to improve occupational health in depressed people

Melatonin for the prevention and treatment of jet lag

Preventing occupational stress in healthcare workers

Psychological debriefing for preventing post-traumatic stress disorder (PTSD)

Psychosocial interventions for prevention of psychological disorders in law
enforcement officers

(Continued)

Table 11.   (*Continued*)

Other
Caffeine for the prevention of injuries and errors in shift workers
Cognitive behavioral therapy for tinnitus
Effectiveness of vocational rehabilitation intervention on the return to work and
    employment of persons with multiple sclerosis
Flexible working conditions and their effects on employee health and well-being
Interventions to promote the wearing of hearing protection
Interventions in the workplace to support breastfeeding for women in employment
Preventive staff support interventions for health workers

Source: Finnish Institute of Occupational Health (2010).

A review of evaluations of economic incentives to promote occupational safety and health showed that economic incentive schemes were feasible and reasonably effective. The few cases that were reviewed delivered positive results for large samples. However, analysis regarding the efficiency of such schemes was generally scarce and there were also deficits in the quality of evaluations in many instances (Esler *et al.*, 2010).

An evaluation of a program could comprise comparison of pre- and post-intervention health outcomes, as the case study below demonstrates.

Case Study 6

A preventive program, which emphasized skin and respiratory protection, workplace cleanliness and beryllium migration control in lowering beryllium sensitization, was evaluated. Sensitization prevalence and incidence were 8.9% and 3.7/1000 person-months for the Pre-Program Group compared to 2.1% and 1.7/1000 person-months for the Program Group.

After adjusting for potential selection and information bias, sensitization prevalence for the Pre-Program Group was found to be 3.8 times higher (95% CI = 1.5 to 9.3) than the Program Group. The sensitization incidence rate ratio of the Pre-Program Group to the Program Group was 1.6 (95% CI = 0.8 to 3.6).

It was concluded that the preventive program reduced the prevalence but did not eliminate beryllium sensitization (Bailey et al., 2010).

Conclusion

This chapter addresses the issue of health promotion as well as the prevention of work-related and occupational diseases in the working population. In the prevention of occupational diseases the priority should be to effect primary prevention. However, when this fails, secondary and tertiary prevention activities are undertaken to contain damage.

References

ACGIH. (2009) *Threshold Limit Values and Biological Exposure Indices.* Cincinnati: ACGIH.

ACOM, ACRM. (1987) *Occupational Rehabilitation. Guidelines and Practice.* A report prepared by the joint working party of the Australian College of Occupational Medicine and Australian College of Rehabilitation Medicine.

Bailey RL, Thomas CA, Deubner DC, *et al.* (2010) Evaluation of a preventive program to reduce sensitization at a beryllium metal, oxide, and alloy production plant. *J Occup Environ Med* **52**(5): 505–512.

Elsler D, Treutlein D, Rydlewska I, *et al.* (2010) A review of case studies evaluating economic incentives to promote occupational safety and health. *Scand J Work Environ Health* **36**: 289–298.

Finnish Institute of Occupational Health. (2010) *Cochrane Occupational Health Field.* http://www.ttl.fi/partner/cohf/cochrane_reviews/topic_list/pages/default.aspx (accessed 27 April 2010).

Hosgood HD III, Berndt SI, Qing L. (2007) GST genotypes and lung cancer susceptibility in Asian populations with indoor air pollution exposures: A meta-analysis. *Mutation Research* **636**: 134–143.

Koh D, Seow A, Ong CN. (1999) New techniques in molecular epidemiology and their relevance to occupational medicine. *Occup Environ Med* **56**: 725–729.

Koh D, Sng J. (2009) Occupational health and safety in newly industrializing countries. *Occupational Health Southern Africa* **15** (special ICOH issue): 12–16.

Ministry of Manpower, Singapore. (2010) *Health and Environmental Surveillance.* http://www.mom.gov.sg/publish/momportal/en/communities/ workplace_safety_and_health/maintaining_a_safe_workplace/health_and_ environmental.html (accessed 20 June 2010).

OSHA. (1995) Personal protective equipment. US Dept of Labor. Occupational Safety and Health Administration. OSHA 3077.

United Nations Environment Programme. *Harmful Substances.* http://www. unep.org/hazardoussubstances (accessed 28 December 2009).

Pilger A, Rüdiger HW. (2006) 8-Hydroxy-2-deoxyguanosine as a marker of oxidative DNA damage related to occupational and environmental exposures. *Int Arch Occup Environ Health* **80**: 1–15.

Vlaanderen J, Moore LE, Smith MT, *et al.* (2010) Application of OMICS technologies in occupational and environmental health research; current status and projections. *Occup Environ Med* **67**(2): 136–143.

Index

595

Neurotoxicity, 35, 175
Newcastle virus, 385
n-hexane, 168, 174, 183, 185
Nickel, 108, 115, 125, 136, 287,
    424
Nitroaniline, 154
Nitrobenzene, 156, 267, 270
Nitroglycerin, 54
Nitroglycerine, 54
Nitroglycol, 54
Nitrous oxide, 282, 421, 426
Noise, 430, 431
Noise reduction rate, 326
Noise-induced hearing loss
    (NIHL), 295, 297, 307, 308,
    317, 327, 329

Obsessive-compulsive disorder,
    202
Occupational and environmental
    medicine, 3
Occupational asthma, 67, 77, 79,
    98
Occupational dermatitis, 110, 116,
    137, 139
Occupational dermatoses, 101,
    104, 106, 107, 109, 110, 125,
    131, 136
Occupational respiratory diseases,
    59
Ocular injury, 338–340
Ocular trauma, 335, 337, 341,
    342
Ocular Trauma Score (OTS),
    345
Office politics, 214, 217

Oil acne, 122
Oil folliculitis, 108
Oligospermia, 444
Open globe injuries, 342
Optic atrophy, 356
Orbital fractures, 340
Organic lead, 31, 148, 164, 173
Organic mercury, 32
Organic solvents, 27, 34, 164,
    167, 168, 174, 186, 189, 262,
    278, 418–420, 425, 435,
    449
Organochlorine, 170
Organophosphate, 183, 286
Ornithosis, 385
Otoacoustic emission, 327

Painful arc syndrome, 239
Pancreatic cancer, 286, 287
Pancreatitis, 286
Panic disorder, 202, 203
Paraphenylenediamine, 122
Paraquat, 171, 267
Parkinson's disease, 169
Parkinsonian, 165
Patch testing, 113, 116, 121, 133
Patent foramen ovale, 52
Peak expiratory flow rate (PEFR),
    61, 75, 77
Penicillamine, 153
Peptic ulcers, 285
Perchloroethylene, 35, 183, 279
Periodic medical examination, 78,
    150, 177, 189
Peripheral neuropathy, 164, 166,
    169, 174, 190